PHARMACOLOGY - RESEARCH, SAFETY TESTING AND REGULATION

PRODRUGS DESIGN

A NEW ERA

PHARMACOLOGY - RESEARCH, SAFETY TESTING AND REGULATION

Additional books in this series can be found on Nova's website under the Series tab.

Additional e-books in this series can be found on Nova's website under the e-book tab.

Pharmacology - Research, Safety Testing and Regulation

Prodrugs Design

A New Era

Rafik Karaman
Editor

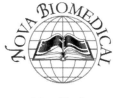

New York

Copyright © 2014 by Nova Science Publishers, Inc.

All rights reserved. No part of this book may be reproduced, stored in a retrieval system or transmitted in any form or by any means: electronic, electrostatic, magnetic, tape, mechanical photocopying, recording or otherwise without the written permission of the Publisher.

For permission to use material from this book please contact us:
Telephone 631-231-7269; Fax 631-231-8175
Web Site: http://www.novapublishers.com

NOTICE TO THE READER

The Publisher has taken reasonable care in the preparation of this book, but makes no expressed or implied warranty of any kind and assumes no responsibility for any errors or omissions. No liability is assumed for incidental or consequential damages in connection with or arising out of information contained in this book. The Publisher shall not be liable for any special, consequential, or exemplary damages resulting, in whole or in part, from the readers' use of, or reliance upon, this material. Any parts of this book based on government reports are so indicated and copyright is claimed for those parts to the extent applicable to compilations of such works.

Independent verification should be sought for any data, advice or recommendations contained in this book. In addition, no responsibility is assumed by the publisher for any injury and/or damage to persons or property arising from any methods, products, instructions, ideas or otherwise contained in this publication.

This publication is designed to provide accurate and authoritative information with regard to the subject matter covered herein. It is sold with the clear understanding that the Publisher is not engaged in rendering legal or any other professional services. If legal or any other expert assistance is required, the services of a competent person should be sought. FROM A DECLARATION OF PARTICIPANTS JOINTLY ADOPTED BY A COMMITTEE OF THE AMERICAN BAR ASSOCIATION AND A COMMITTEE OF PUBLISHERS.

Additional color graphics may be available in the e-book version of this book.

Library of Congress Cataloging-in-Publication Data

ISBN: 978-1-63117-701-9

Library of Congress Control Number: 2014939488

Published by Nova Science Publishers, Inc. † New York

Contents

Preface		**vii**
About the Editor		**ix**
Chapter I	Prodrugs Design Based on Inter- and Intramolecular Processes *Rafik Karaman*	**1**
Chapter II	Prodrug Overview *Ala' Abu-Jaish, Salma Jumaa* *and Rafik Karaman*	**77**
Chapter III	Chemical Approaches Used in Prodrugs Design *Beesan Fattash and Rafik Karaman*	**103**
Chapter IV	Targeted Prodrugs *Maryam Bader, Ameen Thawabteh* *and Rafik Karaman*	**139**
Chapter V	Virus Directed Enzyme Prodrug Therapy (VDEPT) *Nidaa Habbabeh and Rafik Karaman*	**177**
Chapter VI	Gene Directed Enzyme Prodrug Therapy (GDEPT) *Jawna' Sirhan and Rafik Karaman*	**211**
Chapter VII	Antibody Directed Enzyme Prodrug Therapy (ADEPT): A Promising Cancer Therapy Approach *Wajd Amly and Rafik Karaman*	**233**
Index		**279**

Preface

This book is a collaborative effort by the editor and many of his graduate students as coauthors to address the concept of prodrugs and their utilities in the pharmaceutical and medicinal fields. "Prodrug" (pro-agent, pre-drug) is a term that was first introduced in 1958 by Albert in his article in *Nature* to signify a pharmacologically inactive chemical moiety that can be used to temporarily alter the physicochemical properties of a drug to increase its usefulness and decrease its associated toxicity. Recently, the terms "drugability" and "druglike" commenced to be frequently used to describe physicochemical properties that required for a certain molecule to be clinically tested and potentially marketed as a drug.

Over the past two decades, an increase in the recognition that the discovery of potent therapeutics involves a design of entities that possess "drug-like" properties and high binding affinity for their biological targets has been established. The drug-like properties consist of solubility, permeation across barriers and metabolic and excretory clearance.

An important approach that has been used to impart good pharmaceutical properties is a design of a prodrug moiety that transiently modifies physicochemical properties of a drug candidate to overcome a shortcoming. Hence, it becomes much more feasible to modify and improve the properties of existing drugs through exploring the prodrug approach in order to eliminate the undesirable properties and to increase the commercial life-cycle and patentability of the concerned drugs.

The prodrug approach is a promising and well established strategy for the development of new entities that possess superior efficacy, selectivity and reduced toxicity. Hence an optimized therapeutic outcome can be accomplished using this approach. Approximately, about 10% of all worldwide marketed medicines can be categorized as prodrugs, and in 2008 alone, about 33% of all approved small molecular weight drugs were prodrugs, and this signifies the success of the prodrug approach.

A complete understanding of the physicochemical and biological behavior of the drug candidate is required when utilizing the approach to modify the drug's absorption, distribution, metabolism and elimination (ADME) properties. This approach consists of comprehensive evaluation of drug-likeness involving prediction of ADME properties which can be accomplished using *in vitro* and *in vivo* data obtained from tissue or recombinant material from humans and pre-clinical species, and *in silico* or computational predictions *in vitro* or *in vivo* data, involving the evaluation of various ADME properties, using computational methods such as quantitative structure activity relationship (QSAR) or molecular modeling.

Recent advances in molecular biology provide direct availability of enzymes and carrier proteins, including their molecular and functional characteristics. Prodrug design is becoming more elaborate in the development of efficient and selective drug delivery systems. The targeted prodrug approach, in combination with gene delivery and controlled expression of enzymes and carrier proteins, is a promising strategy for precise and efficient drug delivery and enhancement of the therapeutic effect.

There are two major prodrug design approaches that are considered as widely used among all other approaches to minimize or eliminate the undesirable drug physicochemical properties while maintaining the desirable pharmacological activity. The first approach is the targeted drug design approach by which prodrugs can be designed to target specific enzymes or carriers by considering enzyme-substrate specificity or carrier-substrate specificity in order to overcome various undesirable drug properties. This type of "targeted-prodrug" design requires considerable knowledge of particular enzymes or carriers, including their molecular and functional characteristics. An example for such approach is the antibody-directed enzyme prodrug therapy (ADEPT) or antibody-directed catalysis, antigens expressed on tumors cells are utilized to target enzymes to the tumor site. Alternative approaches designed to overcome the limitations of ADEPT are gene-directed enzyme prodrug therapy (GDEPT) and virus-directed enzyme prodrug therapy (VDEPT). In these approaches, genes encoding prodrug-activating enzymes are targeted to tumor cells followed by prodrug administration. In GDEPT, nonviral vectors that contain gene-delivery agents, such as peptides, cationic lipids or naked DNA, are used for gene targeting. In VDEPT, gene targeting is achieved using viral vectors, with retroviruses and adenoviruses being the most commonly used viruses. For both GDEPT and VDEPT, the vector has to be taken up by the target cells, and the enzyme must be stably expressed in tumor cells. This process is called transduction.

GDEPT and VDEPT effectiveness has been limited to date by insufficient transduction of tumor cells *in vivo*.

The second approach is a chemical design based on intramolecular processes that has been utilized to understand enzyme's catalysis. The tool used in the design is a computational approach consisting of quantum mechanics calculations and correlations between experimental and calculated reaction rates. In this approach no enzyme is needed for the activation of the prodrug to its parent drug.

Therefore, in the seven chapters of this book, we attempt to present the past and present prodrug concept and its many applications and successes in overcoming the formulation and delivery of problematic drugs.

We hope our enthusiasm for this topic is obvious and infective with a full recognition of the challenges that prodrugs can face.

Rafik Karaman, Ph.D.
Editor

About the Editor

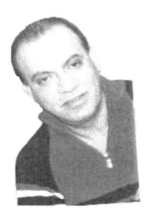

Born: November 1957, Um El-Fahim City
Work: College of Pharmacy, Al-Quds University, Jerusalem
Palestine. Tel. and Fax +972-2-2790413
Home: Ramallah, Palestine
Nationality: USA and Israel
Affiliation: Al-Quds University, Abu-Dies, Jerusalem, P.O. Box 20002, Palestine

Professor Rafik Karaman is currently a Distinguished professor of pharmaceutical sciences, College of Pharmacy, Al-Quds University, Jerusalem, Palestine. He received his Ph.D. degree in bioorganic chemistry from the Hebrew University in 1987, his MS degree in Pharmaceutical Sciences from the Hebrew University in 1983, and his bachelor's degree in Pharmacy from the Hebrew University in 1981. He was an Assistant Professor at the University of Toledo and University of California at Santa Barbara for 5 years where he worked with Professor T.C.Bruice in the bioorganic chemistry field. Professor Karaman is broadly interested in the design and synthesis of prodrug systems to be used for the delivery of certain drugs that have poor water solubility or/and have low bioavailability as well as synthesis of prodrugs for masking the bitter taste of the corresponding parent drugs. The design will be executed using ab initio, DFT, semiempirical, molecular mechanics as well as molecular dynamics and conformational dynamics methods. The overarching goal of his research activities is to establish a method for obtaining prodrugs that their interconversion rates will be controlled or programmed by the linker nature attached to their parent drugs. Professor Karaman has more than 120 peer-reviewed manuscripts and book chapters; 60 of them were published in the recent 6 years. He is currently an editor and an editorial board member of 15 international journals in the areas of pharmaceutical sciences.

In: Prodrugs Design – A New Era
Editor: Rafik Karaman

ISBN: 978-1-63117-701-9
© 2014 Nova Science Publishers, Inc.

Chapter I

Prodrugs Design Based on Inter- and Intramolecular Processes

Rafik Karaman[1,2]*

[1]Pharmaceutical Sciences Department, Faculty of Pharmacy
Al-Quds University, Jerusalem, Palestine
[2]Department of Science, University of Basilicata, Potenza, Italy

Abstract

In this chapter we have presented the past and current status of the prodrug approach and its applications and highlighted its many successes in solving problems associated with drug delivery. The two main prodrugs approaches that are presented in this chapter are the traditional approach by which a prodrug interconversion occurs *via* enzyme catalysis and the second approach is based on enzyme models that have been advocated to understand enzyme catalysis. In the latter approach, a design of prodrugs is accomplished using computational calculations based on molecular orbital and molecular mechanics methods. Correlations between experimental and calculated rate values for some intramolecular processes opened the door widely to predict thermodynamic and kinetic parameters for other processes that can be utilized as prodrugs linkers. This approach does not require any enzyme to catalyze the prodrug interconversion. The interconversion rate is solely dependent on the factors govern the limiting step of the intramolecular process. It is believed that the use of this approach might eliminate many disadvantages related to prodrug interconversion by the metabolic approach. For example, the activity of many prodrug activating enzymes may be varied due to genetic polymorphisms, age-related physiological changes, or drug interactions, leading to undesired pharmacokinetic, pharmacodynamics, and clinical effects. Furthermore, there are wide interspecies variations in both the expression and function of the major enzymes activating prodrugs, and these can pose some obstacles in the preclinical optimization phase.

---

* Corresponding author: Rafik Karaman, e-mail: dr_karaman@yahoo.com; Tel and Fax +972-2-2790413.

Keywords: Predrugs, prodrugs, molecular orbital calculations, molecular mechanics calculations, intramolecular reactions, prodrugs design, enzyme models, aza-nucleosides, Kirby's enzyme model, statins, Bruice's enzyme model, Menger's enzyme model, paracetamol, dopamine, tranexamic acid, DFT calculations

Abbreviations

ADME	Absorption, Distribution, Metabolism and Excretion.
QSAR	Quantitative Structure Activity Relationship
HLB	Hydrophilic Lipophilic Balance
ADEPT	Antibody-directed enzyme prodrug therapy
VDEPT	Virus-direct enzyme prodrug therapy
GDEPT	Gene-directed enzyme prodrug therapy
CYP	Cytochrome P450
GI	Gastro Intestinal.
NSAIDs	Non-steroidal Anti-inflammatory Drugs
PEG	Polyethylene glycol
QM	Quantum Mechanics
MM	Molecular Mechanics.
DFT	Diffused Functional Theory .
HF	Hartree-Fock
IGAC	Intramolecular General Acid Catalysis .
GAC	General Acid Catalysis
EM	Effective Molarity

Introduction

A drug is a chemical entity which is used in the diagnosis, cure, relief, treatment or prevention of disease, or intended to affect the structure or function of the body. Evidence of the use of medicines and drugs can be found three thousand years back. For long time, drug discovery has been a trial-and-error process. The conventional drug development has relied on blind screening approach, which was very time-consuming and labor costly. The disadvantages of conventional drug development and discovery as well as the desire for finding a more deterministic approach to combat disease have led to the concept of "Rational drug design" starting in the sixties of the past century. The process of drug discovery is very complex and requires an interdisciplinary effort to design effective and commercially effective drugs. The objective of drug design is to find a chemical entity that can fit to an active site of a receptor or enzyme. After passing the in vivo animal tests and human clinical trials, this entity becomes a drug available in the drug market. The conventional drug design methods were based on random screening of natural compounds or synthesized natural analogs in the laboratory. The main disadvantages of this method are time consuming cycle and high cost. Modern approach utilizing structure-based drug design with the aid of informatics technologies and a variety of computational methods has accelerated the drug development and discovery process in more efficient manner. Significant achievement has been made during the last decade in most areas concerned with drug design and discovery. A new generation of soft-wares with easy operation and super computers to provide chemically stable compounds with a potential to have therapeutic efficiency has been developed. These tools can tap into cheminformation to shorten the cycle of drug discovery, and thus make drug discovery more cost-effective.

In the last twenty years, a great attention has been paid to a design of chemical compounds that possess "drug-like" properties and high binding affinity for their biological targets. The drug-like properties include solubility, permeation across barriers and metabolic and excretory clearance [1-7].

Balanced physicochemical properties are crucial factors for attaining and maintaining a required systemic concentration of a drug to achieve its therapeutic effect. This can be achieved by optimizing the drug's absorption, distribution, metabolism, and excretion (ADME). Poorly absorbed, rapidly metabolized or quickly excreted drugs will not provide efficient therapeutic profiles. The drug's pharmaceutical properties are generally optimized by *de novo* design which involves selections of appropriate physicochemical attributes into the drug entity or via formulation of the drug with pharmaceuticals or biochemicals that can stabilize and improve the physicochemical properties.

A comprehensive study of the drug's physicochemical and biological behavior is a must when utilizing the absorption, distribution, metabolism and elimination (ADME) approach [8-12]. This approach involves an evaluation of drug-likeness involving prediction of ADME properties using *in vitro and in vivo* data obtained from tissue or recombinant material from human and pre-clinical species, and *in silico* or computational predictions. *In vitro* or *in vivo* data, involving the evaluation of various ADME properties, using computational methods such as quantitative structure activity relationship (QSAR) or molecular modeling are required for achieving a comprehensive evaluation on the drug under study [1-7]. Several studies have revealed that high attrition rates in the drug development process are attributed to poor pharmacokinetics and toxicity. Therefore, these issues should be heavily considered as early as possible in drug development and discovery to improve the drug's therapeutic efficiency and cost effectiveness [13].

In order to achieve a drug's success in reaching its biological target the following drug's physical and chemical properties should be fulfilled: (i) chemical stability in aqueous solution such as stomach, intestine and blood circulation environments, (ii) metabolic stability; the drug must survive digestive and metabolic enzymes (liver) and any metabolites (product of drug metabolism) should not be toxic or lose activity, and (iii) successful absorption; diffusion across membrane (solubility and permeability; size, hydrogen bonding) [3-4].

An important approach that has been utilized for improving a drug's pharmaceutical properties is a prodrug design which based on transiently modified physicochemical properties of a drug to overcome a shortcoming. The prodrug approach is a promising and well established strategy for the development of new entities that possess superior efficacy, selectivity and reduced toxicity. Approximately, about 10% of all worldwide marketed therapeutics can be classified as prodrugs, and in 2008 alone, about 33% of all approved small-molecular weight medicines were prodrugs, and this signifies the success of the prodrug approach [5-7].

Therefore, implementing of one or more of the strategies described in the following sections can lead to a drug with optimum pharmacokinetics properties.

Improving Hydrophilic/Lipophilic Balance (Absorption)

Among the important factors that determine the drug's absorption is the drug's hydrophilic hydrophobic balance (HLB) value, a measure which depends on polarity and ionization. Too polar or strongly ionized drugs, having high HLB values, cannot efficiently cross the cell membranes of the gastrointestinal (GI) barrier. Therefore, they are administered by the I.V. route, however, being rapidly eliminated is considered to be disadvantage. Lipophilic (non-polar) drugs, on the other hand, have low HLB values and poor aqueous solubility, therefore, their absorption into membranes is limited. If to be given by injection, they will be retained in fat tissues [14-22].

The drug's polarity and/or ionization can be modified by altering one or more of its functional groups. Examples for such alteration: (1) variation of alkyl or acyl substituents and polar functional groups to vary polarity, (2) variation of N-alkyl substituents to vary pK_a. Use of amines with $pK_a = 6$-9. If the pK_a is out of range, changing the structure of the amine will provide change in the pK_a. Drugs with a pK_a outside the range 6-9 tend to be ionized and are poorly absorbed through membrane tissues, (3) variation of aromatic substituents to vary pK_a; the pKa of carboxylic acid can be varied by adding electron donating or electron withdrawing groups to the ring. The position of the substituent, *ortho*, *meta* or *para*, is important too if the substituent interacts with the ring through resonance, (4) bioisosteres are substituents with similar physical or chemical properties which produce relatively similar biological properties to a drug moiety. The purpose of exchanging one bioisostere for another is to improve the desired biological or physical properties of a given biological moiety without making significant changes in its chemical structure. Bioisostere is used to reduce toxicity or improve the activity of the lead compound, and may alter the metabolism of the lead compound. Among examples of bioisosteres: (i) the replacement of a hydrogen atom with a fluorine atom at a site of metabolic oxidation (such as cytochromes) in a drug to inhibit or slow such metabolism from taking place, thus the drug candidate may have a longer half-life. This approach is generally successful because the fluorine atom is similar in size to the hydrogen atom and thus the overall topology and size of the molecule is not significantly affected, leaving the desired biological activity almost untouched, (ii) the replacement of oxygen atom with a nitrogen atom; a successful example for such replacement is procainamide, an amide, has a longer duration of action than procaine, an ester, (iii) changing the position of a double bond such as in the case of alloxanthine which is an inhibitor of xanthine oxidase and an isostere of xanthine, the normal substrate for the enzyme, (iv) another example is aromatic rings, a phenyl ring can often be replaced by a different aromatic ring such as thiophene or naphthalene which may either improve efficacy or change specificity of binding and (v) carboxylic acid is a highly polar group which can be ionized and hence decreases the absorption of any drug containing it. To overcome this problem blocking the free carboxyl group by making the corresponding ester prodrug or replacing it with a bioisostere group, which has similar physiochemical properties and has advantage over carboxylic acid in regards to its pK_a, such as 5-substituted tetrazoles, is essential; 5-substituted tetrazole ring contains acidic proton like carboxylic acid and is ionized at pH 7.4. On the other hand, most of the alkyl and aryl carboxylic group have a pK_a in the range of 2-5. Other examples of bioisosteres, which may be equivalent in some cases but not in others depending on what factors are important in binding (electronegativity, size, polarity etc.). For example, a chlorine group may often be replaced by a trifluoromethyl group, or by a cyano group, but depending on the particular biological moiety used the substitution may result in little change in activity, or either increases or decreases affinity or efficacy depending on what factors are important for target binding, (5) use of carrier proteins to deliver drugs; this approach utilizes the advantage of carrier proteins in cell membranes that transport sugars, amino acids, neurotransmitters, and metal ions. If a drug resembles the above mentioned biological substances, it might be the drug that can be transported across membranes. Examples of use of carrier proteins to deliver drugs: levodopa is transported by phenylalanine transporter (Figure 1), fluorouracil is transported by thymine and uracil transporters and lisinopril (antihypertensive) is transported by dipeptide transporters (Figure 2), and (6) use of medicinal chemistry to improve hydrophobic hydrophilic balance; change functional groups: alcohol (ROH) versus ether (ROR') or ester (RO2R'), change the number or size of alkyl groups. Change of rings; an example for ring change is tioconazole, a non-polar antifungal agent, which is used in topical treatment and fluconazole which is more polar compound due to the presence of more polar groups in its moiety and it is used as antifungal for systemic use (Figure 3) [14-30].

Figure 1. Chemical structures of levodopa and phenylalanine.

Figure 2. Chemical structure of lisinopril.

**Ticonazole (topical antifungal)
Non-polar**

**Fluconazole (systemic antifungal)
Polar**

Figure 3. Chemical structures of the antifungal agents, tioconazole and fluconazole.

Improving Metabolism

Metabolism of drugs occurs in liver, kidneys, intestine, lungs, blood and skin. It is mostly catalyzed by enzymes. Generally, metabolic products (metabolites) are more water soluble than their corresponding parent drugs, so they may be readily excreted. Drug metabolism can occur by two phases: phase I by which metabolic reactions include oxidations (cytochrome P450 enzymes, flavinmonooxygenase and others), reductions, and hydrolyses, and phase II which involves metabolic reactions as a result of the conjugation of metabolic products or parent drugs to other small molecules via carboxyl, hydroxyl, thiol and amino groups. Conjugated products are even more water soluble than the drug metabolites and have no toxicity or pharmacological activity.

Strategies to Make Drugs More Resistant to Hydrolysis and Metabolism, Prolonging Reactivity

The strategies that are taken to make drugs more resistant to hydrolysis and metabolism are:

(1) Steric shields; some functional groups are more susceptible to chemical and enzymatic degradation than others. For example, esters and amides are much more affordable to hydrolysis than other organic compounds such as carbamates and oximes. Placing steric shields to these drugs increases their stability. Steric shields, designed to hinder the approach of a nucleophile or an enzyme having nucleophilic moiety to the susceptible group. These usually involve the addition of a bulky alkyl group like t-butyl in close proximity to the functional group: one of such examples is shown in Figure 4.

Steric sheilds block hydrolysis of peptide link

Figure 4. An illustration of how steric shields block a peptide hydrolysis.

(2) Isosteric/bioisostere replacement: changing a more reactive ester to a less reactive amide. Such an example is acetylcholine and carbachol shown in Figure 5.

Acetylcholine (neurotransmitter)

Carbachole (cholinergic agonist) more resistant to hydrolysis

Figure 5. Chemical structures of acetylcholine and carbachol.

In this example the methyl groups on the phenyl ring impose steric shielding, while replacing the ester (procaine) to a less reactive amide (lidocaine) slows the enzymatic hydrolysis reaction (Figure 6).

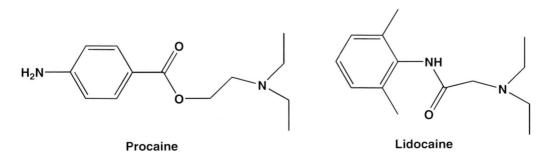

Procaine

Lidocaine

Figure 6. An illustration of a combination of both effects; steric shields and isosteric effect; procaine is a short-lasting anesthetic because of ester hydrolysis.

(3) Removal of functional group that is susceptible to metabolic enzymes. Aryl methyl groups such as in tolbutamide are oxidized to carboxylic acids and eliminated from the body. Replacing the toluene methyl group in tolbutamide with a chloro group makes the drug (chlorpropamide) more resistant to metabolism and as a result a long duration of the drug's action (Figure 7). Other common metabolic reactions include aliphatic and aromatic C-hydroxylation, O and S-dealkylations, N- and S-oxidations and deamination.

Tolbutamide (antidiabetic)

Chlorpropoamide
Longer-lasting

Figure 7. Chemical structures of tolbutamide and chlorpropamide.

(4) Electronic effects of bioisosteres. This approach is used to protect a labile functional group by electronical stabilization. For example: replacing the methyl group of an ethanolate ester with an amine group gives a urethane functional group which is more stable than its corresponding ester. The amine group has the same size and valence as the methyl group, however, it has no steric effect, but it has totally different electronic properties, since it can donate electrons into the carbonyl group resulting in reducing the electophilicity of the carbonyl carbon and hence hydrolysis stabilization.

Carbachol, a cholinergic agonist, and cefoxitin, an antibacterial cephalosporin, are stabilized by this way.

(5) Metabolic blockers; some drugs are easily metabolized since they have certain polar functional groups at particular positions in their skeleton. For instance, megestrol acetate, a cortisone derivative used as an oral contraceptive, is readily oxidized at position 6 to yield a hydroxyl group, when replacing the hydrogen at position 6 with methyl group its metabolism is blocked and consequently it increases its duration of action (Figure 8).

Megestrol acetate

Figure 8. Chemical structure of megestrol acetate.

Prodrugs Design Based on Inter- and Intramolecular Processes   9

(6) Group shifts; removing or replacing a metabolically vulnerable group is feasible when the group concerned is not engaged in the binding interactions with the active site of the receptor or enzyme. If the group is important, then different strategy should be considered, either by masking the vulnerable group by making a prodrug or placing the vulnerable group within the molecule skeleton. An example for such approach is salbutamol (Figure 9) which was developed from its analogue neurotransmitter, noradrenaline (Figure 9). The Noradrenaline metabolism is via methylation of one of its phenolic groups by catechol O-methyl transferase. The other phenolic group is crucial for the neurotransmitter binding interaction with the receptor. Replacing the hydroxyl group with a methyl group or removing it prevents metabolism but also prevent hydrogen bonding interaction with the receptor binding site. On the other hand, placing the vulnerable hydroxyl group out from the ring by one carbon unit as in salbutamol makes this compound unrecognizable by the enzyme involved in the metabolism, but not to the receptor binding site (prolonged action) and

Salbutamol   **Noradrenaline**

Figure 9. Chemical structures of salbutamol and noradrenaline.

(7) ring variation; a number of biological systems some having cyclic rings are often found to be susceptible to enzymatic metabolism, hence, replacing those rings with more stable ones can often improve the drug metabolic stability. For example, replacement the imidazole ring which is susceptible to metabolism in tioconazole with 1, 2, 4-triazole ring gives fluconazole which is relatively much resistant to enzymatic metabolism (Figure 3).

Strategies to Make Drugs Less Resistant to Metabolic Enzymes

If a drug is too resistant to metabolism, it can pose problems as well (toxicity, long-lasting side effects). Therefore, designing drugs with decreased chemical and metabolic stability can sometimes be beneficial. Methods for applying such strategy are: (a) introducing groups that are susceptible to metabolism is a good way of shorting the lifetime of a drug. For example, addition of functional groups such as a methyl on aromatic ring provides a drug with adequate duration of action (Figure 10).

Figure 10. Chemical structures of anti-asthmatic drugs.

(b) A self-destruct drug is one which is chemically stable under one set of conditions but becomes unstable and spontaneously cleaved under another set of conditions. The advantage of a self-destruct drug is that inactivation does not depend on the activity of metabolic enzymes, which could vary from patient to patient. For example, atracurium, a neuromuscular blocking agent, is stable at acidic pH but self-destruct when it is exposed to the slightly alkaline conditions of the blood (pH 7.4). Thus, the drug has a short duration of action, allowing anesthetists to control its blood concentration levels during surgery by providing it as a continuous intravenous drip [23-30].

Reducing Toxicity

One way to measure the dangers of various drugs is to examine how toxic the drug is at various levels. The most toxic recreational drugs, such as gamma-hydroxybutyrate and heroin, have a lethal dose less than 10 times their typical effective dose. The largest cluster of substances has a lethal dose that is 10 to 20 times the effective dose; these include cocaine, methylenedioxymethamphetamine, often called "ecstasy" and alcohol. A less toxic group of substances, requiring 20 to 80 times the effective dose to cause death, include flunitrazepam and mescaline. The least physiologically toxic substances, those requiring 100 to 1,000 times the effective dose to cause death, include psilocybin mushrooms and marijuana, when ingested. The above mentioned drugs have found their way in the drug market however there are many that did not succeed to enter the market because they failed the clinical trials stage due to their toxic adverse effects.

In most cases the toxic side effects of those drugs might be attributed to their toxic metabolites, in those cases the drug should be made more resistant to metabolism. It is well known that functional groups such as aromatic nitro groups, aromatic amines, bromoarenes, hydrazines, hydroxylamines, or polyhalogenated groups are generally metabolized to toxic metabolites. Replacing such groups with harmless substituents or shifting them from the drug metabolism center might reduce or eliminate their side effects.

For example, addition of a fluorine atom to UK 47265, antifungal agent, gives the less toxic antifungal, fluconazole (Figure 3) [30-35].

Targeting Drugs

The principle of targeting drugs was advocated by Paul Ehrlich who developed antimicrobial drugs that were selectively toxic for microbial cells over human cells. Today, targeting tumor cells is considered one of the most important issues that under concern among the health community. The main goal in cancer chemotherapy is to target drugs efficiently against tumor cells rather than normal cells. Cancer chemotherapeutics are toxic and nonselective which limit its use for cancer. Their selectivity depends on that rapidly dividing cells are more prone to the toxic effect, so they are toxic for rapidly proliferating normal tissue such as hair follicles, gut epithelia, bone marrow, and red blood cells. Therefore, to improve toxicity and efficacy chemotherapy prodrugs were designed to target tumor cells. This targeting is achieved by binding drugs to a ligand that has high affinity to specific antigens, receptors, or transporters that are over expressed in tumor cells. One important method for targeting cancer cells without affecting normal cells is to design drugs which make use of specific molecular transport systems. The idea is to link the anti-cancer active drug to an important building block molecule that is needed in large amounts by the rapidly divided tumor cells. The block molecule could be an amino acid or a nucleic acid base such as uracil mustard. In the cases where the drug is intended to target against gastrointestinal tract infections it must be prevented from being absorbed into the blood circulation system. This can be accomplished by using a fully ionized drug which is incapable of crossing cell membrane barriers. For example, highly ionized sulfonamides are used against gastrointestinal tract infections because they cannot cross the gut wall. It is often possible to target drugs such that they act peripherally and not in the central nervous system (CNS). By increasing the polarity of drugs, they are less likely to cross the blood-brain barrier and thus they are less likely to give CNS adverse effects [36-38].

Prodrugs

The term "prodrug" or "prodrug" was first introduced by Albert to signify pharmacologically inactive chemical moiety that can be used to temporarily alter the physicochemical properties of a drug in order to increase its usefulness and decrease its associated toxicity. The use of the term usually implies a covalent link between a drug and a chemical entity. Generally, prodrugs can be enzymatically or chemically degraded *in vivo* to furnish the parent active drug which exerts a therapeutic effect. Ideally, the prodrug should be converted to the parent drug and non-toxic moiety as soon as its goal is achieved, followed by the subsequent rapid elimination of the released linker group [30-42].

Targeted drugs are drugs or prodrugs that exert their biological action only in specific cells or organs such as in the cases of omeprazole and acyclovir. The active metabolite term refers to the degradation of the drug by the body into a modified form that has a biological effect. Usually these effects are similar to those of the parent drug but are weaker yet still significant. Examples of such metabolites are 11-hydroxy-THC and morphine-6-glucuronide. In certain drugs, such as codeine and tramadol, the corresponding metabolites (morphine and O-desmethyltramadol, respectively) are more potent than the parent drug [43-45].

The rationale behind the use of prodrugs is to optimize the absorption, distribution, metabolism, and excretion properties (ADME). In addition, the prodrug strategy has been used to increase the selectivity of drugs for their intended target. Development of a prodrug with improved properties may also represent a life-cycle management opportunity.

The prodrug approach is a very versatile strategy to increase the utility of biologically active compounds, because one can optimize any of the ADME properties of potential drug candidates. In most cases, prodrugs contain a promoiety (linker) that is removed by an enzymatic or chemical reaction, while other prodrugs release their active drugs after molecular modification such as an oxidation or reduction reaction. The prodrug candidate can also be prepared as a double prodrug, where the second linker is attached to the first promoiety linked to the parent drug molecule. These linkers are usually different each from other and are cleaved by different mechanisms. In some cases, two biologically active drugs can be linked together in a single molecule called a codrug. In a codrug, each drug acts as a promoiety for the other [46-47].

The prodrug approach has been used to overcome various undesirable drug properties and to optimize clinical drug application. Recent advances in molecular biology provide direct availability of enzymes and carrier proteins, including their molecular and functional characteristics. Prodrug design is becoming more elaborate in the development of efficient and selective drug delivery systems. The targeted prodrug approach, in combination with gene delivery and controlled expression of enzymes and carrier proteins, is a promising strategy for precise and efficient drug delivery and enhancement of the therapeutic effect.

The prodrug design can be utilized in the following:

(i) Improving active drug solubility and consequently bioavailability; dissolution of the drug molecule from the dosage form may be the rate-limiting step to absorption [47]. It has been reported that more than 30% of drug discovery compounds have poor aqueous solubility [48]. Prodrugs are an alternative way to increase the aqueous solubility of the parent drug molecules by improving dissolution rate via attached ionizable or polar neutral functions, such as phosphates, amino acids, or sugar moieties [15, 40, 47, 49]. These prodrugs can be used not only to enhance oral bioavailability but also to prepare parenteral or injectable drug delivery.

(ii) Increasing permeability and absorption; membrane permeability has a significant effect on drug efficacy [41]. In oral drug delivery, the most common absorption routes are unfacilitated and largely nonspecific passive transport mechanisms. The lipophilicity of poorly permeable drugs can be enhanced by hydrocarbon moiety modification. In such cases, the prodrug strategy can be an extremely valuable option. Improvement of lipophilicity has been the most widely investigated and successful field of prodrug research. It has been achieved by masking polar ionized or nonionized functional groups to enhance either oral or topical absorption [50].

An example of such approach is esterification of enalprilate (polar and not permeable) to the less polar and permeable antihypertensive enalapril (Figure 11). Another example of increasing lipophilicity via a prodrug approach is a barbitone prodrug, hexabarbitone: since N-demethylation is a common liver metabolic reaction, amines may be methylated to increase hydrophobicity. These N-methyl groups will be removed in the liver (Figure 12).

Figure 11. Chemical structures of the prodrug enalapril and its parent drug enalprilate.

**Enalapril (prodrug)
can cross membrane**

Enalaprilate (anti-hypertensive agent)

Hexobarbital (prodrug)

Figure 12. Chemical structures of barbitone and its prodrug hexabarbitone.

(iii) Modifying the distribution profile; before the drug reaches its physiological target and exerts the desired effect, it has to bypass several pharmaceutical and pharmacokinetic barriers.

Today, one of the most promising site-selective drug delivery strategies is the prodrug approach that utilizes target cell- or tissue-specific endogenous enzymes and transporters. One of the few examples that were designed to increase the efficiency of a drug by accumulation into a specific tissue or organ is the antiParkinson agent L-DOPA. Because of its hydrophilic nature, the neurotransmitter dopamine is not able to cross the blood-brain barrier and distribute into brain tissue. However, the prodrug of dopamine, L-DOPA, enables the uptake and accumulation of dopamine into the brain via the L-type amino acid transporter 1 [40, 51]. After L-type amino acid transporter 1-mediated uptake, L-DOPA is bio activated by aromatic L-amino acid decarboxylase to hydrophilic dopamine, which is concentrated in dopaminergic nerves (Figure 13). Because L-DOPA is extensively metabolized in the peripheral circulation, DOPA decarboxylase inhibitors (carbidopa, benserazide and methyldopa) and/or catechol-*O*-methyltransferase inhibitors (entacapone, tolcapone and nitecapone) are co administered with levodopa to prevent the unwanted metabolism [52-53].

Dopamine
Too Polar
Cannot cross blood brain barrier

Levodopa
Non-polar
Can cross blood brain barrier

Figure 13. Chemical structures of the neurotransmitter dopamine and levodopa.

(iv) Prevention fast metabolism and excretion; the first-pass effect in the gastrointestinal tract and liver may greatly reduce the total amount of active drug reaches the systemic circulation and consequently its target. This problem has been overcome by sublingual or buccal administration or by controlled release formulations. Fast metabolic drug degradation can also be prevented by a prodrug strategy. This is usually done by masking the metabolically labile but pharmacologically essential functional group(s) of the drug. In the case of the bronchodilator and β$_2$-agonist terbutaline, sustained drug action has been achieved by converting its phenolic groups, which are susceptible to fast and extensive first pass metabolism, into bis-dimethylcarbamate. The prodrug bambuterol is slowly bio activated to terbutaline predominantly by nonspecific butyrylcholinesterases outside the lungs [54-56]. As a result of the slower release and prolonged action, once-daily administration of bambuterol provides relief of asthma with a lower incidence of adverse effects than terbutaline (Figure 14) [57].

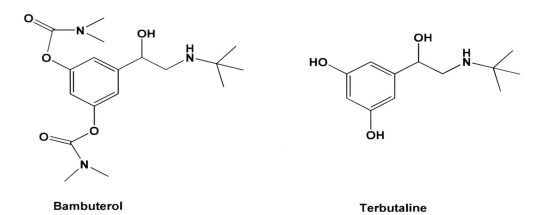

Figure 14. Chemical structures of bambuterol and terbutaline.

(v) Reducing toxicity; adverse drug reactions can change the structure or function of cells, tissues, and organs and can be detrimental to the organism. Reduced toxicity can sometimes be accomplished by altering one or more of the ADME barriers but more often is achieved by targeting drugs to desired cells and tissues via site-selective drug delivery. A successful site-selective prodrug must be precisely transported to the site of action, where it should be selectively and quantitatively transformed into the active drug, which is retained in the target tissue to produce its therapeutic effect [40, 58]. The ubiquitous distribution of most of the endogenous enzymes that are responsible for bioactivating prodrugs diminishes the opportunities for selective drug delivery and targeting. Therefore, exogenous enzymes are selectively delivered via antibody-directed enzyme prodrug therapy or as genes that encode prodrug activating enzymes. This approach is particularly used with highly toxic compounds such as anticancer drugs to reduce the toxicity of the drugs at other sites in the body [59-60].

Another type of prodrugs to mask toxicity and/or side effects is aspirin: salicylic acid is a pain killer, but phenolic -OH causes gastric bleeding. Aspirin has an ester to mask this toxic group until it is hydrolyzed (Figure 15).

Figure 15. Chemical structures of aspirin and salicylic acid.

Similarly, Antiviral drugs such as AZT and acyclovir are nontoxic until they are converted to toxic triphosphates by viral enzymes in infected cells. These phosphorylated compounds are both competitive inhibitors and chain terminators (Figure 16).

Figure 16. Chemical structures of the anti-viral drug AZT and its phosphorylated derivative.

(vi) Prolong drug activity; 6-mercaptopurine is used to suppress the immune system (organ transplants), but is eliminated from the body quickly. A prodrug that slowly is converted to the drug allows a sustained activity (Figure 17).

Azathioprine (prodrug)

6-Mercaptopurine

Figure 17. Chemical structures of the prodrug azathioprine and its active moiety 6-mercaptopurine.

There are two major challenges facing the prodrug approach strategy: (1) hydrolysis of prodrugs by esterases; the most common approaches for prodrug design are aimed at prodrugs undergoing *in vivo* cleavage to the active drug by catalysis of hydrolases such as peptidases, phosphatases, and carboxylesterases [50]. The less than complete absorption observed with several hydrolase-activated prodrugs of penicillins, cephalosporins, and angiotensin-converting enzyme inhibitors highlights yet another challenge with prodrugs susceptible to esterase hydrolysis. These prodrugs typically have bioavailabilities around 50% because of their premature hydrolysis during the absorption process in the enterocytes of the gastrointestinal tract [50]. Hydrolysis inside the enterocytes releases the active drug, which in most cases is more polar and less permeable than the prodrug and is more likely to be effluxes by passive and carrier-mediated processes back into the lumen than to proceed into blood, therefore limiting oral bioavailability.

(2) Bioactivation of the prodrug by cytochrome P450 enzymes. The P450 enzymes are superfamily enzymes that account for up to 75% of enzymatic metabolism of drugs, including several prodrugs. There is accumulating evidence that genetic polymorphisms of prodrug-activating P450s contribute substantially to the variability in prodrug activation and thus to the efficacy and safety of drugs using this bioactivation pathway [61-62].

Bioconversion of prodrugs is perhaps the most vulnerable link in the chain, because there are many intrinsic and extrinsic factors that can influence the process. For example, the activity of many prodrug activating enzymes may be decreased or increased due to genetic polymorphisms, age-related physiological changes, or drug interactions, leading to adverse pharmacokinetic, pharmacodynamics, and clinical effects. In addition, there are wide interspecies variations in both the expression and function of the major enzyme systems activating prodrugs, and these can pose challenges in the preclinical optimization phase.

Nonetheless, developing a prodrug can still be a more feasible and faster strategy than searching for an entirely new therapeutically active agent with suitable ADMET properties.

An ideal drug candidate needs to have specific properties, including chemical and enzymatic stability, solubility, and low clearance by the liver or kidney, permeation across biological membranes, potency, and safety.

The conversion of a prodrug to the parent drug at the target site is crucial for the prodrug approach to be successful. Generally, activation involves metabolism by enzymes that are distributed throughout the body [10-11, 50]. The major problem with these prodrugs is the difficulty in predicting their bioconversion rates, and thus their pharmacological or toxicological effects. Moreover, the rate of hydrolysis is not always predictable, and bioconversion can be affected by various factors such as age, health conditions and gender [63-65].

There are two major prodrug design approaches that are considered as widely used among all other approaches to minimize or eliminate the undesirable drug physicochemical properties while maintaining the desirable pharmacological activity. The first approach is the targeted drug design approach by which prodrugs can be designed to target specific enzymes or carriers by considering enzyme-substrate specificity or carrier-substrate specificity in order to overcome various undesirable drug properties. This type of "targeted-prodrug" design requires considerable knowledge of particular enzymes or carriers, including their molecular and functional characteristics [66-77]. An example for such approach is the antibody-directed enzyme prodrug therapy (ADEPT) or antibody-directed catalysis, antigens expressed on tumors cells are utilized to target enzymes to the tumor site. In this approach, at the beginning, an enzyme-antibody conjugate is administered and given sufficient time to interact with tumor cells and to be eliminated from the circulation. Subsequently, a prodrug is given and selectively activated extracellular at the tumor site.

Alternative approaches designed to overcome the limitations of ADEPT are gene-directed enzyme prodrug therapy (GDEPT) and virus-directed enzyme prodrug therapy (VDEPT). In these approaches, genes encoding prodrug-activating enzymes are targeted to tumor cells followed by prodrug administration. In GDEPT, nonviral vectors that contain gene-delivery agents, such as peptides, cationic lipids or naked DNA, are used for gene targeting. In VDEPT, gene targeting is achieved using viral vectors, with retroviruses and adenoviruses being the most commonly used viruses. For both GDEPT and VDEPT, the vector has to be taken up by the target cells, and the enzyme must be stably expressed in tumor cells. This process is called transduction [66-77].

GDEPT and VDEPT effectiveness has been limited to date by insufficient transduction of tumor cells *in vivo*.

The second approach is the chemical design approach by which the drug is linked to inactive organic moiety which upon exposure to physiological environment releases the parent drug and a non-toxic linker which should be eliminated without affecting the clinical profile.

The prodrug chemical approach can be classified into two sub-classes (1) carrier-linked prodrugs; contains a group that can be easily removed enzymatically, such as an ester or labile amide, to provide the parent drug. Ideally, the group removed is pharmacologically inactive and nontoxic, while the linkage between the drug and promoiety must be labile for *in vivo* efficient activation. Carrier-linked prodrugs can be further subdivided into (a) bipartite which is composed of one carrier group attached to the drug, (b) tripartite which is a carrier group that is attached *via* linker to drug, and (c) mutual prodrugs consisting of two drugs linked together and (2) bioprecursors; chemical entities that are metabolized into new compounds that may be active or further are metabolized to active metabolites, such as amine to aldehyde to carboxylic acid [15, 31, 41-42, 78].

The suitability of a number of functional groups like carboxyl, hydroxyl, amine, phosphate, phosphonate and carbonyl groups for undergoing different chemical modifications, facilitate their utilization in prodrug design [40, 78] In the past few decades a variety of prodrugs based on the chemical approach have been designed, synthesized and tested. Among those are:

Ester Prodrugs

The main trend in prodrug research is toward developing ester prodrugs. This is owing to their acceptable *in vitro* chemical stability, and so reducing formulation problems, along with their susceptibility to the action of esterases, which allows subsequent release of the active drug once it enters the body. Carboxylic acid (-COOH), hydroxyl (-OH), phosphate (-PO_4) and thiol groups (-SH) can easily undergo esterification. Ester prodrugs undergo a rapid conversion into the parent drug via the action of esterases that present everywhere in the body including liver, blood, and other tissues, or via oxidative cleavage catalyzed by cytochrome P450 (CYP) [79-81].

Carboxyl esterases, acetylcholinesterases, butyrylcholinesterases, paraoxonases, arylesterases and biphenyl hydrolase-like protein (BPHL) are some examples of enzymes that are responsible for the hydrolysis catalysis of ester prodrugs [81]. For example, biphenyl hydrolase-like protein (BPHL) is known to catalyze the hydrolysis of prodrugs like valacyclovir and ganciclovir (Figure 18) [81], as well as a number of other amino acid esters of nucleoside analogues including valyl-AZT, prodrugs of floxuridine (5-fluoro-20-deoxyuridine or FUdR) and gemcitabine [82-86].

Ester prodrugs are commonly used to enhance lipophilicity, thus increasing membrane permeation through masking the charge of polar functional groups [79]. For example, acyclovir aliphatic ester prodrugs were prepared by esterification of the hydroxyl group with lipophilic acid anhydride or acyl chloride, thus an enhanced lipophilicity can be achieved. Utilizing lipophilic ester acyclovir prodrugs showed an enhanced nasal and skin absorption [79, 82-86]. It has been revealed that an increase in the length of the alkyl chain can result in an easy cleavage of the ester bond. Therefore, it can be concluded that improved binding to the hydrophobic pocket of carboxylesterase can be accomplished by increasing the length of the alkyl chain, while branching the alkyl chain can result in reduced hydrolysis due to steric hindrance [79].

Other examples of ester prodrugs that were investigated and synthesized for different purposes are thioester of erythromycin, palmitate ester of clindamycin [83], a number of angiotensin converting enzyme inhibitors that are presently marketed as ester prodrugs such as enalapril, ramipril , benazepril and fosinopril for the treatment of hypertension [80, 83] and ibuprofen guiacol ester which was reported to have fewer GI side effects with similar anti-inflammatory/antipyretic action to the parent drug when given in equimolar doses [87].

Figure 18. Chemical structures of acyclovir, valacyclovir, gancyclovir.

Benorylate is a mutual prodrug of aspirin and paracetamol (Figure 19), coupled through an ester linkage, which is postulated to have reduced gastric irritancy with synergistic analgesic effect [88, 89]. Besides, Mutual prodrugs of ibuprofen with paracetamol and salicylamide have been reported with better lipophilicity and diminished gastric toxicity than their parent drugs. Naproxen-propyphenazone mutual prodrugs were synthesized to prevent GI irritation and bleeding. Esterification of naproxen with different alkyl esters and thioesters led to prodrugs with retained anti-inflammatory activity and exhibited greatly reduced GI erosive properties and analgesic potency, but esterification with ethyl piperazine showed that analgesic activity was conserved, whereas anti-inflammatory activity was generally reduced [88].

Figure 19. Chemical structure of benorylate.

Another strategy in mutual prodrugs is linking NSAIDs with histamine H_2 antagonist in order to reduce gastric damage like flurbiprofen, histamine H_2 antagonist conjugate, that have been reported [90].

In addition to reduced GI toxicity achieved using NSAIDs mutual prodrugs, an antiarthritic activity and enhanced analgesic/anti-inflammatory activity can be accomplished using the same approach. For example, mutual prodrugs of ketoprofen, ibuprofen, diclofenac and flurbiprofen with an antiarthritic nutraceutical D-glucosamine [90-92].

Mutual prodrugs approach can also be applied to other therapeutic groups. For instance, sultamicillin in which the irreversible β-lactamase inhibitor sulbactam has been joined chemically via ester linkage with ampicillin (Figure 20); this mutual prodrug possesses a synergistic effect and upon oral administration, sultamicillin is completely hydrolyzed to equimolar proportions of sulbactam and ampicillin, thereby acting as an efficient mutual prodrug [93].

Sultamicillin

Figure 20. Chemical structure of sultamicillin.

Amide Prodrugs

This approach can be exploited to enhance the stability of drugs, to provide targeted drug delivery and to change lipophilicity of drugs like acids and acid chlorides [94]. Drugs that have carboxylic acid or amine group can be converted into amide prodrugs. Generally they are used to a limited extent due to high *in vivo* stability. However, prodrugs using facile intramolecular cyclization reactions have been exploited to overcome this obstacle [95].

In similar to mutual ester prodrugs, mutual amide prodrugs, where the two active drugs are linked together by an amide linkage, such as, atorvastatin-amlodipine which has been synthesized and has shown *in vivo* fast amide hydrolysis to provide the active parent drugs. Amide prodrugs can be converted back to the parent drugs either by nonspecific amidases or specific enzymatic activation such as renal γ-glutamyl transpeptidase. Dopamine double prodrug; γ-glutamyl-L-dopa (gludopa) undergoes specific activation by renal γ-glutamyl transpeptidase where it achieves relatively 5-fold increase in dopamine level compared to L-dopa prodrug. However, since gludopa has low oral bioavailability, docarpamine [*N*-(*N*-acetyl-L-methionyl)-*O*,*O*-*bis*(ethoxycarbonyl)dopamine), a pseudopeptide prodrug of dopamine, was developed and has shown improved oral absorption , hence, it is given orally and is used in the treatment of renal and cardiovascular diseases (Figure 21). Basically, dopamine prodrugs are developed due to dopamine inactivation by COMT and MAO when administered by the oral route [96-97].

Figure 21. Chemical structures of docarpamine [N-(N-acetyl-L-methionyl)-O, O-bis (ethoxycarbonyl) dopamine), a pseudopeptide prodrug of dopamine and dopamine.

A respected number of amine conjugates with amino acids through amide linkage have been considered for providing active drugs with remarkable enhancement in solubility such as dapsone [98].

Other examples of amide based prodrugs are allopurinol N-acyl derivatives which were found to be more lipophilic than allpurinol itself [99].

Carbonates and Carbamates Prodrugs

Generally, carbonates and carbamates are more stable than their corresponding esters but less stable than amides [100]. Carbamates and carbonates have no specific enzymes for their hydrolysis reactions; however, they are degraded by esterases to give the corresponding active parent drugs [100-101]. Co-carboxymethylphenyl ester of amphetamine is an example of carbamate prodrug that can be hydrolyzed by esterase to yield amphetamine [101]. Another example of carbamate prodrug is the one obtained by linking phosphorylated steroid, an estradiol, to normustard, an alkylating agent, through a carbamate linkage which yields estramustine prodrug. The latter is used in the treatment of prostate cancer. The steroid moiety has an anti-androgenic action and acts to concentrate the prodrug in the prostate gland where prodrug hydrolysis takes place and normusard action can then be exerted [89]. Carbamate prodrugs can also be used to increase the solubility of active drugs like cephalosporins [102]. In addition, carbamate prodrugs have been exploited in targeted therapy such as ADEPT. In this case, the carbamate group is susceptible to the action of tyrosinase enzyme present in melanomas. This approach is usually utilized in cancer targeted therapy [94].The list of carbamate prodrugs is long, among other examples is the nonsedating antihistamine loratadine, an ethylcarbamate, that undergoes in vivo interconversion to its active form, desloratadine, through the action of CYP450 enzymes (Figure 22) [95], and capecitabine, an anticancer agent, that undergoes a multistep activation, to finally yield 5-flurouracil in the liver [96-98].

Loratadine

Desloratadine

Figure 22. Chemical structures of loratadine and its active form desloratidine.

Oxime Prodrugs

These prodrugs serve to increase the permeability of the corresponding active drugs and they are converted back to their parent drugs by microsomal cytochrome P450 enzymes (CYP450) [79].

Dopaminergic prodrug 6-(*N,N*-Di-*n*-propylamino)-3,4,5,6,7,8-hexahydro-2*H*-naphthalen-1-one is a representative example for such approach [103].

N- Mannich Bases, Enaminones and Schiff -Bases (Imines)

N- Mannich base formation is another approach which can be utilized to enhance drug's solubility. Rolitetracycline is the Mannich derivative of tetracycline, and it is the only one available for intravenous administration (Figure 23) [104]. N-Mannich bases of dipyrone (metamizole), the methane sulfonic acid of the analgesic 4-(methylamino) antipyrine, is water soluble and suitable for parenteral route and when given orally it is hydrolyzed in the stomach to give the parent active drug [105].

Despite the success of N-Mannich base prodrugs to improve bioavailability of active drugs there still some stability/formulation problems arise from poor *in vitro* stability of some of the prodrugs [104]. In addition, the *in vivo* formation of formaldehyde upon enzymatic breakdown [106-109] of these prodrugs is considered a limitation of these prodrug approach.

Tetracycline

Rolitetracycline

Figure 23. Chemical structures of tetracycline and Rolitetracycline.

Phosphate and Phosphonite Prodrugs

Phosphorylation offers increased aqueous solubility to the parent drugs. A traditional example of phosphate prodrugs is prednisolone sodium phosphate, a water soluble prodrug of prednisolone, its water solubility exceeds that of its active form, prednisolone, by 30 times [3], it is often used as an immunosuppressant and it is formulated as a liquid dosage form [3]. Another common phosphate prodrug is fosamprenavir. In similar to prednisolone; the phosphate promoiety in fosamprenavir is linked to a free hydroxyl group and the prodrug is 10-fold more water soluble than amprinavir. An enhanced patient compliance is achieved when using this antiviral prodrug; instead of administering the drug 8 times daily, dosage regimen is reduced into 2 times per day [110]. In the gut and *via* the action of alkaline phosphatases, phosphate prodrugs are cleaved back to their corresponding active drugs and then absorbed into the systemic circulation [3]. Another application of this approach is fosphenytoin a prodrug of the anticonvulsant agent pheytoin. Fospheytoin has an enhanced solubility over its parent drug [111].

Azo Compounds

Colonic bacteria can be exploited in prodrug approach as an activator for prodrugs through the action of azo reductases; this approach is applied specially in targeted drug release [104]. Sulfasalazine (Figure 24) a prodrug of 5-aminosalycilic acid and sulfapyridine is used in the treatment of ulcerative colitis [112]. Upon reaching the colon, sulfasalazine undergoes a cleavage at the azo bond which results in a release of the active moieties [89]. Osalazine, a dimer of 5-aminosalycilic acid, balsalazide and ipsalazide in which 5-aminosalicylic acid moiety is conjugated to 4-aminobenzoyl-β-alanine and 4-aminobenzoylglycine, respectively [113], are other examples of prodrugs that are activated by azo reductases. A prodrug by which 5-aminosalicylic acid is linked to L-aspartic acid is another example for such class that has shown a desirable colon specific delivery and a 50% release of 5-aminosalicylic acid from the administered dose [114]. Usually this approach is limited to aromatic amines, since azo compounds of aliphatic amines exhibits significant instability [115].

Sulfasalazine

Figure 24. Chemical structure of sulfasalazine.

Poly Ethylene Glycol (PEG) Conjugates

PEG can be linked to drugs either to increase drug solubility or to prolong drug plasma half-life [115]. An ester, carbamate, carbonate or amide spacer can be used to link the drug to PEG. Upon enzymatic breakdown of the spacer the resultant ester or carbamate drug can be liberated by 1,4- or 1,6-benzyl elimination [116].

Dounorobicine conjugated to PEG is an example of this kind of prodrugs. In this prodrug system PEG is conjugated to the phenol group of the open lactone *via* a spacer. Controlling the active drug's release can be accomplished by manipulation of the substituents on the aromatic ring [117].

Intramolecular Processes Used for the Design of Potential Prodrugs

The striking efficiency of enzyme catalysis has inspired many organic chemists and biochemists to explore enzyme mechanisms by investigating particular intramolecular processes such as enzyme models which proceed faster than their intermolecular counterparts. This research brings about the important question of whether enzyme models will replace natural enzymes in the conversion of prodrugs to their parent drugs.

Enzymes are mandatory for the interconversion of many prodrugs to their active parent drugs. Among the most important enzymes in the bioconversion of prodrugs are those for amides, such as, trypsin, chymotrypsin, elastase, carboxypeptidase, and aminopeptidase, and for esters, such as paraoxonase, carboxylesterase, cetylcholinesterase and cholinesterase. Most of these enzymes are hydrolytic enzymes, however, non-hydrolytic ones, including all cytochrome P450 enzymes, are also capable of catalyzing the bioconversion of ester and amide-based prodrugs.

In this chapter, the novel prodrug approach discusses the design, synthesis and in vitro kinetics of prodrugs based on intramolecular processes (enzyme models), that were advocated to assign the factors playing dominant role in enzyme catalysis. The design of the studied prodrugs is based on computational calculations using different molecular orbital and molecular mechanics methods, and correlations between experimental and calculated rate values for some intramolecular processes.

This approach does not require enzyme catalysis of the intraconversion of a prodrug to its active parent drug. The release rate of the active drug is determined only by the factors playing dominant role in the rate limiting step of the intraconversion process. Knowledge gained from the mechanisms of the previously studied enzyme models was used in the design.

Using this approach might have a potential to eliminate all disadvantages associated with prodrug interconversion by enzymes. As discussed before, prodrug bioconversion is perhaps the most vulnerable link in the chain, since many intrinsic and extrinsic factors can affect the interconversion process

Enzyme Models Used in the Prodrug Design

Several organic chemists and biochemists, such as Bender, Jencks, Bruice, Menger, Kirby and Walesh have extensively studied a variety of intramolecular systems (enzyme models) for understanding how enzymes catalyze biochemical reactions [118-121].

Today, the consensus is that the catalytic activity of enzymes is based on the combined effects of catalysis by functional groups and the ability to reroute intermolecular reactions through alternative pathways by which substrates bind to preorganized active sites. Rate acceleration by enzymes can be due to (1) covalently enforced proximity, as in chymotrypsin, (2) non-covalently enforced proximity, as in the catalytic activity of metallo-enzymes, (3) covalently enforced strain, and (4) non-covalently enforced strain, which has been heavily studied in models that mimic the enzyme lysozyme.

The rate constants for a large majority of enzymatic reactions exceed 10^{10} to 10^{18}-fold the non-enzymatic bimolecular counterparts. For example, reactions catalyzed by cyclophilin are enhanced by 10^5 and those by orotidine monophosphate decarboxylase are enhanced by 10^{17}. The significant rate of acceleration achieved by enzymes is brought about by the binding of the substrate within the confines of the enzyme pocket called the active site. The binding energy of the resulting enzyme-substrate complex is the dominant driving force and the major contributor to catalysis. It is believed that in all enzymatic reactions, binding energy is used to overcome prominent physical and thermodynamic factors that create barriers for the reaction (ΔG) [118-122].

The similarity between intramolecularity and enzymes has promoted a design of enzyme models based on intramolecular processes by which two reactive centers interaction might reveal to the mode and mechanism of enzymes catalysis. In the past five decades proposals have been made from attempts to interpret changes in reactivity versus structural variations in intramolecular systems. Among these proposals: (i) Koshland ''orbital steering'' which suggests a rapid intramolecularity arises from a severe angular dependence of organic reactions, such as in the lactonization of rigid hydroxy acids [123]; (ii) ''proximity'' in intramolecular processes (near attack conformation) model as proposed by Bruice and demonstrated in the lactonization of di-carboxylic acids semi-esters[124-126]; (iii) ''stereopopulation control'' based on the concept of freezing a molecule into a productive rotamer as advocated by Cohen [127-129], (iv) Menger's ''spatiotemporal hypothesis'' which postulates that the rate of reaction between two reactive centers is proportional to the time that the two centers reside within a critical distance [130-134] and (v) Kirby's proton transfer models on the acid-catalyzed hydrolysis of acetals and N-alkylmaleamic acids which demonstrated the importance of hydrogen bonding formation in the products and transition states leading to them [135-143].

Investigation on intramolecularity have played a fundamental role in elucidating the chemistry of functional groups involved in enzyme catalysis as well as in unraveling the mechanisms proposed for particular processes. Thus, it is highly believed that these investigations have the potential to provide an adequate understanding of how efficiency depends on structure in intramolecular catalysis which in turns could shed light on related problems in enzyme catalysis. In addition, understanding these intramolecular processes can provide a basis for a design of prodrugs that are able to release their active parent drugs in predicted rates.

Computational Methods Background

In the past sixty years, the use of computational chemistry for calculating molecular properties of ground and transition states has been a progressive task of organic, bioorganic and medicinal chemists alike. Computational chemistry uses principles of computer science to assist in solving chemical problems. It uses the theoretical chemistry results, incorporated into efficient computer programs, to calculate the structures and physical and chemical properties of molecules.

Reaction rates and equilibriums energy-based calculations for biological systems that have pharmaceutical and bio medicinal interests are a very important challenge to the health community. Nowadays, quantum mechanics (QM) such as *ab initio*, semi-empirical and density functional theory (DFT), and molecular mechanics (MM) are increasingly being used and broadly accepted as reliable tools for providing structure-energy calculations for an accurate prediction of potential drugs and prodrugs alike [144].

The above mentioned computational methods can handle both static and dynamic situations. In all cases the computer time, memory and disk space increase drastically with the studied system's size. *Ab initio* methods generally are useful only for small systems. They are based entirely on theory from first principles. The *ab initio* molecular orbital methods (QM) such as HF, G1, G2, G2MP2, MP2, MP3 and MP4 are based on rigorous use of the Schrodinger equation with a number of approximations. *Ab initio* electronic structure methods have the advantage that they can be made to converge to the exact solution, when all approximations are sufficiently small in magnitude and when the finite set of basis functions tends toward the limit of a complete set. The disadvantage of *ab initio* methods is their time-consuming cost [145-146].

Other less accurate methods are the semi-empirical because they make many approximations and obtain some parameters from empirical data. The semi-empirical quantum chemistry methods are based on the Hartree–Fock formalism and they are very important in computational chemistry for treating large molecules where the full Hartree–Fock method without the approximations is too expensive. Semi-empirical calculations are much faster than their *ab initio* counterparts. Their results, however, can be very wrong if the molecule being computed is not close enough to the molecules in the data base used to parameterize the method. The most used semiempirical methods are MINDO, MNDO, MINDO/3, AM1, PM3 and SAM1 [147-150].

Another quantum mechanical method that is commonly utilized in chemistry and physics to calculate the electronic structure, especially the ground state of variety of systems, in particular atoms, molecules, and the condensed phases is the density functional theory (DFT). With this theory, the properties of many systems can be predicted by using functionals, i.e., functions of another function, which in this case is the spatially dependent electron density. Therefore, the name density functional theory comes from the use of functionals of the electron density. The DFT method is used to calculate geometries and energies for medium-sized systems (up to 60 atoms depending on the basis set used) of biological and pharmaceutical interest and is not restricted to the second row of the periodic table [151-153].

On the other hand, molecular mechanics is a mathematical approach used for the computation of structures, energy, dipole moment, and other physical properties. It is widely used in calculating many diverse biological and chemical systems such as proteins, large crystal structures, and relatively large solvated systems. However, this method is limited by the determination of parameters such as the large number of unique torsion angles present in structurally diverse molecules [154].

Ab initio is an important tool to investigate functional mechanisms of biological macromolecules based on their 3D and electronic structures. The system size which *ab initio* calculations can handle is relatively small despite the large sizes of biomacromolecules surrounding solvent water molecules. Accordingly, isolated models of areas of proteins such as active sites have been studied in *ab initio* calculations. However, the disregarded proteins and solvent surrounding the catalytic centers have also been shown to contribute to the regulation of electronic structures and geometries of the regions of interest.

To overcome these discrepancies, quantum mechanics/molecular mechanics (QM/MM) calculations are utilized, in which the system is divided into QM and MM regions where QM regions correspond to active sites to be investigated and are described quantum mechanically. MM regions correspond to the remainder of the system and are described molecular mechanically. The pioneer work of the QM/MM method was accomplished by Warshel and Levitt, and since then, there has been much progress on the development of a QM/MM algorithm and applications to biological systems [155-157].

In similar to that utilized for drug discovery, modern computational methods such as those based on QM and MM methods could be exploited for the design of innovative prodrugs for common used drugs having functional groups, such as hydroxyl, phenol, or amine. For example, mechanisms of intramolecular processes for a number of enzyme models that have been previously studied by others to understand enzyme catalysis have been recently computed by us and were used for a design of some novel prodrug linkers [158-176]. Using DFT, molecular mechanics and *ab initio* methods, several enzyme models were explored for assigning the factors govern the intramolecular reaction rate in such models. Among the enzyme models that have been investigated: (i) proton transfer between two oxygens and proton transfer between nitrogen and oxygen in Kirby's acetals [135-143]; (ii) intramolecular acid-catalyzed hydrolysis in maleamic acid amide derivatives [135-143]; (iii) proton transfer between two oxygens in rigid systems as investigated by Menger [130-134]; (iv) acid-catalyzed lactonization of hydroxy-acids as researched by Cohen [127-129] and Menger [130-134]; and (v) SN2-based ring-closing as studied by Bruice [124-126].

In the past seven years a respected number of studies by our group on the above mentioned enzyme models (intramolecular processes) revealed the necessity to further explore the intramolecular processes mechanisms the following: (1) The driving force for enhancements in rate for intramolecular processes are both entropy and enthalpy effects. In the cases by which enthalpic effects were predominant such as ring-cyclization and proton transfer reactions proximity or/and steric effects were the driving force for rate accelerations. (2) The nature of the reaction being intermolecular or intramolecular is determined on the distance between the two reactive centers. (3) In S_N2-based ring-closing reactions leading to three-, four- and five-membered rings the *gem*-dialkyl effect is more dominant in processes involving the formation of an unstrained five-membered ring, and the need for directional flexibility decreases as the size of the ring being formed increases. (4) Accelerations in the rate for intramolecular reactions are a result of both entropy and enthalpy effects, and (5) an efficient proton transfer between two oxygens and between nitrogen and oxygen in Kirby's acetal systems were affordable when strong hydrogen bonds are developed in the products and the corresponding transition states leading to them [158-176].

Unraveling the reaction mechanisms has provided better design of efficient chemical devices to be utilized as a prodrug promoiety to be covalently linked to a drug which can chemically and not enzymatically be cleaved to release the active drug in a programmable manner. For example, exploring the proton transfer mechanism of Kirby's acetals has led to a design and synthesis of novel prodrugs of aza-nucleosides for the treatment of myelodysplastic syndromes [177], atovaquone prodrugs to treat malaria [178, 179], bitterless paracetamol prodrugs to be used by pediatrics and geriatrics as antipyretic and pain killer [180], statin prodrugs for lowering cholesterol levels in the blood [181] and prodrugs of phenylephrine as decongestant [182]. In these examples, the prodrug promoiety was covalently linked to the active drug hydroxyl group such that the drug-linker entity (prodrug) has a potential to intraconvert upon exposure into physiological environments such as stomach, intestine, and/or blood circulation, with rates that are solely dependent on the structural features of the pharmacologically inactive promoiety (Kirby's enzyme model) [136-143]. Other different linkers such as Kirby's N-alkylmaleamic acids enzyme model was also explored for the design of a respected number of prodrugs such as those for masking the bitter sensation of the antibacterial, cefuroxime [183], tranexamic acid prodrugs as antibleeding agents [184], acyclovir prodrugs as anti-viral for the treatment of Herpes Simplex [185] and atenolol prodrugs for treating hypertension with enhanced stability and bioavailability [186, 187]. Menger's Kemp acid amide enzyme model was utilized for the design of dopamine prodrugs to treat Parkinson's disease as well [188]. Details on the design and synthesis of the above mentioned prodrugs are discussed in the following sections.

Calculation Methods Used for the Prodrugs Design

The Becke three-parameter, hybrid functional combined with the Lee, Yang, and Parr correlation functional, denoted B3LYP, were employed in the calculations using density functional theory (DFT). All calculations were carried out using the quantum chemical package Gaussian-2003 and Gaussian-2009 [189]. Calculations were carried out based on the restricted Hartree-Fock method [189].

The starting geometries of all calculated molecules were obtained using the Argus Lab program [190] and were initially optimized at the HF/6-31G level of theory, followed by optimization at the B3LYP/6-31G(d,p) and B3LYP/6-311 + G(d,p) levels. Total geometry optimizations included all internal rotations. Second derivatives were estimated for all 3N-6 geometrical parameters during optimization. An energy minimum (a stable compound or a reactive intermediate) has no negative vibrational force constant. A transition state is a saddle point which has only one negative vibrational force constant [191]. Transition states were located first by the normal reaction coordinate method [192] where the enthalpy changes was monitored by stepwise changing the interatomic distance between two specific atoms.

The geometry at the highest point on the energy profile was re-optimized by using the energy gradient method at the B3LYP/6-31G(d,p) level of theory [189]. The "reaction coordinate method" [192] was used to calculate the activation energy in the studied processes. In this method, one bond length is constrained for the appropriate degree of freedom while all other variables are freely optimized. The activation energies obtained from the DFT for all molecules were calculated with and without the inclusion of water. The calculations with the incorporation of a water molecule were performed using the integral equation formalism model of the Polarizable Continuum Model (PCM) [193-196]. In this model the cavity is created via a series of overlapping spheres. The radii type employed was the United Atom Topological Model on radii optimized for the PBE0/6-31G (d) level of theory. The MM2 molecular mechanics strain energy calculations were done using Allinger's MM2 program [154].

In this chapter, the mechanisms of some enzyme models that have been advocated to understand how enzymes work were computationally explored. The tool used in the study is computational approach consisting of calculations using a variety of different molecular orbital and molecular mechanics methods and correlations between experimental and calculated reactions rates [166-184].

Kirby's Enzyme Model Based on Intramolecular Proton Transfer in acetals [135, 136, 138-143]

Intramolecular processes are faster and more efficient than their intermolecular counterparts because of the two reacting centers proximity orientation which mimics that of functional groups when brought together in the enzyme active site [118-143].

For assessing the factors determining the rate-limiting step in Kirby's enzyme, using molecular orbital methods, we have investigated the mode and scope of the proton transfers efficiency in Kirby's enzyme models 1-18 (Figures 25- 27) [135, 136, 138-143].

The aim of this study was to: (i) assign the driving force(s) for the high extreme efficiency of the intramolecular general acid catalysis (IGAC) in 1-15 (Figures 25 and 26), and (ii) to locate possible intramolecular hydrogen bonding along the reaction pathway (in reactants, transition state and products) and to evaluate their role in the intramolecular process efficiency.

Using ab initio at HF/6-31G (d,p) and DFT at B3LYP/6-31G (d,p) basis sets the kinetic and thermodynamic parameters for the IGAC in processes 1-15 (Figures 25 and 26) were calculated.

The intermolecular processes 16 and 17 (Figure 27) were selected as intermolecular proton transfer processes for calculating the effective molarity (EM) values of the corresponding intramolecular processes 1-8 and 9-15, respectively. Process 18 (Figure 27) was calculated to represent a proton transfer process driven by "classical" general catalysis (GAC) for comparisons with IGAC.

The calculation results demonstrated that the structural features required for a system to achieve an efficient intramolecular proton transfer are: (1) the distance between the two reactive centers (r_{GM}, see Figure 28) in the ground state (GM) should be short which subsequently results in strong intramolecular hydrogen bonding, and (2) the attack angle α (Figure 28) in the ground state should be about 180° for maximizing the orbital overlap of the two reactive centers upon their engagement along the reaction pathway. Among the first set of systems, 1-8, that were calculated, systems 4 and 8 were the most reactive ones because they both fulfill, to a high extent, the two requirements (α= 170° and r_{GM} = 1.7 Å). On the other hand, system 6 was found to be with the lowest rate as a result of having an attack angle and distance between the two reactive centers far away from the optimal values (α=48° and r_{GM} = 3.7 Å, see Table 1).

In order to examine whether the reaction mechanism for systems such as 4 occurs via an efficient intramolecular general acid catalysis (IGAC) or via "classical" general acid catalysis (GAC), calculations for processes 16 and 18 were conducted; where process 16 involves intermolecular proton transfer from acetic acid to the acetal, and process 18 is similar to that of 4 except that an acetic acid molecule is replaced with a water molecule as a proton donor to the acetal (Figure 27).

Comparison of the calculated DFT activation energy values for processes 16 and 18 with that of 4 indicates that IGAC for 4 is much more efficient than that of 16 and 18 ($\Delta G^{\ddagger}$ value for 4 is 24.15 kcal/mol, and for 16 and 18 are 38.55 kcal/mol and 53.14 kcal/mol, respectively).

This result confirms that catalysis of the acetal cleavage in 4 must be supplied by the proton of the carboxyl group. Thus the mechanism in systems such as 4 is via IGAC and not via GAC. The EM values depicted in Table 1 show that 4 and 8 are the most efficient processes among 1-15 (log EM 10-13) and among the least efficient processes are 2, 11 and 13-15 with log EM <1. In addition, the calculations revealed that the proton transfer rate in systems 1–15 is quite responsive to geometric disposition, especially in relation to the distance between the two reactive centers, r_{GM}, and the attack angle, α. Requirements for a system to achieve a high intramolecular proton transfer rate are: (a) a short distance between the two reactive centers (r_{GM}) in the ground state which subsequently results in strong intramolecular hydrogen bonding, and (b) a hydrogen bonding angle (α_{GM}) close to linearity in order to maximize orbitals overlapping.

Table 1. DFT (B3LYP/6-31G (d,p)) calculated kinetic and thermodynamic properties for the proton transfer in 1-15

System	H2-O3 r_{GM} (Å)	α	$\Delta H^{\ddagger}$	$T\Delta S^{\ddagger}$	$\Delta G^{\ddagger}$	log EM (calc.)	log EM [135, 143] (exp.)
1	1.69	143	33.09	-1.25	34.34	7.40	-----
2	3.60	48	48.29	-2.23	46.52	-1.52	-----
3	1.74	147	34.32	-3.42	37.74	5.17	4.00
4	1.70	170	21.47	-2.68	24.15	10.58	10.00
5	1.69	149	26.64	-3.71	30.35	6.04	3.45
6	3.66	48	40.15	1.04	39.11	-0.41	------
7	1.74	147	26.22	-5.12	31.34	5.30	3.98
8	1.72	171	21.22	0.03	21.19	12.72	12.60
9	1.72	146	23.62	0.07	23.55	1.67	-----
10	2.04	125	24.73	-3.34	28.07	-1.65	-----
11	3.33	123	25.41	-4.15	29.56	-2.75	-----
12	1.73	144	22.54	0.90	21.64	3.07	-----
13	3.33	124	23.59	-4.15	27.74	-1.41	-----
14	1.92	122	29.33	0.61	28.72	-2.13	-----
15	2.51	107	34.71	-2.00	36.71	-8.01	-----

$\Delta H^{\ddagger}$ is the activation enthalpic energy (kcal/mol). $T\Delta S^{\ddagger}$ is the activation entropic energy in kcal/mol. $\Delta G^{\ddagger}$ is the activation free energy (kcal/mol). α is the hydrogen bonding angle in the ground state structure (For H2O3 (r_{GM}), see Figure 28). ln EM =-($\Delta G^{\ddagger}_{intra}$- $\Delta G^{\ddagger}_{inter}$)/RT.

Figure 25. Chemical structures of 1-8.

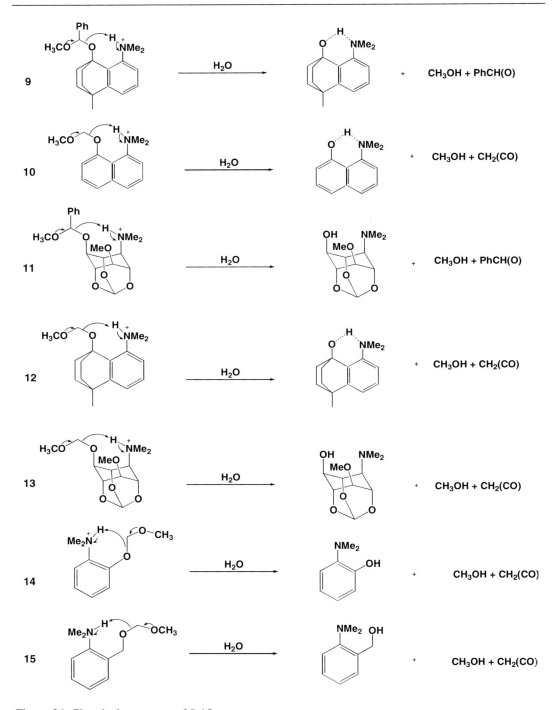

Figure 26. Chemical structures of 9-15.

Prodrugs Design Based on Inter- and Intramolecular Processes

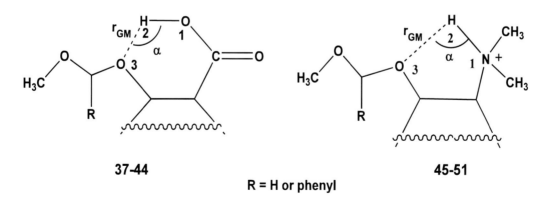

Figure 27. Chemical structures of 16-18.

Figure 28. Schematic representation for the cleavage in 1-15 showing the distance between the reacting centers (r_{GM}) and the angle of attack (α).

The strong correlation found between the calculated $\Delta G^{\ddagger}$ values, which reflect the experimental reaction rate, and geometrical parameters such as r^2_{GM} and α provides a mathematical tool ($\Delta G^{\ddagger}$ vs. $r^2_{GM} \times (1 + \sin(180 - \alpha))$) which can predict reaction rate based on a calculated GM for a certain system. The equation slope can be used as an indicator of the mode by which the two reactive centers are orchestrated in an intramolecular process.

Aza nucleosides prodrugs based on Intramolecular proton transfer in Kirby's acetals [177]

The myelodysplastic syndromes are a diverse collection of hematological conditions united by ineffective production of blood cells and varying risks of transformation to acute myelogenous leukemia (AML) which requires chronic blood transfusion [197].

With the exception of allogeneic blood stem cell transplantation, there is no current treatment, with high rate of cure, of patients with high-risk MDS. However, because the median age at diagnosis of a MDS is 60 - 75 years, and allogeneic transplantation is performed in only subset of these patients, the majority of older MDS patients are offered best supportive care and low-dose chemotherapy such as low dose cytarabine.

The three MDS agents approved by the U.S. Food and Drug Administration are: 5-azacitidine, decitabine and cytarabine (Figure 29). Chemotherapy with the hypomethylating agents, 5-azacytidine and decitabine resulted in a decrease of blood transfusion requirements and progression retard of MDS to AML. All three nucleoside agents have a short terminal elimination ($t_{1/2}$). Design and synthesis of a slow degrading prodrug can provide sustained exposure to the drug during the treatment of MDS patients. This might result in better clinical outcome, more convenient dosing regimens and potentially less side effects.

For instance, SC injection of azacitidine results in peak plasma concentration. However, if a slow release prodrug can be provided, then C_{max} related side effects may be avoided and longer duration exposure and more efficient clinical profile may be achieved. Another example, decitabine has to be administered by continuous IV infusion, if a prodrug is designed to be cleaved in a controlled manner by SC route, optimum MDS maintenance treatment could be imminent [198- 202].

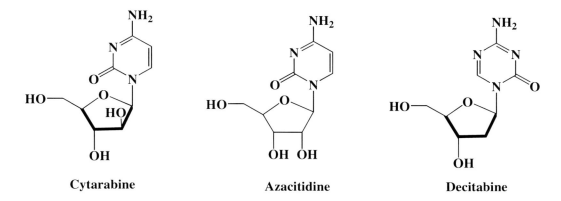

Figure 29. Chemical structures of cytarabine, azacitidine and decitabine.

By improving azacitidine, cytarabine and decitabine pharmacokinetic properties the drug absorption *via* a variety of administration routes, especially the SC injection route, can be facilitated. Utilizing a carrier-linked prodrug strategy by linking the aza nucleoside drugs to a carrier moiety can provide a chemical device capable of penetrating the membrane tissues and releasing the aza nucleoside in a programmable manner.

Based on our reported DFT calculations on a proton transfer reaction in some of Kirby's enzyme models (Figures 26), three prodrugs of aza nucleoside were proposed. As shown in Figure 30, the aza nucleoside prodrugs **ProD 1- ProD 3** have N, N-dimethylanilinium group (hydrophilic moiety) and a lipophilic moiety (the rest of the prodrug), where the combination of both moieties secures a moderate HLB. Furthermore, in a physiologic environment of pH 5.5, SC, aza nucleoside prodrugs **ProD 1- ProD 3** may have a better bioavailability than their parent drug due to improved absorption. In addition, those prodrugs may be used in different dosage forms (i.e., enteric coated tablets) because of their potential solubility in organic and aqueous media due to the ability of the anilinium group to be converted to the corresponding aniline group in a physiological pH of 6.5.

It should be emphasized that at pH 5.5-6.5 (SC and intestine physiologic environments) the anilinium form of the three prodrugs (**ProD 1- ProD 3**) will equilibrate with the free aniline form. Subsequently, the former will undergo proton transfer reaction (rate limiting step) to yield the anti-preleukemia aza nucleoside drug and the inactive carrier as by-product.

It should be emphasized, that our proposal is to exploit prodrugs **ProD 1 – ProD 3** for S.C. use. The physiological environment of the skin has a pH of 5.5. At pH 5.5, prodrugs **ProD 1 – ProD 3** are predicted to exist in the unionized (free base) and ionized (ammonium) forms where the equilibrium constant for the exchange between both forms is dependent on the pK_a of the given prodrug. The experimental determined pK_a for N, N-dimethylanilin is 5.15 [203] hence it is expected that the pK_a values for prodrugs **ProD 1 – ProD 3** will be in the same range. Since the pH for the skin lies in the range around 5.5, the calculated ionized (ammonium) /unionized (free base) ratio will be 69/31.

It is quite safe to assume that the unionized forms for prodrugs **ProD 1 – ProD 3** will be more lipophilic than their parent drug due the presence of a relatively bulky group (Kirby's enzyme model linker). Therefore, their absorption through the skin membranes and the efficiency for delivering their parent drug are expected to be increased. If the prodrugs, **ProD 1 – ProD 3**, are intended to be administered by *per os* dosage form, for example as an enteric coated tablets, the absorption and consequently the efficiency of those prodrugs will be relatively reduced compared to the SC route.

This is because the calculated percentage of the unionized form, in the case where the absorption is taking place in the small intestine (pH = 6.5), is predicted in the range of 5%-31%.

The selection of Kirby's enzyme model to be utilized as carriers to aza nucleosides is based on the fact that those carriers undergo proton transfer reaction to yield an aldehyde, an alcohol and a hydroxy amine (Figures 26 and 30). The rate-limiting step in these processes (**9-15** in Figure 26) is a proton transfer from the anilinium group into the neighboring ether oxygen. Furthermore, the proton transfer rate is strongly dependent on the strength of the hydrogen bonding in the products and in the transition states leading to them. Therefore, it will be safe to assume that the reaction rate will be greatly affected by the structural features of Kirby's enzyme model system as evident from the different experimental rate values determined for the different processes (Table 1) [135-143].

Replacing the methoxy group in **9-15** (Figure 26) with aza nucleoside drug, as shown for **ProD 1- ProD 3** in Figure 30, is not expected to have any significant effect on the relative rates of these processes. Therefore, computational calculations of the kinetic and thermodynamic properties for these models will shed light on the rates for the intraconversion of prodrugs **ProD 1 – ProD 3** to their active aza nucleoside drug.

Figure 30. Intraconversion of aza-nucleoside prodrugs ProD 1-ProD 3 to their active drug.

DFT calculation results for intramolecular proton transfer reactions in Kirby's enzyme models **9-15** (Figure 26) demonstrate that the reaction rate is quite responsive to geometric disposition, especially to the distance between the two reactive centers, r_{GM}, and the angle of attack, α (the hydrogen bonding angle, see Figure 28).

Hence, the study on the systems reported herein could provide a good basis for a design of aza nucleoside prodrugs that are less hydrophilic than their parent drugs and can be used, in different dosage forms, to release the parent drug in a controlled manner. For example, based on the calculated log EM (Table 1), the cleavage process for prodrug **ProD 1** is predicted to be about 10^{10} times faster than for prodrug **ProD 2** and about 10^4 times faster than prodrug **ProD 3**:rate$_{ProD1}$> rate$_{ProD3}$> rate $_{ProD2}$. Hence, the rate by which the prodrug releases the aza nucleoside can be determined according to the structural features of the linker (Kirby's enzyme model).

Statin Prodrugs Based on Intramolecular Proton Transfer in Kirby's Acetals [181]

Hyperlipidemia is a common heterogeneous group of disorders, most commonly treated with statin medications. Statins are selective and competitive inhibitors of HMG-CoA reductase, rate-limiting enzyme that converts 3-hydroxy-3-methylglutaryl coenzyme A to mevalonate, a precursor of cholesterol [204]. Statins are hepatoselective and the mechanisms contributing to this are governed by their solubility profiles. Passive diffusion through hepatocellular membranes is the key for effective first pass uptake for hydrophobic statins, which can also be diffused to non-hepatocellular parts, whereas extensive carrier-mediated uptake is the major uptake route [205]. This can prove that hydrophilic statins acquire greater hepatoselectivity. All satin are absorbed rapidly after administration, reaching peak plasma concentration within 4 hours [205]. Statins in general have a low bioavailability mostly due to the extensive first pass effect and/or bad solubility.

Simvastatin is a hydrophobic fungal derivative compound [204]; it is administered as a lactone prodrug, simvastatin A (Figure 31) that after oral ingestion undergoes a hydroxylation to yield its corresponding (β)-hydroxy acid form, simvastatin B (Figure 31), an inhibitor of HMG-CoA reductase [206]. The percentage of simvastatin dose retained by the liver is >80% [204].

The solubility of simvastatin is the limiting factor for its bioavailability [207]. Simvastatin undergoes an extensive first pass effect and has a bioavailability of only 5%; it has a poor absorption rate from the gastro-intestinal tract (GIT). Hence, improving its solubility and its dissolution rate is a crucial for enhancing its bioavailability [205, 208].

Many attempts have been made in order to improve simvastatin bioavailability. One strategy was by co-solvent evaporation method, where a hydrophilic, low viscosity grade polymer hydroxypropylmethylcellulose (HPMC) was used to enhance simvastatin solubility and dissolution rate.

The study results revealed a significant enhancement in its solubility by converting simvastatin particles from regular to amorphous form *via* reducing the particle size and increasing wettability [208].

In another study glycerylmonooleate (GMO)/poloxamer 407 cubic nanoparticles was investigated as potential oral drug delivery system to enhance simvastatin bioavailability. The study showed that oral bioavailability of simvastatin cubic nanoparticles was enhanced significantly at 2.41-fold compared to that in micronized crystal powder. In addition, it demonstrated a sustained plasma simvastatin level for over 12 hours [209]. In 2012, developments of stable pellets-layered simvastatin nano-suspensions were tested for simvastatin dissolution and bioavailability. The study revealed an improved dissolution and bioavailability of the drug [206].

Atorvastatin and rosuvastatin (Figure 31) are fully synthetic compounds; atorvastatin is relatively lipophilic [204], whereas rosuvastatin is more hydrophilic due to its polar hydroxyl and methane sulphonamide groups [205]. Atorvastatin has a bioavailability of only 14% and half-life of 14 hours, however, the half-life of its inhibitory activity (HMG-CoA reductase) is 20 - 30 hours due to contribution of its active metabolites [210].

Figure 31. Chemical structures of simvastatin A, simvastatin B, atorvastatin and rosuvastatin.

Solid forms of atorvastatin are unstable when exposed to heat, moisture or light since its hydroxy acid form is converted to the corresponding lactone form. It is worth noting, that atorvastatin hydroxy acid form is about 15 times more soluble than its lactone [207].In addition, atorvastatin is vulnerable to destabilization upon contact with other excipients present in the formulation as they might negatively interact with the drug. Therefore, most of the commercial atorvastatin medications consist of an alkaline metal salt such as calcium carbonate [207]. Atorvastatin instability which leads to poor solubility is the main reason for its low bioavailability [207].One method that was performed in an attempt to improve the oral bioavailability of atorvastatin was using a stabilized gastro-retentive floating dosage form, where floating formulations usually guarantee a complete and constant release of the drug within a period of 12 hours, particularly for drugs absorbed in the gastric region, thereby enhancing bioavailability. The developed formulations were stable during the development process and have a potential to improve the oral bioavailability of atorvastatin [207]. Another approach, was utilizing cyclodextrin complexation to enhance the solubility and stability of atorvastatin, where the *in vitro* studies showed that the solubility and dissolution rate of atorvastatin- Ca were significantly improved by β-CD complexation with respect to the drug alone [211]. Rosuvastatin has a bioavailability of about 20% and is metabolized to its major metabolite; N-desmethylrosuvastatin, and has approximately 1/6–1/2 the HMG-CoA reductase inhibitory activity of rosuvastatin [206]. In an attempt to improve the medication bioavailability, efforts to prepare and optimize micro emulsion of rosuvastatin calcium were made, as micro-emulsions are thermodynamically stable system and can provide higher solubilization.

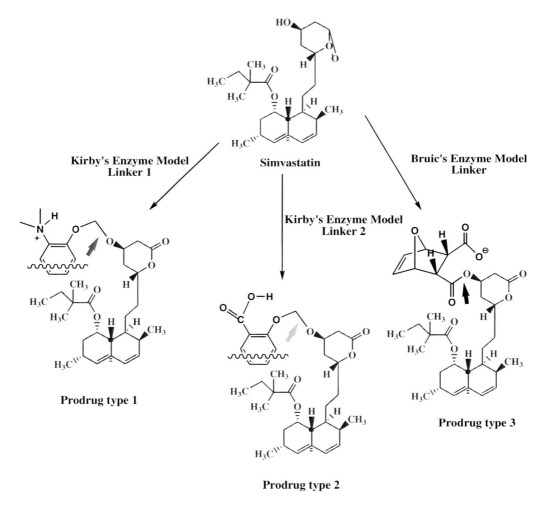

Figure 32. Proposed three types of chemical approaches for simvastatin prodrugs design.

The study demonstrated a potential use of micro emulsion system to enhance the solubility and hence the bioavailability for the poorly water soluble drug, rosuvastatin [212]. The solubility of simvastatin is the limiting factor for its bioavailability due to slow tissue penetration [207], hence, it undergoes an extensive first pass effect; therefore, improving its solubility and hence its dissolution rate is a must to enhance its bioavailability. Therefore, development of more hydrophilic prodrugs that have the capability to release the parent drug in physiological environments such as intestine is a significant challenge.

Figure 33. Intraconversion of simvastatin ProD 1- ProD 3.

In principle, three approaches could be considered to fulfill the requirements mentioned above: (Figure 32): (1) linking the statin free hydroxyl group to Kirby's enzyme model (ammonium linker), (2) blocking the statin hydroxyl group with Kirby's enzyme model (carboxylic acid linker) and (3) attaching the statin free hydroxyl group with Bruice's model (dicarboxylic semi-ester linker.

Based on our DFT calculations on a proton transfer reaction in some of Kirby's enzyme models (**8-15**, Figure 26), three prodrugs of simvastatin are proposed. As shown in Figure 33, the simvastatin prodrugs, **ProD 1- ProD 3**, have N,N-dimethylanilinium group (hydrophilic moiety) and a lipophilic moiety (the rest of the prodrug), where the combination of both moieties secures a moderate hydrophilic lipophilic balance (HLB). Furthermore, in a physiological environment of pH around 6, intestine, prodrugs **ProD 1- ProD 3** may have a better bioavailability than their parent drug due to improved absorption. In addition, those prodrugs may be used in different dosage forms (i.e., enteric coated tablets) because of their potential solubility in organic and aqueous media due to the ability of the anilinium group to be converted to the corresponding aniline group in a physiological pH of 6.5.

DFT calculations at B3LYP 6-31G (d,p) for intramolecular proton transfer in the three simvastatin prodrugs revealed that the interconversion of simvastatin prodrug **ProD 3** to simvastatin is predicted to be about 10 times faster than that of either simvastatin **ProD 1** or simvastatin **ProD 2**. Hence, the rate by which the prodrug releases the statin drug can be determined according to the structural features of the promoiety (Kirby's enzyme model).

Menger's Enzyme Model Based on Intramolecular Proton Transfer in Kemp's Acid Amides [130-134]

Menger's singularity model and its partner the spatiotemporal hypothesis predict that an efficient enzyme model could be achieved using chemical systems that rigidly hold a nucleophile and an electrophile at a distance at or near the critical distance. One of the most interesting enzyme models that obeys the requirements imposed for high efficiency is an intramolecular-catalyzed cleavage of an aliphatic amide (Figure 34) [130-134]. Taking into consideration that an aliphatic amide is very difficult to be hydrolyzed; a 10-hour reflux in concentrated hydrochloric acid is not unusual. However, when a carboxyl group is held in a 1,3-diaxial orientation to the amide, the amide bond cleavage occurs with a half-life of only 8 minutes at neutral pH and 21.5 °C. Although the structure shown in Figure 34 has two carboxyl groups, only a single carboxyl is actually needed for this enzyme-like rate acceleration, the other carboxyl being merely a "spectator". It should be emphasized, that the aliphatic amide reaction occurs *via* the more stable structure B rather than structure A (Figure 34).

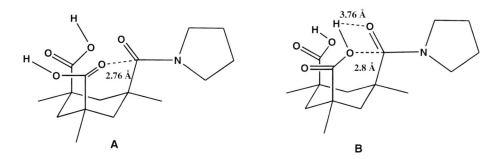

Figure 34. Chemical structures of conformations A and B for Menger's reactive amide, where B is presumably the most reactive conformer.

One striking example of enzyme models that were proposed for understanding enzyme catalysis is the intramolecular cleavage reaction of Kemp's di-acid amide **19** that was exploited by Menger and Ladika to unravel the mechanism of chymotrypsin enzyme catalyzed biotransformation reactions [130-134]. Chymotrypsin cleaves peptide bonds by attacking the unreactive carbonyl group of the peptide with its serine 195 residue located in its active site, which briefly becomes covalently bonded to the substrate, forming an enzyme–substrate intermediate. It was demonstrated that the biotransformation of chymotrypsin with its substrate involves two stages, an initial ''burst'' phase at the start of the reaction and a steady-state phase called ''ping-pong'' stage. Thus the enzyme's mode of action is as hydrolysis takes place in two steps. First acylation of the substrate which involves a proton transfer to form an acyl-enzyme intermediate and in the second step, deacylation in order to return the enzyme to its original state [214, 215]. In the laboratory, the hydrolysis reaction rate of a peptide linkage is too slow; at neutral pH and ambient temperature, the half-life is about 500 years, unless a strong acid catalyst is added [216, 217], yet in the small intestines, where the conditions are about neutral rather than acidic, most of the proteins hydrolysis takes place rather quickly. This is due to the presence of enzymes called peptidases that catalyze the amide cleavage *via* a proton transfer reaction [218].

Molecular orbital calculations using ab initio at HF/6-31G(d,p) and DFT at B3LYP/6-31G (d,p) levels for the amide cleavage reactions of di-carboxylic aliphatic amides **19–29** (Figure 35) were done to unravel the unusual striking rates acceleration brought about when these amides stand in neutral aqueous solution at ambient temperature. The calculations aimed to: (1) determine whether amides **19–29** undergo fast cleavage due to a proton transfer stemming from a proximity orientation of the nucleophile (O6, see Figure 36) to the electrophile (H5, see Figure 36), as was suggested by Menger [130-134], or due to pseudoallylic (pseudo-A) strain relief that occurs upon the cleavage of the distorted amide bond to a less strained tetrahedral intermediate that is formed from the approach of the carboxylic oxygen (O4, see Figure 36) towards the amidic carbonyl carbon (C7, see Figure 36), as was proposed by Curran and others [219, 220].

The mechanistic calculation results shown in Figure 37 and listed in Table 2 revealed: (i) The activation energy barriers for the cleavage of amides **19– 29** at a pH range where the carboxylic group is in its free acid form (not ionized) are much smaller *via* a proton transfer (route b) than *via* an approach of the carboxylic oxygen onto the amide carbonyl carbon (route a). For example, the gas phase B3LYP/6-31G (d,p) calculated activation energy for the hydrolysis of amide **19** *via* a proton transfer (route b) is 45.18 kcal/mol less than that for the cleavage *via* route a. (ii) The calculated activation energy values for the cleavage reactions of amides **19** and **20** are almost the same (~15 kcal when calculated by B3LYP/6-31G (d,p) in the presence of water as a solvent). This result suggests that the presence of only one carboxylic group, such as in amide **20**, is needed to supply a proton transfer for achieving the same acceleration as for the reaction of amide **19**. The calculation results are in accordance with the experimental findings by Menger [130-134]. (iii) The calculated activation energy in the presence of water for the cleavage of amide **21** was found to be ~3 kcal/mol smaller than that of amide **19**. This slight difference in energy might be due to the difference between the calculated distances of the electrophile (carboxylic proton) and the nucleophile (amide carboxylic carbon) in the more strained amide **19** and the less strained amide, **21**; H5—O6 distance (Figure 36) in **19** is 2.9 Å and in **21** is 3.0 Å. This is in accordance with Menger's

Prodrugs Design Based on Inter- and Intramolecular Processes 43

"spatiotemporal hypothesis" and our computational studies on other enzymes models [158-161, 213].

Figure 35. Chemical structures of aliphatic amides 19-29.

Figure 36. Schematic representation for the cleavage of **19-29** showing the distance between the reacting centers (r) and the angle of attack (α).

Table 2. DFT calculated properties for the proton transfers in 19-25, 26-28 and ProD1-2

System	$\Delta H^{\ddagger}$ (GP)	$T\Delta S^{\ddagger}$ (GP)	$\Delta G^{\ddagger}$ (GP)	$\Delta H^{\ddagger}$ (Water)	$\Delta G^{\ddagger}$ (Water)	r_{GM} (Å)	α (degree)	$t_{1/2}$ (hour)
19	27.61	-1.11	28.72	12.55	13.66	3.00	70.90	0.028
20	28.39	-2.92	31.31	14.64	17.56	3.01	75.92	0.03
21	29.50	0.04	29.46	15.06	15.02	3.10	72.18	----
22	32.00	-0.92	32.92	15.69	16.61	3.09	71.55	----
23	29.12	-1.23	30.35	17.69	18.92	3.06	75.23	0.1
24	30.56	-1.28	31.84	28.82	30.10	3.62	56.63	283
25	34.22	-2.73	36.95	27.74	30.47	3.16	75.70	----
27	29.36	-1.88	31.24	29.81	31.69	3.33	73.96	324
28	30.48	-1.44	31.92	17.85	19.31	3.20	67.60	2.2
29	32.57	-1.68	34.25	21.96	23.64	3.20	68.00	90
ProD 1	31.12	-2.22	33.34	24.85	27.07	3.19	75.40	----
ProD 2	28.72	-1.59	30.31	23.00	24.59	3.25	74.88	----

$T\Delta S^{\ddagger}$ is the entropic activation energy (kcal/mol), $\Delta H^{\ddagger}$ is the enthalpic activation energy (kcal/mol), $\Delta G^{\ddagger}$ is the free activation energy (kcal/mol), r_{GM} and α are the H6-O5 distance and the angle O5-H6-O7 in the global minimum structures, respectively (Figure 36). GP and Water refer to calculated in the gas phase and water, respectively. $t_{1/2}$ is the time needed to cleave 50% of the amide to the corresponding amine and carboxylic acid.

Figure 37. Proposed mechanism for the hydrolysis of aliphatic amides 19-29.

Furthermore, the DFT results for the cleavage reactions in Kemp's mono- and di-acid amides **19–29** demonstrate that the rate limiting step in the acylolysis process is a proton transfer from the carboxyl group onto the amide carbonyl oxygen. It is proposed that accelerations in rate are mainly due to the distance between the two reactive centers (r) and the angle of attack (α) (Figure 36). In fact, a linear correlation was found between the activation energy ($\Delta G^{\ddagger}$) and r^2 x sin (180 - α). On the other hand, contrarily to previous studies the ground-state pseudoallylic strain effect has a little contribution if any to the cleavage rates of Kemp's triacid tertiary amides reactions. Further, the calculations suggest a change in the mode and the mechanism of the amide cleavage upon changing the pH of the reaction medium. Thus, peptidases are extremely reactive around neutral pH while their activities diminish under basic medium.

Dopamine Prodrugs Based on a Proton Transfer in Menger's Aliphatic Amide Enzyme Model [188]

Dopamine is a neurotransmitter that is naturally produced in the body. Dopamine is produced in several areas of the brain, including the substantial nigra and the ventral tegmental area and it activates the five types of dopamine receptors D1, D2, D3, D4 and D5. Dopamine is also a neurohormone released by the hypothalamus and its main function to inhibit the release of prolactin from the anterior lobe of the pituitary. Dopamine is present in the regions of the brain that regulate movement, emotion, motivation and the feeling of pleasure. Shortage of dopamine, particularly the death of dopamine neurons in the nigrostriatal pathway, causes Parkinson's disease, in which a person loses the ability to execute smooth, controlled movements. Dopamine can be supplied as a medication that acts on the sympathetic nervous system, producing effects such as increased heart rate and blood pressure. However, because dopamine cannot cross the blood-brain barrier, dopamine given as a drug does not directly affect the central nervous system. To increase the amount of dopamine in the brains of patients with diseases such as Parkinson's disease and dopa-responsive dystonia, L-DOPA (levodopa), a precursor of dopamine, is given because it can cross the blood-brain barrier. Levodopa is used in various forms to treat Parkinson's disease and dopa-responsive dystonia. It is typically co-administered with an inhibitor of peripheral decarboxylation (DDC, dopa decarboxylase such as carbidopa or benserazide (Figure 38) [221, 222]. The main objective of this study was to design and synthesize new prodrugs for the treatment of Parkinson's disease that have the potential to be with a higher bioavailability than the current medications. For achieving this goal, the dopamine prodrugs physicochemical properties are: (i) adequate solubility in physiological environment (ii) a moderate hydrophilic lipophilic balance (HLB) value (iii) providing upon chemical cleavage the parent drug in a controlled manner, and (iv) providing upon cleavage safe and non-toxic by-products. By fulfilling these requirements the following objectives may be achieved: (1) a high absorption and permeability of the prodrug into the body tissues. (2) The possibility to use the anti-Parkinson's drug in different administration routes. (3) A chemically driven system that able to release dopamine in a controlled manner, and (4) a drug with a high bioavailability and efficient clinical profile.

Figure 38. Enzymatic conversion of L-dopa to dopamine along with the chemical structures of carbidopa and benserazide.

Continuing our investigations for utilizing enzyme models as potential linkers for weak amine-drugs, we have researched the driving forces responsible for accelerations in rate of proton transfer reactions in some of Kemp's acid amide derivatives, **19-29**. It is expected that molecules such as **19-29** will have a potential of being appropriate linkers to dopaminergic agents such as dopamine. The proposed dopamine prodrugs based on proton transfer reaction are depicted in Figure 39. Based on our reported DFT calculations on proton transfer reactions in Kemp's acid amide derivatives, **19-29**, two dopamine prodrugs are proposed. As shown in Figure 39, **ProD 1** and **ProD 2** have a carboxylic group as a hydrophilic moiety and the rest of the prodrug as a lipophilic moiety, where the combination of both moieties secures a moderate HLB. Furthermore, in a physiologic environment of the blood circulation (pH 7.4) dopamine is expected to be primary in the ionized forms while its prodrugs **ProD1-2** are expected to equilibrate between the ionic and the free acid forms. Thus, prodrugs **ProD 1-2** may have a better bioavailability than the parent drugs due to improved absorption. In addition, these prodrugs can be used in different dosage forms (i.e., enteric coated tablets) because of their potential solubility in organic and aqueous media due to the ability of the carboxylic group to be converted to the corresponding carboxylate anion in physiological environments of pH 5.0-7.4 (intestine and blood circulation). It is worth noting, that at pH 5.0-7.4 the carboxylic group in prodrugs **ProD 1-ProD 2** will equilibrate with the corresponding carboxylate form. Subsequently, the free acid form will undergo proton transfer reaction (rate limiting step) after being transferred through the membrane to yield dopamine and the inactive linker as a byproduct (Figure 39). The proposed prodrugs **ProD 1-ProD 2** will be exploited for per os use in the form of enteric coated tablets. It is well known, that enteric coated tablets are stable at the high acidic pH found in the stomach, but break down rapidly at a less acidic pH. For example, the enteric coated tablets will not dissolve in the acidic juices of the stomach (pH ~3), but they will in the higher pH (above pH 5.5) present in the small intestine. In the intestine, prodrugs **ProD 1- ProD 2** will exist in the acidic and ionic forms where the equilibrium constant for the exchange between both forms is dependent on the pK$_a$ of the given prodrug. The experimental determined pK$_a$'s for **ProD-1- ProD 2** linkers are in the range of 5.0-6.0. Therefore, it is expected that the pK$_a$'s of the corresponding prodrugs will be in the same range. Since the pH for the small intestine lies in the range of 5.0-7.5, the calculated unionized (acidic) /ionized ratio will be 40-50%. Although the percentage of the acidic form is not significantly high, we anticipate that prodrugs undergoing an efficient proton transfer (rate limiting step) to yield dopamine and Kemp's carboxylic acid by-products (Figure 39) will have the potential to be effective prodrugs. In the blood circulation (pH 7.4), the calculated acidic form for those prodrugs is around 10- 30% and it is expected that the rate for delivering the parental drug will be reduced.

In summary, we conclude that the driving force for rate accelerations witnessed in the cleavage reactions of Kemp's acid amides **19-29** and **ProD 1- ProD 2** under physiological environment is the proximity of the carboxylic proton and the amide carbonyl oxygen. The proximity parameters, r$_{GM}$ and α in the ground state are determined by the strain energy of the reactants (Es). In systems with high strain energies the global minimum structures tend to reside in a conformation by which the distance between the two reactive centers (distance between the nucleophile and the electrophile, r$_{GM}$) is short and the angle of attack α is close to linearity. Thus the activation energy of the system is minimized resulting in an enhancement in the reaction rate due to close resemblance of the ground state to the corresponding transition state (Table 2). Furthermore, the DFT calculation results predict a t$_{1/2}$ value of the cleavage reactions of **ProD 1- ProD 2** in pH 6 to be between 12 to 20 hours, whereas at pH 7 the value is expected to be higher (Table 2). The strategy to achieve desirable prodrugs for the treatment of Parkinson's disease that possess a high bioavailability values are: (1) synthesis of the linker moiety and attaching it with the parent drug Menger's synthetic method [130]; (2) kinetic studies (*in vitro*) of the synthesized prodrugs (**ProD 1- ProD 2**) in physiological environment (37 °C, pH = 6.0 in aqueous medium) and (3) for the prodrugs that show desirable controlled release in the *in vitro* studies, *in vivo* pharmacokinetic studies should be launched in order to determine the bioavailability and the duration of action of the tested prodrugs.

Figure 39. Intraconversion of dopamine prodrugs **ProD 1- ProD 2** to dopamine.

Bruice's Enzyme Model Based on Cyclization of Di-Carboxylic Semi-Esters [125, 126]

Bruice and Pandit have studied the cyclization of di-carboxylic semi-esters 30-35 illustrated in Figure 40 and found that the relative rate (k_{rel}) for 30>31>32>33>34>35. They attributed the discrepancy in rates for these di-carboxylic semi-esters to proximity orientation. Using the observation that alkyl substitution on succinic acid influences rotamer distributions, the ratio between the reactive gauche and the unreactive anti-conformers, they proposed that *gem*-dialkyl substitution increased the probability of the resultant rotamer adopting the more reactive conformation. Therefore, for efficient ring-closing to occur, the two reactive centers must be in the gauche conformation. In the unsubstituted reactant, the reactive centers are almost completely in the anti-conformation in order to minimize steric interactions [124-126].

Menger in his "spatiotemporal" hypothesis developed an equation correlating activation energy with distance and based on this equation, he concluded that significant rate accelerations in reactions catalyzed by enzymes are achieved by imposing short distances between the reacting centers of the substrate and enzyme [130-134]. On the other hand, Bruice attributed enzyme catalysis to favorable 'near attack conformations'. According to Bruice's hypothesis, systems that have a high quota of near attack conformations will have a higher intramolecular reaction rate and *vice versa*. Bruice's idea invokes a combination of distance between the two reacting centers and the angle of attack of the nucleophile towards the electrophile [124-126]. In contrast to the proximity proposal, others suggested that high rate enhancements in intramolecular processes area result of steric effects (strain energy relief of the ground state reactant) [223, 224].

Figure 40. Chemical structures for di-carboxylic semi-esters 30-35.

To test whether the discrepancy in the ring-closing rates of di-carboxylic semi-esters **30–35** is due to proximity orientation (difference in the distance between the nucleophile and the electrophile) or to strain effects, calculations using *ab initio* molecular orbital methods at B3LYP/6-31G (d,p) and HF/6-31G (d,p) levels, of the ground state, intermediate and transition state structures as well as the activation energy values for the cyclization reactions of **30–35** were conducted. The calculations revealed that the ring-closing reaction proceeds by one mechanism, by which the rate-limiting step is the tetrahedral intermediate collapse and not its formation (Figure 41), and the acceleration in rate is due to steric effects rather than to proximity orientation stemming from the "rotamer effect".

Allinger's MM2 strain energy calculations were done to examine whether the discrepancy in the rates of **30–33** and **35** (Figure 40) stems from proximity orientation or due to steric effects (strain energy) [154]. The calculated MM2 strain energy values for the reactants and intermediates in systems **30–33** and **35** are listed in Table 3 and they were correlated with the experimental relative rate (log k_{rel}) values [124-126]. The correlation results revealed strong correlation between the two parameters (equations 1 and 2). Attempts to correlate the distance between the two reacting centers (r_{GM}) and log k_{rel} failed to give any linearity between the two parameters. This suggests that the driving force for acceleration in the cyclization process is driven by strain effects. This is in contrast, to that suggested by Bruice's near attack proximity orientation [224-226]. Further support to this conclusion was obtained by a strong correlation found between the activation energy values ($\Delta G^{\ddagger}_{H2O}$ and $\Delta G^{\ddagger}_{GP}$) for **30–33** and **35** with both log k_{rel} and the MM2strain energy values, ΔEs (TS - AN) (equations 3 and 4).

(eq. 1) $\Delta G^{\ddagger}_{H2O}$ B3LYP/6-31G (d,p) = -2.0657logkrel + 17.653 0.95
(eq. 2) $\Delta G^{\ddagger}_{GP}$ B3LYP/6-31G (d,p) = -1.7747logkrel + 14.729 0.90
(eq. 3) $\Delta G^{\ddagger}_{H2O}$ B3LYP/6-31G (d,p) = -1.0467ΔEs (TS - AN) + 3.262 0.99
(eq. 4) $\Delta G^{\ddagger}_{GP}$ B3LYP/6-31G (d,p) = -0.9101ΔEs (TS -AN) + 3.647 0.98

Figure 41. Proposed mechanism for the ring-closing of 30-35.

The followings summarize the study emerging points: (i) the activation energy values for **30-35** are solely dependent on the strain energies of the transition states and the reactants, and not on the distance between the nucleophile (O1) and the electrophile (C2). (ii) The observation of opening the cyclic ring during the reaction rate limiting step supports the notion that the difference in the strain energies of the reactant and the transition states plays a crucial role in the discrepancy in the rates of cyclization of the di-carboxylic semi-esters **30-**

35, (iii) strained reactants such as **35** are more reactive than the less strained reactants, and the reactivity extent is linearly correlated with the strain energy difference between the transition state and the reactant (ΔEs), and (iv) The energy needed to provide a stable transition state for a strained system is less than that for the unstrained system, since the conformational change from the reactant to the transition state in the strained systems is smaller.

Table 3. DFT calculated properties for the cyclization reactions of 30-33 and 35

System	log k_{rel} [125,126] (exp.)	ES$_{INT-GM}$ (MM2 calc.)	$\Delta G^{\ddagger}$ (GP) B3L	$\Delta G^{\ddagger}$ (H$_2$O) B3L	r_{GM} B3L	$\Delta G^{\ddagger}$ (GP) B3L311	$\Delta G^{\ddagger}$ (H$_2$O) B3L311
30	3.00	8.70	19.09	29.37	4.24	9.26	20.33
31	3.30	9.30	12.22	21.10	4.34	13.13	22.03
32	5.26	8.07	12.83	16.13	4.31	10.27	13.98
33	5.36	4.24	1.43	9.03	4.08	2.76	12.54
35	7.90	2.31	10.48	16.51	2.37	------	------

log krel is the experimental relative rate [125,126]. $\Delta G\ddagger$ is the activation free energy (kcal/mol). rGM is the distance between the nucleophile (O1) and the electrophile (C6) in the reactant. B3L and B3L311 refer to calculated by B3LYP/6-31 G (d,p) and B3LYP/6-311 + G (d,p), respectively. GP and H2O refer to calculated in the gas phase and water, respectively.

Paracetamol Prodrugs without Bitter Sensation Based on Bruice's Enzyme Model [180]

Taste is an important issue for orally administered drugs; one of the most serious problems for drug formulation is the undesirable drug's taste. Drugs bitterness might reduce patient compliance thus decreases therapeutic effect especially in children patients. Therefore, masking the bitter taste of a drug is an important issue in the pharmaceuticals industry [225]. There are five basic tastes; sweet, sour, salt, bitter and umami. When a molecule dissolves in saliva it binds to a taste receptor that is found in taste buds which are distributed throughout the tongue. Sweet receptors are located on the tip of the tongue, sour receptors on the bilateral sides of tongue, salty taste receptors are on the bilateral sides and the tip of the tongue, bitter taste receptors are on the posterior part of the tongue and umami taste receptors are located all over the tongue. When a molecule binds to a receptor, a signal will be transmitted to the brain via facial, glossopharyngeal and vagus cranial nerves.

Chemical molecules dissolve in saliva and bind to taste receptors on the tongue to give a bitter, sweet, salty, sour, or umami sensation. The sensation is a result of signal transduction from taste receptors located in areas known as taste buds. The taste buds contain very sensitive nerve endings, which are responsible for the production and transmission of electrical impulses *via* cranial nerves VII, IX, and X to certain areas in the brain that are devoted to the perception of taste [226]. Molecules with bitter taste [227–231] are very diverse in their chemical structure and physicochemical properties [232, 233]. In humans, bitter taste perception is mediated by 25 G-protein coupled receptors of the hTAS2R gene family. Drugs such as macrolide antibiotics, non-steroidal anti-inflammatory and penicillin derivatives have a pronounced bitter taste [234]. Masking the taste of water soluble bitter drugs, especially those given in high doses, is difficult to achieve by using sweeteners alone.

As a consequence, several approaches were developed for achieving more efficient techniques for masking the bitter taste of molecules. Techniques available for masking drug's bitterness are: (1) taste masking with flavors, sweeteners, and amino acids [235] ; (2) taste masking with lipophilic vehicles such as lipids, lecithin, and lecithin- like substances[236]; (3) coating which is classified based on the type of coating material, coating solvent system, and the number of coating layers [237] ; (4) microencapsulation based on the principle of solvent extraction or evaporation [238]; (5) sweeteners are generally used in combination with other taste masking technologies [239]; (6) taste suppressants and potentiators, such as Linguagen's bitter blockers [240]; (7) resins are utilized to mask pharmaceuticals bitterness by forming insoluble resonates [241, 242]; (8) inclusion complex by which the drug molecule fits into the cavity of a complexing agent and forms a stable complex that masks the bitter taste of a drug by decreasing its oral solubility [243]; (9) pH modifiers [244]; (10) and adsorbates; [245]. All of the developed techniques are based on the physical modification of the formulation containing the bitter tastant. Although these approaches have helped to improve the taste of some drugs formulations, the problem of the bitter taste of drugs in pediatric and geriatric formulations still creates a serious challenge to the health community. Thus, different strategies should be developed in order to overcome this serious problem. Altering the ability of the drug to interact with its bitter taste receptors could reduce or eliminate its bitterness. This could be achieved by an appropriate modification of the structure and the size of a bitter compound. Bitter molecules bind to the G-protein coupled receptor-type T2R on the apical membrane of the taste receptor cells located in the taste buds. In humans, about 25 different T2R's are described. Additionally, several alleles are known and about 1000 different bitter phenotypes exist in human beings [228-234]. Due to the large variation of structural features of bitter taste molecules, it is difficult to generalize the molecular requirements for bitterness. Nevertheless, it was reported that a bitter tastant molecule requires a polar group and a hydrophobic moiety. Structural modifications, such as an increase in the number of amino groups/residues to more than 3 and a reduction in the poly-hydroxyl group/ COOH, have been proven to decrease bitterness. Moreover, changing the configuration of a bitter tastant molecule by making isomer analogues was found to be important for binding affinity to enhance bitterness agonist activity (e.g., L-tryptophan is bitter while D-tryptophan is sweet) [246].

Paracetamol, (N-(4-hydroxyphenyl)ethanamide, is an over the counter analgesic and anti-pyretic drug; it is used as pain killer by decreasing the synthesis of prostaglandin due to inhibiting cyclooxygenases . Paracetamol is favored over aspirin as pain killer in patients who have excessive gastric secretion or prolonged bleeding. It was approved to be used as fever reducer in all ages. Bitter unpleasant taste is one of paracetamol undesired properties. Paracetamol has a strong bitter taste. The bitter unpleasant taste of a drug might reduce patient compliance. Paracetamol was found in the urine of patients who had taken phenacetin and later on, it was demonstrated that paracetamol was a urinary metabolite of acetanilide (Figure 42). Phenacetin (Figure 42), on the other hand, lacks or has a very slight bitter taste. Examination of the structures of paracetamol and phenacetin revealed that the only difference in the structural features is the nature of the group in the *para* position of the benzene ring. While in the case of paracetamol the group is hydroxy, in phenacetin it is ethoxy. Acetanilide has a chemical structure similar to that of paracetamol and phenacetin but lacks the group in the *para* position of the benzene ring, making it lack the bitter taste characteristic of paracetamol. These combined facts suggest that the presence of a hydroxy group on the *para* position is the major contributor for the bitter taste of paracetamol. Therefore, it is expected that blocking the hydroxyl group in paracetamol with a suitable linker could inhibit the interaction of paracetamol with its bitter taste receptors and mask its bitter taste [180]. It is likely that paracetamol binds to the active site of its bitter taste receptor via hydrogen bonding interactions by which its phenolic hydroxyl group is engaged. It is worth noting that linking paracetamol with Bruice's enzyme model linker *via* its phenolic hydroxyl group might hinder paracetamol bitter taste. Based on the DFT calculations on the cyclization of Bruice's **30-35** (Figure 40), three paracetamol prodrugs were proposed (Figure 43). As shown in Figure 43, the paracetamol prodrugs, **ProD 1-3**, have a carboxylic acid group as a hydrophilic moiety and the rest of the prodrug, as a lipophilic moiety, where the combination of both groups provides a moderate HLB. It should be noted that the HLB value will be determined upon the pH of the physiologic environment by which the prodrug is dissolved. For example, in the stomach, the paracetamol prodrugs will primarily exist in the carboxylic acid form whereas in the blood circulation the carboxylate form will be dominant. Since Bruice's cyclization reaction occurs in basic medium paracetamol **ProD 1-3**were obtained as carboxylic free acid form, since this form is expected to be stable in acidic medium such as the stomach.

Figure 42. Chemical structures of paracetamol, phenacetin and acetanilide.

Figure 43. Hydrolysis of paracetamol ProD 1 – ProD 3.

In Vitro Intra-Conversion of Paracetamol Prodrugs to Their Active Drug, Paracetamol

The hydrolysis of paracetamol **ProD 1-ProD 2** was studied in four different media; 1N HCl, buffer pH 3, and buffer pH 7.4. The prodrug hydrolysis was monitored using HPLC analysis. At constant pH and temperature the release of paracetamol from its prodrug was followed and showed a first order kinetics. k_{obs} (h^{-1}) and $t_{1/2}$ values for the intraconversion of paracetamol **ProD 1-ProD 2** was calculated from regression equation obtained from plotting log concentration of residual of the prodrug vs. time. The kinetics results in the different media are summarized in Table 4 and Figure 44.

Table 4. Observed *k* and *t*$_{1/2}$ values for the intraconversion of paracetamol ProD 1-ProD 2 in 1N HCl and buffers pH 3 and 7.4

Medium	ProD 1 k_{obs} (h^{-1})	ProD 2 k_{obs} (h^{-1})	ProD 1 $t_{1/2}$ (h)	ProD 2 $t_{1/2}$ (h)
1N HCl	No reaction	No reaction	No reaction	No reaction
Buffer pH 3	-----------	6.3 x 10^{-5}	Very fast	3
Buffer pH 7.4	-----------	6.1 x 10^{-4}	Very fast	0.3

As shown in Table 4 the hydrolysis rate of paracetamol **ProD 1** at pH 7.4 was the fastest among all media, followed by pH 3 medium. In 1N HCl no conversion of the prodrug to the parent dug was observed.

On the other hand, paracetamol **ProD 2** underwent fast hydrolysis (within seconds) in pH 7.4 whereas in pH 3.0 and in 1N HCl was entirely stable. The discrepancy in the behavior between the two prodrugs is due to the fact that the strain energy of maleic anhydride is higher than that of succinic anhydride. It should be emphasized that the reaction rate in these processes is determined on the strain energy of the system.

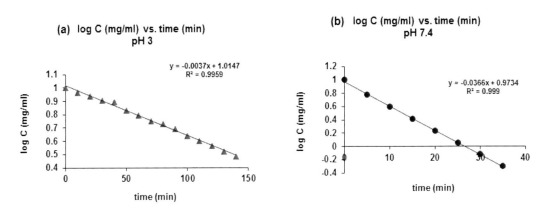

Figure 44. First order hydrolysis plot of paracetamol **ProD 1** in (a) buffer pH 3 and (b) buffer pH 7.4.

Kirby's Enzyme Model Based on the Acid-Catalyzed Hydrolysis of N-Alkylmaleamic Acids [137]

Proton transfer reactions are the most common processes catalyzed by enzymes. Examples for such catalysis are the proton transfers catalyzed by triose phosphate isomerase (k_{cat} = 53,000 s^{-1}) and Δ5-3-ketosteroid isomerase (k_{cat} = 8300 s^{-1}) which involve weakly basic and acid groups to achieve such significant rates. Scientists have encouraged exploiting intramolecularity in modeling enzyme catalysis due to the fact that reactions of an enzyme active site and substrate are between functional groups held in a close proximity. Both, enzymes and intramolecularity are similar in that the reacting centers are held together, non-covalently with the enzymes, and covalently with the intramolecular process. The tremendous high efficiency of enzymes catalysis depends on a combination of some factors that most of them have been recognized but none of them was fully understood. Although the devoted research to the chemistry of enzyme catalysis is growing rapidly a number of several factors remain to be studied [247-252].

Kirby and coworkers have studied the mechanism of the acid-catalyzed hydrolysis of N-alkylmaleamic acids **36-42** to maleamic acid derivatives and amines (Figure 45). Their study revealed that the reaction is remarkably sensitive to the pattern of substitution on the carbon-carbon double bond and the hydrolysis rates range over more than ten powers of ten, and the "effective concentration" of the carboxyl group of the most reactive amide, dimethyl-N-n-propylmaleamic acid, is greater than 10^{10} M. This acid amide was found to be converted into the more stable dimethylmaleic anhydride with a half-life of less than one second at 39 °C below pH 3 [137]. In addition, the results have showed that the amide bond breakdown is due to intramolecular nucleophilic catalysis by the adjacent carboxylic acid group. Furthermore, based on the fact that the tetrahedral intermediate, isomaleimide, was converted quantitatively into N-methylmaleamic acid (Figure 46), the authors suggested that the rate-limiting step is the dissociation of the tetrahedral intermediate [137]. Some years later, Kluger and Chin investigated the intramolecular hydrolysis mechanism of a series of N-alkylmaleamic acids derived from aliphatic amines having a wide range of basicity [253]. Their study demonstrated that the identity of the rate-limiting step is a function of both the basicity of the leaving group and the acidity of the solution. In 1990, based on AM1 semiempirical calculations, Katagi had concluded that the rate- limiting step is the formation of the tetrahedral intermediate and not its dissociation [254].

For determining the factors playing dominant role in proton transfer processes we have computationally studied Kirby's intramolecular acid catalyzed hydrolysis of (4-amino- 4-oxo-2-butenoic) acids (N-alkylmaleamic acids) **36–42**.

The goal of our study was to: (a) determine whether the rate-limiting step in **36-42** is the tetrahedral intermediate formation or collapse, and to assign the driving force(s) responsible for the extremely high rates for the acid-catalyzed hydrolysis of **37**and **40**, and (b) determine the structural features associated with high reactivity in the acid-catalyzed hydrolysis, with the expectation that similar factors will be operative in enzyme catalysis.

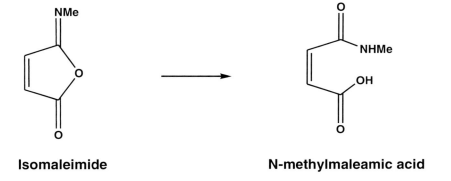

36; R₁=R₂=H
37; R₁=R₂=Me
38; R₁=H; R₂=Me
39; R₁,R₂ Cyclopent-l-ene-1,2-diyl
40; R₁, R₂ Cyclohex-l-ene-1,2-diyl
41; R₁=H; R₂=Et
42; R₁=H; R₂=n-Propyl

Figure 45. Chemical structures of N-alkylmalic acids 36-42.

Figure 46. Conversion of isomaleimide to N-methylmaleamic acid.

Using DFT calculation method at B3LYP/6-31G (d,p) level the acid catalyzed hydrolysis of maleamic (4-amino-4-oxo-2-butenoic) acids (Kirby's N-alkylmaleamic acids) 36-42 (Figure 45) were computed. The results confirmed that the reaction proceeds in three steps: (i) proton transfer from the carboxylic group to the adjacent amide carbonyl carbon followed by, (ii) nucleophilic attack of the carboxylate anion onto the protonated carbonyl carbon and the final step of the reaction involves (iii) dissociation of the tetrahedral intermediate to provide products (Figure 47). In addition, the calculation results demonstrate that the rate-limiting step is dependent on the reaction medium. In the gas phase the rate-limiting step was the formation of the tetrahedral intermediate, whereas in the presence of water the dissociation of the tetrahedral intermediate was the rate-limiting step. Further, when the leaving group (CH₃NH₂) in 36-42 was replaced with a group having a low pK$_a$ value the rate-limiting step was the formation of the tetrahedral intermediate, such as in the case where CH₃NH₂ was replaced with CF₃NH₂ (see Figure 47).The results revealed that the efficiency of the intramolecular acid-catalyzed hydrolysis by the carboxyl group is remarkably sensitive to the pattern of substitution on the carbon-carbon double bond. The rate of hydrolysis was found to be linearly correlated with the strain energy of the tetrahedral intermediate or the product

(Table 5). Systems having strained tetrahedral intermediates or products were found to be with low rates and *vice versa* [164, 183,185].

NHR = atenolol, acyclovir, cefuroxime, tranexamic acid or methyl
R1 and R2; H, methyl or trifluoromethyl

Figure 47. Proposed mechanism for the hydrolysis of N-alkylmaleamic acids 30-36.

Table 5. DFT (B3LYP) calculated kinetic and thermodynamic properties for the acid catalyzed hydrolysis of 36-42

System	$\Delta G_{bGP}^{\ddagger}$ (kcal/mol)	$\Delta G_{bW}^{\ddagger}$ (kcal/mol)	$\Delta G_{fGP}^{\ddagger}$ (kcal/mol)	$\Delta G_{fW}^{\ddagger}$ (kcal/mol)	$\log k_{rel}$ [137]	log EM [137, 255] (Exp)	log EM (Calc)	Es (INT$_2$) (kcal/mol)	Es (GM) (kcal/mol)
36	28.08	33.06	33.53	26.10	0	7.724	8.52	20.55	10.16
37	16.42	20.05	27.08	17.90	4.371	15.86	18.08	16.16	10.82
38	24.90	28.42	32.57	24.80	1.494	7.742	11.93	17.32	9.40
39	36.77	38.11	45.37	32.16	-4.377	1.255	4.81	27.89	12.30
40	17.41	23.12	26.87	17.89	2.732	15.190	15.82	19.25	9.18
41	23.92	27.28	32.12	23.87	1.516	6.962	12.76	17.59	5.12
42	25.03	27.55	32.3	24.40	1.648	8.568	12.57	18.55	6.20

B3LYP refers to values calculated by B3LYP/6-31G (d, p) method. $\Delta G^{\ddagger}$ is the calculated activation free energy (kcal/mol). Es refers to strain energy calculated by Allinger's MM2 method. GM and INT_2 refer to reactant and intermediate 2, respectively. EM = e $^{-(\Delta G \ddagger inter-}$ $^{\Delta G \ddagger intra)/RT}$. BW and FW refer to tetrahedral intermediate breakdown and tetrahedral intermediate formation calculated in water, respectively. Exp refers to experimental value. Calc refers to DFT calculated values.

The linear correlation between the calculated EM values and the experimental EM values (Table 5) demonstrates the credibility of using DFT methods in predicting energies as well as rates for reactions of the type described herein [164, 183,185, 186].

Designed Tranexamic Acid Prodrugs Based On Intramolecular Acid-Catalyzed Hydrolysis of Kirby's N-Alkylmaleamic Acids [184]

Tranexamic acid (trans-4 (aminomethyl) cyclohexanecarboxylic acid) is a synthetic lysine amino acid derivative. It is used to prevent and reduce excessive hemorrhage in hemophilia patients and reduce the need for replacement therapy during and following tooth extraction. It is often prescribed for excessive bleeding. The mechanism by which tranexamic acid exerts its antifibrinolytic activity is by it is competitive inhibition of plasminogen that prevents the activation of plasminogen to plasmin; plasmin is an enzyme used to degrade fibrin clot. Tranexamic acid has roughly 8 times the antifibrinolytic activity of an older analogue, ε-aminocaproic acid. Over the past few years, the use of tranexamic acid has been expanding beyond the small number of hemophilia patients; it is an important agent in decreasing mortality rate due to bleeding in trauma patients. It can be used safely in women whom undergo lower segment cesarean section, in this operation it was found that tranexamic acid reduces the blood loss during and after surgery, and it is pharmacologically active in reducing intra-operative using of blood heart surgery, hip and knee replacement surgery and liver transplant surgery.

Recently, a new oral formulation of tranexamic acid was shown to be safe and effective for treatment of heavy menstrual bleeding. Oral administration of tranexamic acid results in a 45% oral bioavailability. The total oral dose recommended in women with heavy menstrual bleeding was two 650 mg tablets three times daily for 5 days. Accumulation following multiple dosing was reported to be minimal. Post-partum hemorrhage is a leading cause of maternal mortality, accounting for about 100000 maternal deaths every year. In third world countries, availability of blood and fluid replacement may be an issue. One approach to decrease the risk of maternal hemorrhage may be to improve the availability of blood and fluid replacement. An alternative approach is to decrease the likelihood of maternal hemorrhage. Furthermore, all the treatment options mentioned above are intended for intravenous administration; this may not be a viable option in under-developed countries. Therefore, a cheaper oral alternative may be better suited for such circumstances.

Oral tranexamic acid dosage form was found to be effective and safe in treating malesma, a hypermelanosis disease that occurs in Asian women. Since tranexamic acid is an amino acid derivative and undergoes ionization in physiologic environments its oral bioavailability is expected to be low due to inefficient absorption through membranes. Note the log P (partition coefficient) for tranexamic acid is -1.6. Hence, there is a necessity to design and synthesis relatively more lipophilic tranexamic acid prodrugs that can provide the parent drug in a sustained release manner which might result in better clinical outcome, more convenient dosing regimens and potentially fewer side effects than the original medication. For example, tranexamic acid is given by continuous IV infusion resulting in peak plasma concentration following administration. If a slow release prodrug can be prepared, then C_{max} related side effects may be avoided and longer duration exposure may be achieved resulting in potentially better maintenance paradigm. Improvement of tranexamic acid pharmacokinetic properties and hence its effectiveness may increase the absorption of the drug *via* a variety of administration routes, especially the oral and SC injection routes [256- 261].

Based on DFT calculations for the acid-catalyzed hydrolysis of several N-alkylmaleamic acid derivatives (Figure 45) four tranexamic acid prodrugs were designed (Figure 48). The DFT results on the acid-catalyzed hydrolysis demonstrated that the reaction rate-limiting step is determined on the nature of the amine leaving group. When the amine leaving group was a primary amine or tranexamic acid moiety, the tetrahedral intermediate collapse was the rate-limiting step, whereas in the cases where the amine leaving group was aciclovir or cefuroxime the rate-limiting step was the tetrahedral intermediate formation. Based on the DFT calculated rates the predicted $t_{1/2}$ (a time needed for 50% of the prodrug to be converted into drug) values for tranexamic acid prodrugs ProD 1- ProD 4 (Figure 48)at pH 2 were 556 hours, 253 hours, 70 seconds and 1.7 hours, respectively.

The kinetic study for the acid-catalyzed hydrolysis of tranexamic acid **ProD 1**was carried out in aqueous buffer in the same manner as that done by Kirby on Kirby's enzyme model **36-42**. This is in order to explore whether the prodrug hydrolyzes in aqueous medium and to what extent or not, suggesting the fate of the prodrug in the system. Acid-catalyzed hydrolysis kinetics of the synthesized tranexamic acid **ProD 1** was studied in four different aqueous media: 1 N HCl, buffer pH 2, buffer pH 5 and buffer pH 7.4. Under the experimental conditions the target compounds hydrolyzed to release the parent drug (Figure 49) as evident by HPLC analysis. At constant pH and temperature the reaction displayed strict first order kinetics as the k_{obs} was fairly constant and a straight plot was obtained on plotting log concentration of residual prodrug verves time. The rate constant (k_{obs}) and the corresponding half-lives ($t_{1/2}$) for tranexamic acid prodrug **ProD 1** in the different media were calculated from the linear regression equation correlating the log concentration of the residual prodrug verses time. The kinetic data are listed in Table 6. The 1N HCl, pH 2 and pH 5 were selected to examine the interconversion of the tranexamic acid prodrug in pH as of stomach, because the mean fasting stomach pH of adult is approximately 1-2 and increases up to 5 following ingestion of food. In addition, buffer pH 5 mimics the beginning small intestine pathway. Finally, pH 7.4 was selected to examine the interconversion of the tested prodrug in blood circulation system. Acid-catalyzed hydrolysis of the tranexamic acid **ProD 1** was found to be higher in 1N HCl than at pH 2 and 5 (Figure 49). At 1N HCl the prodrug was hydrolyzed to release the parent drug in less than one hour. On the other hand, at pH 7.4, the prodrug was entirely stable and no release of the parent drug was observed. Since the pK_a of tranexamic acid **ProD1** is in the range of 3-4, it is expected at pH 5 the anionic form of the prodrug will be dominant and the percentage of the free acidic form that undergoes the acid-catalyzed hydrolysis will be relatively low. At 1N HCl and pH 2 most of the prodrug will exist as the free acid form and at pH 7.4 most of the prodrug will be in the anionic form. Thus, the difference in rates at the different pH buffers.

Figure 48. Acid-catalyzed hydrolysis of tranexamic acid prodrugs ProD 1 –ProD 4.

Comparison between the calculated $t_{1/2}$value (556 h) for tranexamic acid **ProD 1** to the experimental value (23.9 h) indicates that the calculated value is about 23 times larger than the experimental. This discrepancy between the calculated and the experimental values might be attributed to the fact that the PCM model (calculations in presence of solvent) is not capable for handling calculations in acidic aqueous solvent (medium) since the dielectric constant for pH 2 aqueous solutions is not known. The $t_{1/2}$ experimental value at pH 5 was 270 hours and at pH 7.4 no interconversion was observed. The lack of the reaction at the latter pH might be due to the fact that at this pH tranexamic acid **ProD 1** exists solely in the ionized form (pK_a about 4). As mentioned before the free acid form is a mandatory requirement for the reaction to proceed. On the other hand, tranexamic acid **ProD 4** has a higher pK_a than tranexamic acid **ProD 1** (about 6 vs. 4). Therefore, it is expected that the interconversion rate of tranexamic acid **ProD 4** to its parent drug, tranexamic acid, at all pHs studied will be higher (log EM for **ProD 4** is 14.33 vs. 9.53 for **ProD 1**). Future study to achieve desirable tranexamic acid prodrugs capable of releasing tranexamic acid in a controlled manner and enhancing the parent drug bioavailability is: (i) synthesis of tranexamic acid **ProD 4**; (ii) kinetic studies (*in vitro*) on **ProD 4** at pH 6.5 (intestine) and pH

7.4 (blood circulation system) (iii) in vivo pharmacokinetic studies to determine the bioavailability and the duration of action of the tested prodrug. Furthermore, based on the in vivo pharmacokinetics characteristics of tranexamic acid **ProD 4** new prodrugs may be designed and synthesized.

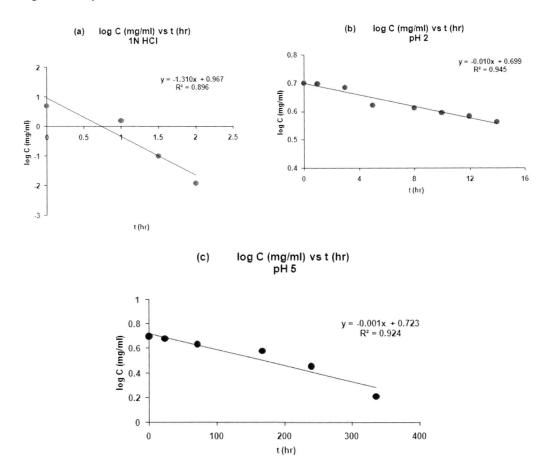

Figure 49. First order hydrolysis plots of tranexamic acid ProD1 in (a) 1N HCl, (b) buffer of pH 2 and (c) buffer pH 5.

Table 6. The observed k value and $t_{1/2}$ of tranexamic acid prodrug (ProD 1) in 1N HCl and at pH 2, 5 and 7.4

Medium	k_{obs} (h^{-1})	$t_{1/2}$ (h)
1N HCl	5.13 x 10^{-3}	0.9
Buffer pH 2	3.92 x 10^{-5}	23.9
Buffer pH 5	3.92 x 10^{-6}	270
Buffer pH 7.4	No reaction	No reaction

Conclusion

Unraveling the mechanisms of a number of enzyme models has allowed for the design of efficient chemical devices having the potential to be utilized as prodrug linkers that can be covalently attached to commonly used drugs which can chemically, and not enzymatically, be converted to release the active drugs in a programmable manner. For instance, exploring the mechanism for a proton transfer in Kirby's N-alkylmaleamic acids (enzyme model) has led to the design of a number of prodrugs such as tranexamic acid for bleeding conditions, acyclovir as antiviral drug for the treatment for herpes simplex [185], atenolol for treating hypertension with enhanced stability and bioavailability, and lacks a bitter sensation [186, 187]. In addition, prodrugs for masking the bitter sensation of paracetamol and some antibacterial drugs, such as cefuroxime, amoxicillin and cephalexin were also designed and synthesized [183]. The role of the linkers in atenolol, paracetamol and the antibacterial prodrugs is to block the free hydroxyl or amine, which is responsible for the drug bitterness, and to enable the release of the drug in a controlled manner. Menger's Kemp acid enzyme model was utilized for the design of dopamine prodrugs for the treatment for Parkinson's disease [188]. Prodrugs of dimethyl fumarate for the treatment psoriasis was also designed, synthesized and studied [262]. Furthermore, unraveling the mechanism of Kirby's acetals has led to the design and synthesis of novel prodrugs of aza-nucleosides for the treatment for myelodysplastic syndromes [177], atovaquone prodrugs for the treatment for malaria [178, 179], less bitter paracetamol prodrugs to be administered to children and elderly as antipyretic and pain killer [180], statin prodrugs [181] and prodrugs of phenylephrine as decongestant [182]. In these examples, the prodrug moiety was linked to the hydroxyl group of the active drug such that the drug-linker moiety (prodrug) has the potential to interconvert when exposed into physiological environments such as stomach, intestine, and/or blood circulation, with rates that are solely dependent on the structural features of the pharmacologically inactive promoiety (Kirby's enzyme model). Further details on this approach could be found in references [263-269].

Acknowledgments

The author would like to acknowledge funding by the German Research Foundation (DFG, ME 1024/8-1).

References

[1]   DiMasi, J.A.; Hansen, R.W. & Grabowski, H.G. (2003) The price of innovation: new estimates of drug development costs. *J. Health Econ. 22*, 151–185.

[2]   DiMasi, J.A. (2002) The value of improving the productivity of the drug development process: faster times and better decisions. *Pharmacoeconomics20*, 1–10.

[3]   Huttunen, K.M.; Raunio, H. & Rautio, J. (2011) Prodrugs from serendipity to rational design. *Pharmacol. Rev. 63*, 750–771.

[4] Stella, V.J. & Nti-Addae, K.W. (2007) Prodrug strategies to overcome poor water solubility. *Adv. Drug Deliv. Rev. 59*, 677–694.

[5] Dahan, A.; Khamis, M.; Agbaria, R. & Karaman, R. (2012) Targeted prodrugs in oral delivery: the modern molecular biopharmaceutical approach. *Expert Opinion on Drug Delivery9*, 1001–1013.

[6] Karaman, R.; Fattash B. & Qtait A. (2013) The future of prodrugs – design by quantum mechanics methods. *Expert Opinion on Drug Delivery10*, 713–729.

[7] Karaman, R. (2013) Prodrugs design based on inter- and intramolecular processes. *Chem. Biol. Drug. Des. 82*, 643–668.

[8] Gonzalez, F.J. & Tukey, R.H. (2006) Drug metabolism. In: Brunton, L.L., Lazo, J.S. & Parker, K.L., editors. Goodman & Gilman's The Pharmacological Basis of Therapeutics. New York: The McGraw-Hill Companies, Inc.; p. 71–91.

[9] Testa, B. & Kramer, S.D. (2007) The biochemistry of drug metabolism–an introduction: part 2. Redox reactions and their enzymes. *Chem. Biodivers. 4*, 257–405.

[10] Gangwar, S.; Pauletti, G.M.; Wang, B.; Siahaan, T.J.; Stella, V.J. & Borchardt, R.T. (1997) Prodrug strategies to enhance the intestinal absorption of peptides. *DDT2*, 148–155.

[11] Wang W.; Jiang J.; Ballard C.E. & Wang B. (1999) Prodrug approaches to the improved delivery of peptide drugs. *Curr. Pharm. Des. 5*, 265–287.

[12] Chan, O.H. & Stewart, B.H. (1996) Physicochemical and drug-delivery considerations for oral drug bioavailability. *Drug. Discov. Today1*, 461–473.

[13] Ohlstein, E. H.; Ruffolo, R. R. Jr. & Elliott, J. D. (2000) Drug discovery in the next millennium. *Annu. Rev. Pharmacol.Toxicol.40*, 177-91.

[14] Stella, V.J. (2010) Prodrugs: some thoughts and current issues. *J. Pharm. Sci. 99(12)*, 4755–4765.

[15] Muller, C.E. (2009) Prodrug approaches for enhancing the bioavailability of drugs with low solubility. *Chem. Biodivers. 6*, 2071–2083.

[16] Tunek, A.; Levin, E. & Svensson, L.A. (1988) Hydrolysis of 3H-bambuterol, a carbamate prodrug of terbutaline, in blood from humans and laboratory animals in vitro. *Biochem. Pharmacol. 37*, 3867–3876.

[17] Browne, T.R.; Kugler, A.R. & Eldon, M.A. (1996) Pharmacology and pharmacokinetics of fosphenytoin. *Neurology 46*, S3–S7.

[18] Wolff, M.E. (editor) (1995) Medicinal Chemistry and Drug Discovery, 5th edn. New York: *John Wiley & Sons.*

[19] Williams, D.A., Foye, W.O. & Lemke, T.L. editors. (2002) Foye's Principles of Medicinal Chemistry. *Baltimore, MD: Wolters Kluwer Health;* p. 26–53.

[20] Kenny, B.A.; Bushfield M.; Parry-Smith D.J.; Fogarty S. & Trehene M. (1998) The application of high throughput screening to novel lead discovery, *Prog. Drug Res 41*, 246–269.

[21] Blundell, T. (1996) Structure-based drug design. *Nature384*, 23–26.

[22] Williams, M. (1993) Strategies for drug discovery. *NIDA Res.Monogr.132*, 1–22.

[23] Beaumont, K.; Webster, R.; Gardner, I. & Dack, K. (2003) Design of ester prodrugs to enhance oral absorption of poorly permeable compounds: challenges to the discovery scientist. *Curr. Drug Metab.4*, 461–485.

[24] Bellott, R.; Le Morvan, V.; Charasson, V.; Laurand, A.; Colotte, M.; Zanger, U.M. & Robert, J. (2008) Functional study of the 830C >G polymorphism of the human carboxylesterase 2 gene. *Cancer Chemother Pharmacol 61*, 481–488.

[25] Reddy, K.R.; Matelich, M.C.; Ugarkar, B.G.; Gomez- Galeno, J.E.; DaRe, J.; Ollis, K. & Erion, M.D. (2008) Pradefovir: a prodrug that targets adefovir to the liver for the treatment of hepatitis B. *J. Med. Chem. 51*, 666–676.

[26] Kumpulainen, H.; Mahonen, N.; Laitinen, M.L.; Jaurakkaj, J.; Jarvinen, T. & Rautio, J. (2006) Evaluation of hydroxyimine as cytochrome P450 selective prodrug structure. *J. Med. Chem. 49*, 1207–1211.

[27] Saunders, M.P.; Patterson, A.V.; Chinje, E.C.; Harris, A.L. & Stratford, I.J. (2000) NADPH: cytochrome c (P450) reductase activates tirapazamine (SR4233) to restore hypoxicandoxic cytotoxicity in anaerobic resistant derivative of the A549 lung cancer cell line. *Br. J. Cancer82*, 651–656.

[28] Dobesh, P.P. (2009) Pharmacokinetics and pharmacodynamics of prasugrel, a thienopyridine P2Y12 inhibitor. *Pharmacotherapy29*, 1089–1102.

[29] Pereillo, J.M.; Maftouh, M.; Andrieu, A.; Uzabiaga, M.F.; Fedeli, O.; Savi, P. & Picard, C. (2002) Structure and stereochemistry of the active metabolite of clopidogrel. *Drug Metab. Dispos. 30*, 1288–1295.

[30] Svensson, L.A. & Tunek, A. (1988) The design and bioactivation of presystemically stable prodrugs. *Drug Metab. Rev. 19*, 165–194.

[31] Stella, V.J. (2007) A case for prodrugs. In: Stella, V.J.; Borchardt, R.T.; Hageman, M.J.; Oliyai, R.; Magg, H. & Tilley, J.W., editors. Prodrugs: Challenges and Rewards. Part 1. New York, NY: *AAPS Press/Springer;* p. 3–33.

[32] Albert, A. (1958) Chemical aspects of selective toxicity. *Nature182*, 421–422.

[33] Harper, N.J. (1959) Drug latentiation. *J. Med. Pharm. Chem. 1*, 467–500.

[34] Harper, N.J. (1962) Drug latentiation. *Prog. Drug Res. 4*, 221–294.

[35] Sinkula, A.A. & Yalkowsky, S.H. (1975) Rationale for design of biologically reversible drug derivatives: prodrugs. *J. Pharm. Sci. 64*, 181–210.

[36] Schrama, D,; Reisfeld, R.A. & Becker, J.C. (2006) Antibody targeted drugs as cancer therapeutics. *Nature reviews Drug discovery 5(2)*, 147-59.

[37] Mahato, R.; Tai, W. & Cheng, K. (2011) Prodrugs for improving tumor targetability and efficiency.*Advanced drug delivery reviews 63(8)*, 659-70.

[38] Singh, Y.; Palombo, M. & Sinko, P.J. (2008) Recent trends in targeted anticancer prodrug and conjugatedesign. *Current medicinal chemistry.* 15(18), 1802-26.

[39] Niculescu-Duvaz, I.; Niculescu-Duvaz, D. & Friedlos, F. (1999) Self-immolative anthracycline prodrugs for suicide gene therapy. *Journal of clinical investigation.* 13, 2485-2489.

[40] Stella, V.J.; Borchardt, R.T.; Hageman, M.J.; Oliyai, R.; Maag, H. & Tilley, J.W. (2007) Prodrugs: Challenges and Rewards Part 1 and 2, *Springer Science + Business Media,* New York.

[41] Stella, V.J.; Charman, W.N. & Naringrekar, V.H. (1985) Prodrugs. Do they have advantages in clinical practice? *Drugs 29*, 455-473.

[42] Banerjee, P.K. & Amidon, G.L. (1985) Design of prodrugs based on enzymes-substrate specificity. In: Bundgaard, H., ed. Design of Prodrugs. New York: *Elsevier;* 93-133.

[43] Haffen, E.; Paintaud, G.; Berard, M.; Masuyer, C.; Bechtel, Y. & Bechtel, P.R. (2000). On the assessment of drug metabolism by assays of codeine and its main metabolites. *Therapeutic Drug Monitoring 22 (3)*, 258–65.

[44] Raffa, R.B. (1996). A novel approach to the pharmacology of analgesics. *The American Journal of Medicine 101 (1A)*, 40S–46S.

[45] Zhou, S. F.; Zhou, Z. W.; Yang, L. P. & Cai, J. P. (2009). Substrates, inducers, inhibitors and structure-activity relationships of human Cytochrome P450 2C9 and implications in drug development. *Current medicinal chemistry 16(27)*, 3480-3675.

[46] Huttunen, K.M.; Raunio, H. & Rautio, J. (2011) Prodrugs -- from serendipity to rational design. *Pharmacol Rev. 63*, 750-71

[47] Higuchi, T. & Stella, V. J. (1975). Pro-drugs as novel drug delivery systems.

[48] Di, L. & Kerns, E.H. (2007) Solubility issues in early discovery and HTS, in Solvent Systems and Their Selection in Pharmaceutics and Biopharmaceutics (Augustijins, P. & Brewster, M. eds) pp 111–136, *Springer Science + Business Media,* New York.

[49] Fleisher, D.; Bong, R. & Stewart, B.H. (1996) Improved oral drug delivery: solubility limitations overcome by the use of prodrugs. *Adv Drug Deliv Rev* 19, 115–130.

[50] Beaumont, K.; Webster, R.; Gardner, I. & Dack, K. (2003) Design of ester prodrugs to enhance oral absorption of poorly permeable compounds: challenges to the discovery scientist. *Curr. Drug Metab.* 4, 461–485.

[51] del Amo, E.M.; Urtti, A. & Yliperttula, M. (2008) Pharmacokinetic role of L-type amino acid transporters LAT1 and LAT2. *Eur J Pharm Sci* 35, 161–174.

[52] Khor, S.P. & Hsu, A. (2007) The pharmacokinetics and pharmacodynamics of levodopa in the treatment of Parkinson's disease. *Curr. Clin. Pharmacol.* 2, 234–243.

[53] Hornykiewicz, O. (2010) A brief history of levodopa. *J. Neurol.* 257 (Suppl 2), S249–S252.

[54] Svensson, L.A. & Tunek, A. (1988) The design and bioactivation of presystemically stable prodrugs. *Drug Metab. Rev.* 19, 165–194.

[55] Tunek, A.; Levin, E. & Svensson, L.A. (1988) Hydrolysis of ^{3}H-bambuterol, a carbamate prodrug of terbutaline, in blood from humans and laboratory animals in vitro. *Biochem. Pharmacol.* 37, 3867–3876.

[56] Sitar, D.S. (1996) Clinical pharmacokinetics of bambuterol. *Clin.Pharmacokinet.*31, 246–256.

[57] Persson, G.; Pahlm, O. & Gnosspelius, Y. (1995) Oral bambuterol versus terbutaline in patients with asthma. *Curr. Ther. Res.* 56, 457–465.

[58] Ettmayer, P.; Amidon, G.L.; Clement, B. & Testa, B. (2004) Lessons learned from marketed and investigational prodrugs. *J. Med. Chem.* 47, 2393–2404.

[59] Denny, W.A. (2010) Hypoxia-activated prodrugs in cancer therapy: progress to the clinic. *Future Oncol* 6, 419–428.

[60] Shanghag, A.; Yam, N. & Jasti, B. (2006) Prodrugs as drug delivery systems, in Design of Controlled Release Drug Delivery Systems (Li, X. & Jasti, B.R. eds) pp75–106, *The McGraw-Hill Company,* Inc., New York.

[61] Gonzalez, F.J. & Tukey, R.H. (2006) Drug metabolism, in Goodman and Gilman's The Pharmacological Basis of Therapeutics (Brunton, L.L.;, Lazo, J.S. & Parker, K.L. eds) pp 71–91, *The McGraw-Hill Companies,* Inc., New York.

[62] Testa, B. & Krämer, S.D. (2007) The biochemistry of drug metabolism–an introduction: Part 2. Redox reactions and their enzymes. *Chem. Biodivers.* 4, 257–405.

[63] Draganov, D.I. & La Du, B.N. (2004). Pharmacogenetics of paraoxonases: A brief review. *Naunyn Schmiedebergs Arch Pharmacol 369*, 78–88.

[64] Ngawhirunpat, T.; Kawakami, N.; Hatanaka, T.; Kawakami, J. & Adachi, I. (2003). Age dependency of esterase activity in rat and human keratinocytes. *Biol. Pharm. Bull. 26*, 1311–1314.

[65] Moser, V.C.; Chanda, S.M.; Mortensen, S.R. & Padilla, S. (1998). Age- and gender-related differences in sensitivity to chlorpyrifos in the rat reflect developmental profiles of esterase activities. *Toxicol. Sci. 46*, 211–222.

[66] Stella, V.J. (1975) Pro-drugs: an overview and definition. In: Higuchi, T. & Stella, V., editors. Prodrugs as Novel Drug Delivery Systems. ACS Symposium Series. Washington, DC: *American Chemical Society;* p. 1–115.

[67] Amidon, G.L.; Leesman, G.D. & Elliott, R.L. (1980) Improving intestinal absorption of water-insoluble compounds: a membrane metabolism strategy. *J. Pharm. Sci. 69*, 1363–1368.

[68] Fleisher, D.; Stewart, B.H. & Amidon, G.L. (1985) Design of prodrugs for improved gastrointestinal absorption by intestinal enzyme targeting. *Methods Enzymol. 112*, 360–381.

[69] Bai, J.P. & Amidon, G.L. (1992) Structural specificity of mucosal-cell transport and metabolism of peptide drugs: implication for oral peptide drug delivery. *Pharm. Res. 9*, 969–978.

[70] Stella, V.J. & Himmelstein, K.J. (1980) Prodrugs and site-specific drug delivery. *J. Med. Chem. 23*, 1275–1282.

[71] Stella, V.J. & Himmelstein, K.J. (1982) Critique of prodrugs and site specific delivery. In: Bundgaard, H., editor. Optimization of Drug Delivery. *Alfred Benzon Symposium Copenhagen: Munksgaard;* p. 134–155.

[72] Friend, D.R. & Chang, G.W. (1984) A colon-specific drug-delivery system based on drug glycosides and the glycosidases of colonic bacteria. *J. Med. Chem. 27*, 261–266.

[73] Philpott, G.W.; Shearer, W.T.; Bower, R.J. & Parker, C.W. (1973) Selective cytotoxicity of hapten-substituted cells with an antibody-enzyme conjugate. *J. Immunol. 111*, 921–929.

[74] Deonarain, M.P.; Spooner, R.A. & Epenetos, A.A. (1996) Genetic delivery of enzymes for cancer therapy. *Gene Ther. 2*, 235–244.

[75] Singhal, S. & Kaiser, L.R. (1998) Cancer chemotherapy using suicide genes. *Surg. Oncol. Clin. North Am. 7*, 505–536.

[76] Aghi, M.; Hochberg, F. & Breakefield, X.O. (2000) Prodrug activation enzymes in cancer gene therapy. *J. Gene Med. 2*, 148–164.

[77] Greco, O. & Dachs, G.U. (2001) Gene directed enzyme/ prodrug therapy of cancer: historical appraisal and future prospectives. *J. Cell. Physiol. 187*, 22–36.

[78] Roche, E.B. Design of Biopharmaceutical Properties through Prodrugs and Analogs. Washington, DC: American Pharmaceutical Association; 1977.

[79] Li, F.; Maag, H. & Alfredson, T. (2008) Prodrugs of nucleoside analogues for improved oral absorption and tissue targeting. *J. Pharm. Sci. 97*, 1109–1134.

[80] Tammara, V.K.; Narurkar, M.M.; Crider, A.M. & Khan, M.A. (1994) Morpholinoalkyl ester prodrugs of diclofenac: synthesis, in vitro and in vivo evaluation. *J. Pharm. Sci. 83*, 644–648.

[81] del Amo, E.M.; Urtti, A. & Yliperttula, M. (2008) Pharmacokinetic role of L-type amino acid transporters LAT1 and LAT2. *Eur. J. Pharm. Sci. 35*, 161–174.

[82] Kim, I.; Song, X.; Vig, B.S.; Mittal, S.; Shin, H.C.; Lorenzi, P.J. & Amidon, G.L. (2004) A novel nucleoside prodrug activating enzyme: substrate specificity of biphenyl hydrolase-like protein. *Mol. Pharm. 1*, 117–127.

[83] Hu, L. (2004) Prodrugs: effective solutions for solubility, permeability and targeting challenges. *Drugs 7*, 736– 742.

[84] Kim, I.; Chu, X.Y.; Kim, S.; Provoda, C.J.; Lee, K.D. & Amidon, G.L. (2003) Identification of a human valacyclovirase: biphenyl hydrolase-like protein as valacyclovir hydrolase. *J. Biol. Chem. 278*, 25348–25356.

[85] Bronson, J.J.; HO, H.T.; Boeck, H.D.; Woods, K.; Ghazzouli, I.; Martin, J.C. & Hitchcock, M.J. (1990) Biochemical pharmacology of acyclic nucleotide analogues. *Ann. N. Y. Acad. Sci. 616*, 398–407.

[86] Cundy, K.C.; Barditch-Crovo, P.; Walker, R.E.; Collier, A.C.; Ebeling, D.; Toole, J. & Jaffe, H.S. (1995) Clinical pharmacokinetics of adefovir in human immunodeficiency virus type 1-infected patients. *Antimicrob. Agents Chemother. 39*, 2401–2405.

[87] Cioli, V.; Putzolu, S.; Rossi, V. & Corradino, C. (1980) A toxicological and pharmacological study of ibuprofen guaiacol ester (AF 2259) in the rat. *Toxicol. Appl. Pharmacol. 54*, 332–339.

[88] Croft, D.N.; Cuddigan, J.H. & Sweetland, C. (1972) Gastric bleeding and benorylate, a new aspirin. *Br. Med. J. 3*, 545–547.

[89] Bhosle, D.; Bharambe, S.; Gairola, N. & Dhaneshwar, S.S. (2006) Mutual prodrug concept: fundamentals and applications. *Indian J. Pharm. Sci. 68*, 286–294.

[90] Muscara, M.N.; McKnight, W.; Soldato, P.D. & Wallace, J.L. (1998) Effect of a nitric oxide-releasing naproxen derivative on hypertension and gastric damage induced by chronic nitric oxide inhibition in the rat. *Life Sci. 62*, PL235–PL240.

[91] Burgaud, J.L.; Riffaud, J.P. & Del Soldato, P. (2002) Nitric-oxide releasing molecules: a new class of drugs with several major indications. *Curr. Pharm. Des.8*, 201–213.

[92] Shanbhag, V.R.; Crider, A.M.; Gokhale, R.; Harpalani, A. & Dick, R.M. (1992) Ester and amide prodrugs of ibuprofen and naproxen: synthesis, anti-inflammatory activity, and gastrointestinal toxicity. *J. Pharm. Sci. 81*, 149–154.

[93] English, A.R.; Girard, D. & Haskell, S.L. (1984) Pharmacokinetics of sultamicillin in mice, rats, and dogs. *Antimicrob. Agents Chemother.25*, 599–602.

[94] Jordan, A.M.; Khan, T.H.; Malkin, H. & Osborn, H.M.I. (2002) Synthesis and analysis of urea and carbamate prodrugs as candidates for melanocyte-directed enzyme prodrug therapy (MDEPT). *Bioorg. Med. Chem. 10*, 2625–2633.

[95] Yumibe, N.; Hule, K.; Chen, K.-J.; Snow, M.; Clement, R.P. & Cayen, M.N. (1996) Identification of human liver cytochrome P450 enzymes that metabolize the nonsedating antihistamine loratadine. Formation of descarboethoxyloratadine by CYP3A4 and CYP2D6. *Biochem. Pharmacol. 51*, 165–172.

[96] Shimma, N.; Umeda, I.; Arasaki, M.; Murasaki, C.; Masubuchi, K.; Kohchi, Y.; Miwa, M.; Ura, M.; Sawada, N.; Tahara, H.; Kuruma, I.; Horii, I. & Ishitsuka, H. (2000) Thedesign and synthesis of a new tumor-selective fluoropyrimidine carbamate, capecitabine. *Bioorg. Med. Chem. 8*, 1697–1706.

[97] Ajani, J. (2006) Review of capecitabine as oral treatment of gastric, gastroesophageal, and esophagealcancers. *Cancer 107*, 221–231.

[98] Alexander, J.; Carqill, R.; Michelson, S.R. & Schwam, H. (1988) (Acyloxy) alkyl carbamates as novel bioreversible prodrugs for amines: increased permeation through biological membranes. *J. Med. Chem. 31*, 318–322.

[99] Venhuis, B.J.; Dijkstra, D.; Wustrow, D.; Meltzer, L.T.; Wise, L.D.; Johnson, S.J. & Wikstrom, H.V. (2003) Orally active oxime derivatives of the dopaminergic prodrug6-(N,N-di-n-propylamino)-3,4,5,6,7,8-hexahydro-2Hnaphthalen-1-one. Synthesis and pharmacological activity. *J. Med. Chem. 46*, 4136–4140.

[100] Bundgaard, H. (Editor) (1985). *Design of prodrugs.* Elsevier Publishing Company.

[101] Safadi, M.; Oliyai, R. & Stella, V.J. (1993) Phosphoryloxymethylcarbamates and carbonates–novel water-soluble prodrugs for amines and hindered alcohols. *Pharm. Res. 10*, 1350–1355.

[102] Hecker, S.J.; Calkins, T.; Price, M.E.; Huie, K.; Chen, S.; Glinka, T.W. & Dudley, M.N. (2003) Prodrugs of cephalosporin RWJ-333441 (MC-04,546) with improved aqueous solubility. *Antimicrob. Agents Chemother. 47*, 2043–2046.

[103] Venhuis, B.J.; Dijkstra, D.; Wustrow, D.; Meltzer, L.T.; Wise, L.D.; Johnson, S.J. & Wikstrom, H.V. (2003) Orally active oxime derivatives of the dopaminergic prodrug 6-(N,N-di-n-propylamino)-3,4,5,6,7,8-hexahydro-2Hnaphthalen- 1-one. Synthesis and pharmacological activity. *J. Med. Chem. 46*, 4136–4140.

[104] Madsen, U.; Krogsgaard-Larsen, P. & Liljefors, T. (2002) Textbook of Drug Design and Discovery. Washington, DC: Taylor & Francis; p. 410–458.

[105] Testa, B. & Mayer, J.M. (2003) Hydrolysis in Drug and Prodrug metabolism, Chemistry, biochemistry and enzymology 690–695.

[106] Bundgaard, H. & Johansen, M. (1980) Prodrugs as drug delivery systems IV: N-Mannich bases as potential novel prodrugs for amides, ureides, amines, and other NH-acidic compounds. *J. Pharm. Sci. 69*, 44–46.

[107] Caldwell, H.C.; Adams, H.J.; Jones, R.G.; Mann, W.A.; Dittert, L.W.; Chong, C.W. & Swintosky, J.V. (1971) Enamine prodrugs. *J. Pharm. Sci. 60*, 1810–1812.

[108] Murakami, T.; Tamauchi, H.; Yamazaki, M.; Kubo, K.; Kamada, A. & Yata, N. (1981) Biopharmaceutical study on the oral and rectal administrations of enamine prodrugs of amino acid-like beta-lactam antibiotics in rabbits. *Chem. Pharm. Bull. 29*, 1986–1997.

[109] Naringrekar, V.H. & Stella, V.J. (1990) Mechanism of hydrolysis and structure-stability relationship of enaminones as potential prodrugs of model primary amines. *J. Pharm. Sci. 79*, 138–146.

[110] Chapman, T.M.; Plosker, G.L. & Perry, C.M. (2004) Fosamprenavir: a review of its use in the management of antiretroviral therapy-naive patients with HIV infection. *Drugs64*, 2101–2124.

[111] Boucher, B.A. (1996) Fosphenytoin: a novel phenytoin prodrug. *Pharmacotherapy16*, 777–791.

[112] Azadkhan, A.K.; Truelove, S.C. & Aronson, J.K. (1982) The disposition and metabolism of sulphasalazine (salicylazosulphapyridine) in man. *Br. J. Clin. Pharmacol. 13*, 523–528.

[113] Sandborn, W.J. (2002) Rational selection of oral 5-aminosalicylate formulations and prodrugs for the treatment of ulcerative colitis. *Am. J. Gastroenterol. 97*, 2939–2941.

[114] Jung, Y.; Lee, J. & Kim, Y. (2001) Colon-specific prodrug of 5-aminosalicylic acid: synthesis and in vitro/in vivo properties of acidic amino acid derivatives of 5-aminosalicylic acid. *J. Pharm. Sci. 90*, 1767–1775.

[115] Simplicio, A.L.; Clancy, J.M. & Gilmer, J.F. (2008) Prodrugs for amines. *Molecules 13*, 519–547.

[116] Greenwald, R.B.; Pendri, A.; Conover, C.D.; Zhao, H.; Choe, Y.H.; Martinez, A.; Shum, K. & Guan, S. (1999) Drug delivery systems employing 1,4- or 1,6-elimination: poly(ethylene glycol) prodrugs of amine-containing compounds. *J. Med. Chem. 42*, 3657–3667.

[117] Greenwald, R.B.; Choe, Y.H.; McGuire, J. & Conover, C.D. (2003) Effective drug delivery by PEGylated drug conjugates. *Adv. Drug Deliv. Rev. 55*, 217–250.

[118] Hanson, K.R. & Havir, E.A. (1972) The enzymic elimination of ammonia. In: Boyer, P.D., editor. The Enzymes, 3rd edn. vol. 7. New York: *Academic Press;* p 75– 166.

[119] Czarnik, A.W. (1988) Intramolecularity: proximity and strain. In: Liebman, J.F. & Greenberg, A., editors. Mechanistic Principles of Enzyme Activity. New York, NY: *VCH Publishers;* p. 75–117.

[120] Sweigers, G.F. (2008) Mechanical Catalysis. Hoboken, NJ: *John Wiley & Sons.*

[121] Fersht, A. (1979) Structure and Mechanism in Protein Science: A guide to Enzyme Catalysis and Protein Folding. New York: *Freeman,* W. H. and Company.

[122] Nelson, D.L. & Cox, M.M. (2003) Lehninger Principles of Biochemistry. New York: *Worth Publishers.*

[123] Dafforn, A. & Koshland, D.E. Jr (1973) Proximity, entropy and orbital steering. *Biochem. Biophys. Res. Commun. 52*, 779–785.

[124] Lightstone, F. C. & Bruice, T.C. (1997). Separation of ground state and transition state effects in intramolecular and enzymatic reactions. 2. A theoretical study of the formation of transition states in cyclic anhydride formation. *J. Am. Chem. Soc. 119*, 9103-9113.

[125] Bruice, T. C. & Pandit, U. K. (1960) The effect of geminal substitution ring size and rotamer distribution on the intra molecular nucleophilic catalysis of the hydrolysis of monophenyl esters of dibasic acids and the solvolysis of the intermediate anhydrides. *J. Am. Chem. Soc. 82*, 5858–5865.

[126] Bruice, T. C. & Pandit, U. K. (1960) Intramolecular models depicting the kinetic importance of ''Fit'' in enzymatic catalysis. *Proc. Natl. Acad. Sci. USA 46*, 402–404.

[127] Milstein, S. & Cohen, L.A. (1970) Concurrent general-acid and general-base catalysis of esterification. *J. Am. Chem. Soc. 92*, 4377-4382.

[128] Milstein, S. & Cohen, L. A. (1970) Rate acceleration by stereopopulation control: models for enzyme action. *Proc. Natl. Acad. Sci. USA 67*, 1143-1147.

[129] Milstein, S. & Cohen, L. A. (1972) Stereopopulation control I. Rate enhancement in the lactonizations of o-hydroxyhydrocinnamic acids. *J. Am. Chem. Soc. 94*, 9158-9165.

[130] Menger, F. M. & Ladika M. (1988) Fast hydrolysis of an aliphatic amide at neutral pH and ambient temperature. A peptidase model. *J. Am. Chem. Soc. 110*, 6794-6796.

[131] Menger, F. M. (1985) On the source of intramolecular and enzymatic reactivity. *Acc. Chem. Res. 18*, 128-134.

[132] Menger, F. M.; Chow, J. F.; Kaiserman H. & Vasquez P. C. (1983) Directionality of proton transfer in solution. Three systems of known angularity. *J. Am. Chem. Soc. 105*: 4996-5002.

[133] Menger, F. M.; Galloway, A. L. & Musaev D. G. (2003) Relationship between rate and distance. *Chem. Commun.* 2370-2371.

[134] Menger, F. M. (2005).An alternative view of enzyme catalysis. *Pure Appl. Chem. 77*, 1873–187.

[135] Kirby, A. J. & Hollfelder, F. *From Enzyme Models to Model Enzymes, RSC Publishing*, Cambridge UK, 1-273, 2009.

[136] Barber, S. E.; Dean, K. E. S. & Kirby, A. J. (1999) A mechanism for efficient proton-transfer catalysis. Intramolecular general acid catalysis of the hydrolysis of 1-arylethyl ethers of salicylic acid. *Can. J. Chem.77*, 792-801.

[137] Kirby, A. J. & Lancaster, P. W. (1972) structure and efficiency in intramolecular and enzymatic catalysis. Catalysis of amide hydrolysis by the carboxy-group of substituted maleamic acids. . *J. Chem. Soc., Perkin Trans. 2*, 1206-1214.

[138] Kirby, A. J.; de Silva, M. F.; Lima, D.; Roussev, C. D. & Nome, F. (2006) Efficient intramolecular general acid catalysis of nucleophilic attack on a phosphodiester. *J. Am. Chem. Soc.128*, 16944-16952.

[139] Kirby, A. J. & Williams, N. H. (1994) Efficient intramolecular general acid catalysis of enol ether hydrolysis. Hydrogen-bonding stabilization of the transition state for proton transfer to carbon. *J. Chem. Soc., Perkin Trans. 2*, 643-648.

[140] Kirby, A. J. & Williams, N. H. (1991) Efficient intramolecular general acid catalysis of vinyl ether hydrolysis by the neighbouring carboxylic acid group. *J. Chem. Soc. Chem. Commun* 1643-1644.

[141] Kirby, A. J. (1996) Enzyme Mechanisms, Models, and Mimics. *Angewandte Chemie International Edition in English 35*, 706-724.

[142] Fife, T. H. & Przystas, T. J. (1979) Intramolecular general acid catalysis in the hydrolysis of acetals with aliphatic alcohol leaving groups. *J. Am. Chem. Soc.101*, 1202-1210.

[143] Kirby, A. J. (1997) Efficiency of proton transfer catalysis in models and enzymes. *Acc. Chem. Res.30*:290-296.

[144] Reddy, M. R. & Erion, M. D. Free Energy Calculations in Rational Drug Design, *Kluwer Academic/Plenum Publishers,* 379, 2001.

[145] Parr, R. G.; Craig, D. P. & Ross, I. G. (1950) Molecular Orbital Calculations of the Lower Excited Electronic Levels of Benzene, Configuration Interaction included. *Journal of Chemical Physics 18* (12), 1561–1563.

[146] Parr, R. G. (1990) On the genesis of a theory. *Int. J. Quantum Chem 37* (4), 327–347.

[147] Dewar, M. J. S. & Thiel, W. (1977) Ground states of molecules. The MNDO method. Approximations and parameters. *J. Am. Chem. Soc. 99*, 4899-4907.

[148] Bingham, R. C.; Dewar, M. J. S. & Lo, D. H. (1975) Ground states of molecules. XXV. MINDO/3. An improved version of the MNDO semiempirical SCF-MO method. *J. Am. Chem. Soc. 97*, 1285-1293.

[149] Dewar, M. J. S.; Zoebisch, E. G.; Healy, E. F. & Stewart, J. J. P. (1985) AM1: A new general purpose quantum mechanical molecular model. *J. Am. Chem. Soc. 107*, 3902-907.

[150] Dewar, M. J. S.; Jie, C. & Yu, J. (1993) The first of new series of general purpose quantum mechanical molecular models. *Tetrahedron 49*, 5003-5038.

[151] Parr, R. G. & Yang, W. Density Functional Theory of Atoms and Molecules. *Oxford University Press,* Oxford, 1989.

[152] Mourik, T. van & Robert, J.G. (2002). A critical note on density functional theory studies on rare-gas dimers. *Journal of Chemical Physics 116* (22), 9620–9623.

[153] Grimme, S. (2004).Accurate description of van der Waals complexes by density functional theory including empirical corrections. *Journal of Computational Chemistry* 25 (12), 1463–1473. doi:10.1002/jcc.20078. PMID 15224390.

[154] Burker, U. & Allinger, N. L. Molecular Mechanics, American Chemical Society, Washington, DC, USA, 1982.

[155] Warshel, A. & Levitt, M. (1976) Theoretical studies of enzymatic reactions: dielectric, electrostatic and steric stabilization of the carbonium ion in the reaction of lysozyme. *Journal of Molecular Biology 103*(2), 227–249]

[156] Field, M. J. (2002) Simulating enzyme reactions: challenges and perspectives. *Journal of Computational Chemistry 23*(1), 48–58.

[157] Mulholland, A. J. (2005) Modeling enzyme reaction mechanisms, specificity and catalysis. *Drug Discovery Today 10*(20), 1393–1402.

[158] Karaman, R. (2008) Analysis of Menger's spatiotemporal hypothesis. *Tetrahedron Lett 49*, 5998-6002.

[159] Karaman, R. (2009) Cleavage of Menger's aliphatic amide: a model for peptidase enzyme solely explained by proximity orientation in intramolecular proton transfer. *J Mol Struct (THEOCHEM) 910*, 27-33].

[160] Karaman, R. (2010) The efficiency of proton transfer in Kirby's enzyme model, a computational approach. *Tetrahedron Lett 51*, 2130-2135.

[161] Karaman, R. & Pascal, R. A. (2010) Computational Analysis of Intramolecularity in Proton Transfer Reactions. *Org & Bimol Chem 8*, 5174-5178.

[162] Karaman, R. (2010) A General Equation Correlating Intramolecular Rates with Attack' Parameters: Distance and Angle. *Tetrahedron Lett 51*, 5185-5190.

[163] Karaman, R. (2011) Analyzing the efficiency of proton transfer to carbon in Kirby's enzyme model- a computational approach. *Tetrahedron Lett 52*, 699-704.

[164] Karaman, R. (2011) Analyzing the efficiency in intramolecular amide hydrolysis of Kirby's N-alkylmaleamic acids - A computational approach. *Comput Theor Chem 974*, 133-142.

[165] Karaman, R. (2009) A New Mathematical Equation Relating Activation Energy to Bond Angle and Distance: A Key for Understanding the Role of Acceleration in Lactonization of the Trimethyl Lock System. *Bioorganic Chemistry 37*, 11-25.

[166] Karaman, R. (2009) Revaluation of Bruice's Proximity Orientation. *Tetrahedron Lett. 50*, 452-458.

[167] Karaman, R. (2009) Accelerations in the Lactonization of Trimethyl Lock Systems are Due to Proximity Orientation and not to Strain Effects. *Research Letters in Org. Chem.* doi: 10.1155/2009/240253.

[168] Karaman, R. (2009) the *gem*-disubstituent effect- a computational study that exposes the relevance of existing theoretical models. *Tetrahedron Lett. 50*, 6083-6087.

[169] Karaman, R. (2009) Analyzing Kirby's amine olefin – a model for amino-acid ammonia lyases. *Tetrahedron Lett. 50*, 7304-7309.

[170] Karaman, R. (2009) The Effective Molarity (EM) Puzzle in Proton Transfer Reactions. *Bioorganic Chemistry 37*,106-110.

[171] Karaman, R. (2010) Effects of substitution on the effective molarity (EM) for five membered ring-closure reactions- a computational approach. *Journal of Molecular Structure (THEOCHEM) 939*, 69-74.

[172] Karaman, R. (2010) The Effective Molarity (EM) Puzzle in Intramolecular Ring-Closing Reactions. *Journal of Molecular Structure (THEOCHEM) 940*, 70-75.

[173] Menger, F. M. & Karaman, R. (2010) A Singularity Model for ChemicalReactivity. *Eur. J. Chem. 16*, 1420-1427.

[174] Karaman, R. (2010) The Effective Molarity (EM) – a Computational Approach. *Bioorganic Chemistry 38*,165-172.

[175] Karaman, R. (2010) Proximity vs. Strain in Ring-Closing Reactions of Bifunctional Chain Molecules- a Computational Approach. *J. Mol. Phys. 108*, 1723-1730.

[176] Karaman, R. (2011) The role of proximity orientation in intramolecular proton transfer reactions. *Journal of Computational and Theoretical Chemistry 966*, 311-321.

[177] Karaman, R. (2010) Prodrugs of Aza Nucleosides Based on Proton Transfer Reactions. *J. Comput. Mol. Des. 24*, 961-970.

[178] Karaman, R. & Hallak, H. (2010) Computer-assisted design of pro-drugs for antimalarial atovaquone. *Chemical biology & drug design 76* (4), 350-60.

[179] Karaman, R. (2013) Antimalarial Atovaquone Prodrugs Based on Enzyme Models - Molecular Orbital Calculations Approach.in Antimalarial Drug Research and Development, Banet, A C. & Brasier, P. eds.; *Nova Cooperation Publisher,* NY, USA pp 1-67.

[180] Hejaz, H.; Karaman, R. & Khamis, M. (2012) Computer- Assisted Design for paracetamol Masking Bitter Taste Prodrugs. *J. Mol. Model. 18*, 103–114.

[181] Karaman, R.; Amly, W.; Scrano, L.; Mecca, G. & Bufo, S. A. (2013). Computationally designed prodrugs of statins based on Kirby's enzyme model. *J. Mol. Model.* DOI 10.1007/s00894-013-1929-2.

[182] [182] Karaman, R.; Karaman D. & Ziadeh I. (2013) Computationally Designed Phenylephrine Prodrugs- A Model for Enhancing Bioavailability *J. Molecular Physics* 2013,DOI:10.1080/00268976.2013.779395.

[183] Karaman, R. (2013) Prodrugs for Masking Bitter Taste of Antibacterial Drugs- A Computational Approach. *J. Molecular Modeling* 19, 2399–2412.

[184] Karaman, R.; Ghareeb, H.; Dajani, K.K.; Scrano, L.; Hallak, H.; Abu-Lafi, S. & Bufo, S. A. (2013) Design, synthesis and in-vitro kinetic study of tranexamic acid prodrugs for the treatment of bleeding conditions. *J. Molecular Aided Computer Design* 27(7), 615-635.

[185] Karaman, R.; Dajani, K.K.; Qtait, A. & Khamis, M. (2012) Prodrugs of Acyclovir - A Computational Approach. *Chem Biol Drug Des 79*, 819-834.

[186] Karaman, R.; Dajani, K. K. & Hallak, H. (2012) Computer-assisted design for atenolol prodrugs for the use in aqueous formulations. *J Mol Model 18*, 1523-1540.

[187] Karaman, R., Qtait, A., Dajani, K.K. & Abu-Lafi, S. "Design and Synthesis of an Aqueous Stable Atenolol Prodrug"The Scientific World Journal2013, Volume 2014 (2014), Article ID 248651, 13 pages.http://dx.doi.org /10.1155/2014 /248651.

[188] Karaman, R. (2011) Computational aided design for dopamine prodrugs based on novel chemical approach. *Chem. Biol. Drug Design 78*, 853-863.

[189] Gaussian 09, Revision **A.1**, Frisch, M. J.; Trucks, G. W.; Schlegel, H. B.; Scuseria, G. E.; Robb, M. A.; Cheeseman, J. R.; Scalmani, G.; Barone, V.; Mennucci, B.; Petersson, G. A.; Nakatsuji, H.; Caricato, M.; Li, X.; Hratchian, H. P.; Izmaylov, A. F.; Bloino, J.; Zheng, G.; Sonnenberg, J. L.; Hada, M.; Ehara, M.; Toyota, K.; Fukuda, R.; Hasegawa, J.; Ishida, M.; Nakajima, T.; Honda, Y.; Kitao, O.; Nakai, H.; Vreven, T.; Montgomery,

Jr., J. A.; Peralta, J. E.; Ogliaro, F.; Bearpark, M.; Heyd, J. J.; Brothers, E.; Kudin, K. N.; Staroverov, V. N.; Kobayashi, R.; Normand, J.; Raghavachari, K.; Rendell, A.; Burant, J. C.; Iyengar, S. S.; Tomasi, J.; Cossi, M.; Rega, N.; Millam, J. M.; Klene, M.; Knox, J. E.; Cross, J. B.; Bakken, V.; Adamo, C.; Jaramillo, J.; Gomperts, R.; Stratmann, R. E.; Yazyev, O.; Austin, A. J.; Cammi, R.; Pomelli, C.; Ochterski, J. W.; Martin, R. L.; Morokuma, K.; Zakrzewski, V. G.; Voth, G. A.; Salvador, P.; Dannenberg, J. J.; Dapprich, S.; Daniels, A. D.; Farkas, Ö.; Foresman, J. B.; Ortiz, J. V.; Cioslowski, J.; Fox, D. J. Gaussian, Inc., *Wallingford CT*, 2009.

[190] Casewit, C. J.; Colwell, K. S. & Rappe', A. K. (1992) Application of a universal force field to main group compounds. *J. Am. Chem. Soc. 114*, 10046-53.

[191] Murrell, J. N. & Laidler, K. J. (1968) Symmetries of activated complexes. *Trans Faraday Soc. 64*, 371-377.

[192] Muller, K. (1980) Reaction paths on multidimensional energy hypersurfaces. *.Angew. Chem. Int. Ed. Engl. 19*, 1-13.

[193] Cancès, M. T.; Mennucci, B. & Tomasi, J. (1997) A new integral equation formalism for the polarizable continuum model: theoretical background and applications to isotropic and anisotropic dielectrics. *J. Chem. Phys. 107*, 3032-3041.

[194] Mennucci, B. & Tomasi, J. (1997) Coninuum solvation models: A new approach to the problem of solute's charge distribution and cavity boundaries. *J. Chem. Phys. 106*, 5151.

[195] Mennucci, B.; Cancès, M. T. & Tomasi, J. (1997) Evaluation of solvent effects in isotropic and anisotropic dielectrics and in ionic solutions with a unified integral equation method: Theoretical bases, computational implementation, and numerical applications. *J. Phys. Chem. B 101*, 10506-10517.

[196] Tomasi, J.; Mennucci B. & Cancès, M. T. (1997) The IEF version of the PCM solvation method: an overview of a new method addressed to study molecular solutes at the QM ab initio level. *J. Mol. Struct. (Theochem) 464*, 211-226.

[197] Myelodysplastic Syndrome. The Leukemia & Lymphoma Society. *White Plains,* NY. 2001.

[198] Wijermans, P.; Lübbert, M.; Verhoef, G., et al. (2000) Low-dose 5-aza-2'-deoxycytidine, a DNA hypomethylating agent, for the treatment of high-risk myelodysplastic syndrome: a multicenter phase II study in elderly patients. *J. Clin. Oncol. 18*, 956–962.

[199] Silverman, L. R.; Demakos, E. P.; Peterson, B. L., et al. (2002) Randomized controlled trial of azacitidine in patients with the myelodysplastic syndrome: a study of the cancer and leukemia group B. *J. Clin. Oncol. 20*, 2429–2440.

[200] Silverman, L. R; McKenzie, D. R.; Peterson, B. L., et al., (2006) Further analysis of trials with azacitidine in patients with myelodysplastic syndrome: studies 8421, 8921, and 9221 by the Cancer and Leukemia Group B. *J. Clin. Oncol. 24*, 3895–3903.

[201] Kantarjian, H.; Issa, J. P.; Rosenfeld, C. S., et al. (2006) Decitabine improves patient outcomes in myelodysplastic syndromes: results of a phase III randomized study. *Cancer 106*, 1794–1803.

[202] Blum, W.; Klisovic, R. B.; Hackanson. B. et al. (2007) Phase I study of decitabine alone or in combination with valproic acid in acute myeloid leukemia. *J. Clin. Oncol. 25*, 3884–3891.

[203] Perrin, D. D.; Dempsey, B.; Serjeant, E. P. pKa prediction for organic acids and bases, Champan & Hall London, 1981.

[204] Stancu, C. & Sima, A. (2001) Statins: mechanism of action and effects, *Journal of Cellular and Molecular Medicine 5*(4), 378–387.

[205] Schachter, M. (2005) Chemical, pharmacokinetic and pharmacodynamic properties of statins: an update. *Fundam. Clin. Pharmacol. 19*(1), 117-25.

[206] Luo. Y.;Xu, L.; Tao, X.;Xu, M.;Feng, J. & Tang, X. (2012) Characterization, stability and in vitro-in vivo evaluation of pellet-layered Simvastatin nanosuspensions, Drug Development and Industrial Pharmacy; Early Online: 1–11, informa healthcare.

[207] Khan, F.N. & Dehghan, M.H.G. (2011) Enhanced Bioavailability of Atorvastatin Calcium from Stabilized Gastric Resident Formulation. *AAPS Pharm. Sci. Tech. 12*(4), 1077-1086.

[208] Pandya, P.; Gattani, S.; Jain, P.; Khirwal, L. & Surana, S. (2008) Co-solvent Evaporation Method for Enhancement of Solubility and Dissolution Rate of Poorly Aqueous Soluble Drug Simvastatin: In vitro–In vivo Evaluation. *AAPS Pharm. Sci. Tech. 9(4)*, 1247-1257.

[209] Lai, J., Chen, J., Lu, Y., Sun, J., Hu, F., Yin, Z., & Wu, W. (2009).Glycerylmonooleate /poloxamer 407 cubic nanoparticles as oral drug delivery systems: I. In vitro evaluation and enhanced oral bioavailability of the poorly water-soluble drug simvastatin. *AAPS Pharm Sci Tech, 10*(3), 960-966.

[210] http://www.theodora.com/drugs/

[211] Palem, C.R.; Patel, S. & Pokharkar, V.B. (2009) Solubility and stability enhancement of atorvastatin by cyclodextrin complexation. *PDA J. Pharm. Sci. Technol. 63*(3), 217-25.

[212] Patel, Z.B.; Patel, K.S.; Shah, A.S. & Surti, N.I. (2012) Preparation and optimization of microemulsion of Rosuvastatin calcium, *Journal of Pharmacy & Bioallied Sci. 2012 March; 4*(Suppl 1): S118–S119.

[213] Karaman, R. (2011) Analyzing Kemp's amide cleavage: A model for amidase enzymes. *Computational and Theoretical Chemistry 963*(2), 427-434.

[214] Wilcox, P. E. (1970) Chymotrypsinogens—chymotrypsins. *Methods in enzymology, 19*, 64-108.

[215] Appel, W. (1986) Chymotrypsin: molecular and catalytic properties. *Clinical biochemistry, 19*(6), 317-322.

[216] Smith, R. M. & Hansen, D. E. (1998) The pH-rate profile for the hydrolysis of a peptide bond. *J. Am. Chem. Soc. 120*(35), 8910-8913.

[217] Radzicka, A. & Wolfenden, R. (1996) Rates of uncatalyzed peptide bond hydrolysis in neutral solution and the transition state affinities of proteases. *J. Am. Chem. Soc., 118*(26), 6105-6109.

[218] Bender, M. L. (1971) Mechanisms of homogeneous catalysis from protons to proteins. New York: *Wiley-Interscience, 397-455.*

[219] Gerschler, J. J.; Wier, K. A. & Hansen, D. E. (2007) Amide bond cleavage: acceleration due to a 1, 3-diaxial interaction with a carboxylic acid. *J. Org. Chem., 72*(2), 654-657.

[220] Curran, T. P.; Borysenko, C. W.; Abelleira, S. M. & Messier, R. J. (1994) Intramolecular acylolysis of amide derivatives of Kemp's triacid: strain effects and reaction rates. *J. Org. Chem., 59*(13), 3522-3529.

[221] De Stefano, A.; Sozio, P. & Cerasa, L.S. (2008) Antiparkinson prodrugs. *Molecules 13*, 46–68.

[222] Benes, F.M. (2001) Carlsson and the discovery of dopamine. *Trends Pharmacol Sci22*, 46–47.

[223] Houk, K. N.; Tucker, J. A. & Dorigo, A. E. (1990)Quantitative modeling of proximity effects on organic reactivity. *Acc. Chem. Res. 23*,107-113.

[224] Dorigo, A. E. & Houk, K. N. (1987)The origin of proximity effects on reactivity: a modified MM2 model for the rates of acid-catalyzed lactonizations of hydroxy acids. *J. Am. Chem. Soc., 109*(12), 3698-3708.

[225] Reilly, W.J. (2002) Pharmaceutical Necessities in Remington: The Science and Practice of Pharmacy. Balti- more, MD: *Mack Publishing Company;* p. 1018–1020.

[226] Drewnowski, A. & Gomez-Carneros, C. (2000) Bittertaste, phytonutrients, and the consumer: a review. *Am. J. Clin.Nutr.72*, 1424–1435.

[227] Hofmann, T. (2009) Identification of the key bitter compounds in our daily diet is a prerequisite for the understanding of the hTAS2R gene polymorphisms affecting food choice. *Ann. N. Y. Acad. Sci. 1170*, 116–125.

[228] Rodgers, S.; Busch, J.; Peters, H. & Christ-Hazelhof, E. (2005) Building a tree of knowledge: analysis of bitter molecules. *Chem. Senses30*, 547–557.

[229] Rodgers, S.; Glen, R.C. & Bender, A. (2006) Characterizing bitterness: identification of key structural features and development of a classification model. *J. Chem. Inf. Model. 46*, 569–576.

[230] Maehashi, K. & Huang, L. (2009) Bitter peptides and bitter taste receptors. *Cell. Mol. Life Sci. 66*, 1661–1671.

[231] Behrens, M. & Meyerhof, W. (2006) Bitter taste receptors and human bitter taste perception. *Cell Mol. LifeSci. 63*, 1501–1509.

[232] Meyerhof, W.; Born, S.; Brockhoff, A. & Behrens, M. (2011) Molecular biology of mammalian bitter taste receptors. A review. *Flavour Frag, J. 26*, 260–268.

[233] Behrens, M. & Meyerhof, W. (2009) Mammalian bittertaste perception. *Results Probl. Cell Differ. 47*, 203–220.

[234] Ayenew, Z.; Puri, V.; Kumar, L. & Bansal, A.K. (2009) Trends in pharmaceutical taste masking technologies: a patent review. *Recent Pat. Drug Deliv.Formul.3*, 26–39.

[235] Fawzy, A.A. (1998) Pleasant Tasting Aqueous Liquid Composition of a Bitter-Tasting Drug, *PCT Int. Appl.* WO9805312, 2.

[236] Gowan, W.G. (1993) Aliphatic Esters as Solventless Coating pharmaceuticals, *Can. Pat. Appl.* CA2082137, 11.

[237] Gowthamarajan, K.; Kulkarni, G.T. & Kumar, M.N. (2004) Pop the pills without bitterness Taste-Masking technologies for bitter drugs", *resonance*, 25.

[238] Bakan, J.A. (1986) Microencapsulation, Theory and practice of Industrial Pharmacy, Third Edition, 412-429.

[239] Iyer, V.S. & Srinivas, S.C. (2007) WO2007060682.

[240] Bush, L. (2004) Bitter taste bypass need for sugar spoon. Pharm Technol2004.http://pharmtech.findpharma.com/pharmtech/data/articlest and ard //pharmtech/072004/84521/article.pdf.

[241] www.pharmainfo.net., Ion exchange resin complex: an approach to mask the taste of bitter drugs.

[242] Bress, W.S.; Kulkarni, N.; Ambike, S. & Ramsay, M.P. (2006) EP1674078.

[243] Mendes, W.R. (1976) Theory and practice of Industrial pharmacy, Third Edition, 346.

[244] Redondo, A.M.J. & Abanades, L.B. (2003) WO047550.

[245] Kashid, N.; Chouhan, P. & Mukherji, G. (2007) WO2007108010.

[246] Scotti, L.; Scotti, M.T.; Ishiki, H.M.; Ferreira, M.G.P.; Emerenciano, V.P.; Menezes, C.M.S. & Ferreira, E.I. (2007) Quantitative elucidation of the structure-bittereness relationship of cynaropicrin and grosheimin derivatives. *Food Chem. 105*, 77-83.

[247] Bruice, T. C. & Benkovic, S. J. (1966) Bioorganic mechanisms (Vol. 1). New York: *WA Benjamin*.

[248] Walesh, C. (1979) Enzymatic reaction mechanisms (Vol. 868). San Francisco: *WH Freeman*.

[249] Kraut, D. A.; Carroll, K. S. & Herschlag, D. (2003) Challenges in enzyme mechanism and energetics. *Annual review of biochemistry 72*(1), 517-571.

[250] Snider, M. J. & Wolfenden, R. (2000).The rate of spontaneous decarboxylation of amino acids. *J. Am. Chem. Soc. 122*(46), 11507-11508.

[251] Kallarakal, A. T.; Mitra, B.; Kozarich, J. W.; Gerlt, J. A.; Clifton, J. R.; Petsko, G. A. &Kenyon, G. L. (1995) Mechanism of the reaction catalyzed by mandelate racemase: structure and mechanistic properties of the K166R mutant. *Biochemistry 34*(9), 2788-2797.

[252] Wu, Z. R.; Ebrahimian, S.; Zawrotny, M. E.; Thornburg, L. D.; Perez-Alvarado, G. C.; Brothers, P. & Summers, M. F. (1997) Solution structure of 3-oxo-Δ5-steroid isomerase. *Science 276*(5311), 415-418.

[253] Kluger, R. & Chin, J. (1982) Carboxylic acid participation in amide hydrolysis. Evidence that separation of a nonbonded complex can be rate determining. *J. Am. Chem. Soc. 104*, 2891-2897.

[254] Katagi, T. (1990) AM1 study of acid-catalyzed hydrolysis of maleamic (4-amino-4-oxo-2-butenoic) acids. *J. Comp. Chem. 11* (9) 1094-1100.

[255] Kirby, A. J. (2005) effective molarities for intramolecular reactions. *J. Phys. Org. Chem. 18*, 101-278.

[256] CRASH-2 Trial Collaborators (2010) Effects of tranexamic acid on death, vascular occlusive events, and blood transfusion in trauma patients with significant hemorrhage (CRASH-2): a randomized, placebo controlled trial. *Lancet 6736*, 60835–5.

[257] Gohel, M.; Patel, P., Gupta, A. & Desai, P. (2007) Efficacy of tranexamic acid in decreasing blood loss during and after cesarean section: a randomized case controlled prospective study. *J Obstet Gynecol India 57*, 227–230.

[258] Giancarlo, L.; Francesco, B.; Angela, L.; Pierluigi, P. & Gina, R. (2011) Recommendations for the transfusion management of patients in the peri-operative period. II. The intra-operative period. *Blood Transfus 9*, 189–217.

[259] Lukes, A.S.; Kouides, P.A. & Moore, K.A. (2011) Tranexamic acid: a novel oral formulation for the treatment of heavy menstrual bleeding. *Women's Health 7*, 151–158.

[260] Lukes, A.S.; Moore, K.A.; Muse, K.N.; Gersten, J.K.; Hecht, B.R.; Edlund M Richter, H.E.; Eder, S.E.; Attia, G.R.; Patrick, D.L.; Rubin, A. & Shangold, G.A. (2010)Tranexamic acid treatment for heavy menstrual bleeding: a randomized controlled trial. *Obstet Gynecol.116*, 865–875.

[261] Pilbrant, A.; Schannong, M. & Vessman, J. (1981) Pharmacokinetics and bioavailability of tranexamic acid. *Eur. J. Clin. Pharmacol.20*, 65–72.

[262] Karaman, R.; Dokmak, G.; Bader, M.; Hallak, H.; Khamis, M.; Scrano, L. & Bufo, S. A. (2013) Prodrugs of fumarate esters for the treatment of psoriasis and multiple sclerosis (MS)- A computational approach. *J. Molecular Modeling 19*, 439-452.

[263] Karaman, R. (2012) Computationally Designed Enzyme Models to Replace Natural Enzymes In Prodrug Approaches. *Journal of Drug Designing*1:e111] doi:10.4172/2169- 0138.1000e111.

[264] Karaman, R. (2013) Prodrug Design vs. Drug Design. *Journal of Drug Designing*2: e114. doi:10.4172/2169-0138.1000e114

[265] Karaman, R. (2012) The Future of Prodrugs designed by Computational Chemistry. *Journal of Drug Designing* 1:e103. doi:10.4172/ddo.1000e103.

[266] Karaman, R. (2012) Computationally Designed Prodrugs for Masking the Bitter Taste of Drugs. *Journal of Drug Designing,* 1:e106. doi:10.4172/2169-0138.1000e106.

[267] Karaman, R. (2013) Prodrugs Design by Computation Methods- A New Era. *Journal of Drug Designing* 2: e113. doi:10.4172/2169-0138.1000e113.

[268] Karaman, R. (2013) The Prodrug Naming Dilemma. *Journal of Drug Designing 2*: e115.doi:10.4172/2169-0138.1000e115.

[269] Karaman, R. (2013) A Solution to Aversive Tasting Drugs for Pediatric and Geriatric Patients. *Journal of Drug Designingdoi*:10.4172/2169-0138.1000e116.

In: Prodrugs Design – A New Era
Editor: Rafik Karaman

ISBN: 978-1-63117-701-9
© 2014 Nova Science Publishers, Inc.

Chapter II

Prodrug Overview

*Ala' Abu-Jaish[1], Salma Jumaa[1] and Rafik Karaman[1,2]**
[1]Pharmaceutical Sciences Department, Faculty of Pharmacy,
Al-Quds University, Jerusalem, Palestine
[2]Department of Science, University of Basilicata, Potenza, Italy

Abstract

The prodrug term involves chemically modified inert compound which upon administration releases the active parent drug to elicit its pharmacological response within the body. For many years, prodrug strategy has been developed enormously to solve many unwanted drug properties. This approach has several advantages over conventional drug administration and it has the potential to be quite effective method for the treatment of diseases in the future.

In most cases, prodrugs contain a promoiety (linker) that is removed by enzymatic or chemical reactions, while other prodrugs release their active drugs after molecular modification, such as an oxidation or reduction reactions. In some cases, two biologically active drugs can be linked together in a single molecule called a codrug. In a codrug, each drug acts as a linker for the other. It is important to ensure that the prodrug should be pharmacologically inactive, rapidly converted to its active drug and a non-toxic moiety by metabolic reactions.

In this chapter we describe the general terms related to prodrugs, and the ways by which prodrug strategy is used to overcome many pharmaceutical and pharmacokinetic problems such as, low bioavailability by increasing or decreasing lipophilicity of the parent drug, site selectivity for higher absorption and less toxicity, short duration of action to increase patient compliance, rapid metabolism to increase oral bioavailability and masking bitter sensation of commonly used drugs, which is crucial for geriatric and pediatric patient compliance.

Keywords: Prodrugs, Prodrugs history, Physicochemical properties, Chemical reactions, Prodrug metabolism, Permeability, Lipophilicity

---

* Corresponding author: Rafik Karaman, e-mail: dr_karaman@yahoo.com; Tel and Fax +972-2-2790413.

List of Abbreviations

5-	ASA5-Acetyl salicylic acid
I.V	Intravenous
I.M	Intramuscular
GDEPT	Gene directed enzyme prodrug therapy
ADEPT	Antibody directed enzyme prodrug therapy
VDEPT	Virus directed enzyme prodrug therapy
CESs	Carboxylesterases
ER	Endoplasmic reticulum
F-ara-A	2-Fluoroadenosine
mAbs	Monoclonal antibodies
AML	Acute myeloid leukemia
$PepT_1$	Peptide transporters
G.I	Gastrointestinal

Introduction

Generally, a drug is characterized by its biological and physicochemical properties. Some of the used drugs have undesirable properties that result in an inefficient delivery and unwanted side effects. The physicochemical, biological and organoleptic properties of these drugs should be improved in order to increase their usefulness and their utilization in clinical practice [1, 2].

During the last few decades, many methods have been developed in order to facilitate the drug design and discovery phases.

Most of these methods were devoted to find new chemical entities that provide the most meaningful interaction with the desired receptors or enzymes with the potential to have minimal unwanted interactions. However, this strategy is time consuming, costly and requires screening of thousands of molecules for biological activity of which only one might enter the drug market. One of the most attractive and promising method is the prodrug approach, in which the active drug molecule is masked by a promoiety to alter its undesired properties [3, 4].

The prodrug (predrug, proagent) term was introduced for the first time by Albert as a pharmacologically inactive moiety which is converted to an active form within the body [5]. This term has been successfully used to alter the physicochemical, pharmacokinetic properties, (absorption, distribution, excretion and metabolism) of drugs and to decrease their associated toxicity [6].

A prodrug must undergo chemical and/or enzymatic biotransformation in a controlled or predictable manner prior to exert its therapeutic activity [7].

Basically, the use of the term prodrug implies a covalent link between an active drug and a promoiety (Figure 1) [8].

This strategy is designed to overcome barriers through a chemical approach rather than a formulation approach [9].

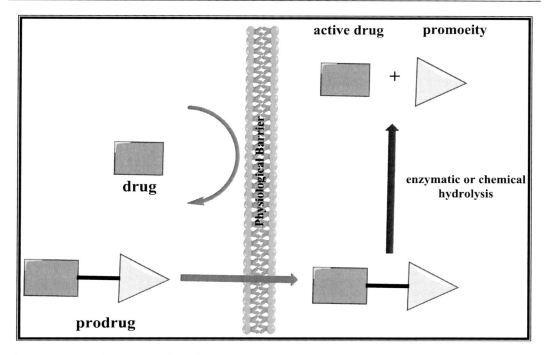

Figure 1. Schematic representation of a prodrug [8].

In general, the imminent goal behind the use of prodrugs is to develop new entities that possess superior efficacy, selectivity, and reduced toxicity [3]. An ideal prodrug should undergo biotransformation rapidly via chemical or enzymatic process to its active form and a non-toxic moiety within the body [7, 10].

The prodrug must release the active drug and the promoiety prior to, during, or after absorption, or in a specific target tissue or organ, depending upon the purpose of which the prodrug has been designed [11].

Nowadays, the prodrug approach is considered as one of the most promising site-selective drug delivery strategies that utilize target cell- or tissue-specific endogenous enzymes and transporters [12].

One of the few examples that were designed to increase the efficiency of a drug by accumulation into a specific tissue or organ is the anti-Parkinson agent L-DOPA. Dopamine is a hydrophilic neurotransmitter, which does not efficiently cross the blood-brain barrier and is rapidly metabolized by oxidative deamination that causes peripheral side effects. However, the prodrug of dopamine, L-DOPA, enables the uptake and accumulation of dopamine into the brain via the L-type amino acid transporter (Figure 2) [6, 13].

Figure 2. L-DOPA prodrug conversion.

//
History

In 1958, Albert introduced the prodrug term for the first time in his book 'selective toxicity'. This term includes any inert compound that undergoes in vivo biotransformation [5]. Others such as Harper also promoted the concept but used the term drug latentiation which includes the prodrug intentionally designed to undergo biotransformation within the body [14]. Few years later, Albert apologized for having invented an inaccurate term, because "pre-drug" would be a more descriptive term [15].

The first prodrug was not originally designed as a prodrug, but its nature was determined later. Earlier examples of compounds fulfill the classical criteria of prodrug were acetanilide and phenacetin, which exhibit their activities after being metabolized within the body [16].

Acetanilide is an antipyretic agent that was in use in 1886. It undergoes metabolism (aromatic hydroxylation) to paracetamol. This is similar to phenacetin which produces paracetamol via O-dealkylation (Figure 3) [17].

Figure 3. Phenacetin and acetanilide metabolism.

In the late nineteenth century a chemist, Felix Hoffman in Bayar Company, synthesized the antipyretic agent Aspirin (acetylsalicylic acid), which was introduced for the first time in clinical practice in 1899; it can be considered a less corrosive prodrug form of salicylic acid to minimize the gastric irritation and ulcerogenicity associated with salicylic acid (Figure 4). However, it remains a matter of debate whether aspirin is a true prodrug or not [18].

Another example of an accidental prodrug and how serendipity aided in prodrug development is methenamine and the first sulfa prodrug, prontosil [6].

Methenamine was discovered in 1899 by Schering as inactive prodrug that delivers the antibacterial formaldehyde. It is useful in the treatment of urinary tract infection, when transported to urinary bladder it becomes acidified to provide a medium in which formaldehyde is generated (Figure 5) [19].

Figure 4. Chemical structure of salicylic acid and its prodrug aspirin.

Figure 5. Methenamine prodrug activation at acidic pH.

Prontosil was found to be effective against microorganisms only in vivo, and not in vitro. When administered in the body it was metabolized by the enzyme azo reductase to sulfanilamide, the first sulfonamide to be discovered (Figure 6) [16].

Figure 6. Prontosil prodrug activation by azo reductase.

Figure 7. Chloramphenicol prodrugs and their conversion to chloramphenicol.

In the mid twentieth century the prodrug concept was intentionally used for the first time when Parke-Davis Company modified the structure of chloramphenicol in order to improve its bitter sensation and poor water solubility. Two prodrugs of chloramphenicol were synthesized, chloramphenicol sodium succinate with a good water solubility for IV, IM, and ophthalmic administration, and chloramphenicol palmitate used in the form of suspension for children (Figure 7) [6, 20].

The prodrug approach has been successfully applied to a wide variety of drugs. It is estimated that currently about 10% of world-wide marketed drugs can be classified as prodrugs, 20% of all small molecular medications approved between 2000-2008 were prodrugs, and in the year 2008, one third of approved drugs were prodrugs [1].

Prodrugs Classification

The conventional method used to classify prodrugs is based on derivatization and the type of carriers attached to the drug. This method classifies prodrugs into two sub-major classes:

(1) Carrier-linked prodrugs, in which the promoiety is covalently linked to the active drug but it can be easily cleaved by enzymes (such as an ester or labile amide) or non-enzymatically to provide the parent drug. Ideally, the group removed is pharmacologically inactive, nontoxic, and non-immunogenic, while the promoiety must be labile for in vivo efficient activation [3, 21].

Carrier-linked prodrugs can be further subdivided into: (a) bipartite which is composed of one carrier (promoiety) attached directly to the drug, (b) tripartite which utilizing a spacer or connect a group between the drug and a promoiety. In some cases bipartite prodrug may be unstable due to inherent nature of the drug-promoiety linkage. This can be solved by designing a tripartite prodrug and (c) mutual prodrugs, which are consisting of two drugs linked together.

(2) Bioprecursors which are chemical entities that are metabolized into new compounds that may be active or further are metabolized to active metabolites (such as amine to aldehyde to carboxylic acid). In this prodrug type there is no carrier but the compound should be readily metabolized to induce the necessary functional groups [6, 9, 22].

In addition, prodrugs can be classified based on cellular site of interconversion into the active drug form. This classification strategy includes two types: Type I: includes prodrugs that are converted to active drug intracellularly (e.g., anti-viral nucleoside analogs, and lipid-lowering statins). Type II: involves prodrugs that are converted extracellularly, especially in digestive fluids or in the systemic circulation (e.g., etoposide phosphate, valganciclovir, fosamprenavir, antibody-directed/gene-directed enzyme prodrugs (ADEP/GDEP) for chemotherapy). Both types are further subdivided into subtypes (Type IA, IB and Type IIA, IIB, and IIC) based on whether or not the intracellular converting location is the site of therapeutic action, or whether the conversion occurs in the gastrointestinal (GI) fluids or systemic circulation (Table 1)[23].

Mutual Prodrug

Mutual prodrugs are a type of carrier linked prodrugs by which two pharmacologically active agents linked together to form a single molecule. Each of these drugs acts as a carrier for the other. Mutual prodrugs approach offers an efficient tool for improving the clinical and therapeutic effectiveness of a drug that is suffering from some undesirable properties hindering its clinical usefulness.

A common example of this approach is benorylate (Figure 8), by which aspirin linked covalently to paracetamol through an ester linkage, which claims to have decreased gastric irritation with synergistic analgesic effect [24].

Table 1. Prodrug classification [23]

Prodrug types	Site of conversion	Subtypes	Tissue/location of conversion	Examples
Type I	Intracellular	A	Therapeutic Target Tissues/Cells	Acyclovir 5-Flurouracil L-Dopa
		B	Metabolic Tissues (Liver, GI mucosal cell, lung, etc…)	Cabamazepine Captopril Suldinac
Type II	Extracellular	A	GI Fluids	Loperamide oxide Oxyphenisatin Sulfasalazine
		B	Systemic circulation and other extracellular fluid compartments	Acetylsalicylate Bacampicillin Fosphenytoin
		C	Therapeutic Target Tissues/Cells	ADEPs GDEPs VDEPs

Figure 8. Mutual prodrug of acetylsalicylic acid and paracetamol.

Another example of mutual prodrug is sulfasalazine. It's a colon selective mutual prodrug, of 5-aminosalicylic acid (5-ASA) and sulfapyridine used in the treatment of ulcerative colitis [25].

Sulfasalazine was the first sulfa drug to be used in inflammatory bowel disease and was developed in 1950. It is composed of 5-aminosalicylic acid (5-ASA) linked to sulfapyridine via a diazo bond (Figure 9). This bond is readily cleaved by bacterial azo-reductases in the colon. Where 5-ASA has been found to be the therapeutically active component, while sulfapyridine is assumed to function solely as a carrier molecule and serves as a delivery system that transports 5-ASA to the affected region of the lower GI [26, 27].

The advantage of this approach is that the cleavage of the azo linkage and generation of 5-ASA prior to the absorption prevents its systemic absorption and helps to concentrate the active drug at the active site. Even though sulfapyridine proved to be a good carrier for targeting 5-ASA to colon, it gave rise to many side effects resulting from its systemic toxicity.

Due to disadvantages related to the use of sulfasalazine, another interesting mutual prodrug of 5-ASA, olsalazine, has been developed. This mutual prodrug is actually a dimer of 5-ASA, where 5-ASA is linked through azo linkage to another molecule of 5-ASA. When it reaches the large intestine, it is cleaved, releasing two molecules of 5-ASA for every molecule of olsalazine administered. This design eliminates the drawbacks of sulfasalazine, targets 5-ASA to the colon, and fulfills all requirements of mutual prodrug as well. Improvement of the bioavailability of 5-ASA was also achieved using this design.

Figure 9. Conversion of the mutual prodrug, sulfasalazine.

Prodrug Activation

Conversion of prodrugs into the active form occurs enzymatically or chemically. Numerous and most commonly carrier linkage prodrugs are designed to be activated via esterases. A wide range of esterases distributed throughout the body, differ in their substrate specificity. Examples of esterases found in the body are acetylcholinesterases, butyrylcholinesterases, carboxylesterases and arylesterases [15].

Therefore, prodrug approach can be employed to control the release of the active compound at a specific site. One of the most important enzymes involved in ester bioactivation are carboxylesterases (CESs). These enzymes are a multi-gene family whose genes are localized in the endoplasmic reticulum (ER) of several tissues. These enzymes efficiently catalyze the hydrolysis of a variety of ester- and amide-containing prodrugs to the corresponding free acids. CESs show ubiquitous tissue expression profiles with the highest levels of CESs activity present in the liver microsomal site [28]. Hence the potential for their substrates to become involved in drug-drug interactions is generally considered to be negligible [29]. Examples of prodrug hydrolyzed by this type of esterases are enalapril (Figure 10) and pivampicillin (Figure 11).

Figure 10. Enalapril conversion via carboxylestrase.

Figure 11. Pivampicillin conversion via carboxylestrase.

Another enzymes involved in the activation of prodrugs are phosphatases [30]. An example of such activation is shown in Figure 12.

Figure 12. Fosphenytoin activation via alkaline phosphatase.

Bioprecursor Activation

Upon administration many compounds are metabolized by molecular modification into new compounds that are active in principle or can be metabolized further into the active drugs.

Five types of reactions can be involved in bioprecursor activation [31]:

1. Oxidative reaction, _catalyzed by CYP450 such as (i) O and N dealkylation; _e.g (bioprecursor prodrug for alprazolam), (ii) oxidative deamination; e.g., (cyclophosphamide activation) and (iii) N-oxidation; e.g., (procarbazine activation).
2. Reductive activation such as (i) disulfide reaction; e.g., (activation of thiamine prodrug) and (ii) bioreductive alkylation; e.g., (activation of anticancer antibiotic, mitomycin c).
3. Nucleotide activation.
4. Phosphorylation activation; e.g., (antiviral drug, acyclovir activation).
5. Decarboxylation activation; e.g., (Nabumetone).

Applications of Prodrugs

Prodrugs are used to overcome pharmacokinetic and pharmaceutical barriers to increase drug biological bioavailability. After overcoming those barriers the prodrug must be converted to the active form in the targeted site of action.

Pharmacokinetic applications:

1. Improvement of bioavailability by alteration of drug's solubility.
2. Prodrugs for site selective drug delivery.
3. Prolongation of action.
4. Minimizing toxicity.
5. Protection from presystemic metabolism.

Improvement of Bioavailability

Chemical modification of drugs is used to improve physicochemical properties solubility, stability, and lipophilicity [32].

Oral drug bioavailability is critical for the development of new drugs, because low oral absorption leads to inter- and intra-patient variability. One of the strategies developed to improve oral bioavailability is prodrugs [33].

Oral bioavailability of lipophilic drugs depends on the dissolution in the gastrointestinal fluids, and polar drug's bioavailability depends on the transport across gastrointestinal mucosa [11]. Therefore, prodrugs are designed to increase or decrease lipophilicity.

Prodrugs to Increase Lipophilicity

Prodrugs are used to increase lipophilicity so that the drugs are available for oral administration, ocular or topical drug delivery.

The main reason for designing prodrugs is to increase oral bioavailability, and the intestinal absorption, which are enhanced by masking the polar moiety of the drug [34]. For example, dabigatran, a potent inhibitor of the active site of thrombin is very polar molecule with a logP of −2.4 (n-octanol/buffer pH 7.4), therefore its oral bioavailability is negligible [35]. Dabigatran etexilate, the first oral alternative to warfarin, was developed as a prodrug of dabigatran (Figure 13). After oral administration, dabigatran etexilate is converted to the active drug dabigatran by esterases. The oral bioavailability of dabigatran etexilate is 6.5% [36].

Dabigatran etexilate

Esterases

Dabigatran

Figure 13. Chemical structures of dabigatran prodrug and its active drug.

Ophthalmic Drug Delivery

Lipophilic prodrugs are also used to enhance ocular absorption. For example latanoprost and travoprost are isopropyl esters of the parent latanoprost and travoprost carboxylic acids (Figure 14). These ester prodrugs have an increased lipophilicity, which enables them to penetrate the cornium epithelium [37].

Figure 14. Chemical structures of travoprost and latanoprost acids, and their corresponding ester prodrugs.

Topical Drug Delivery

Another use of lipophilic prodrugs is to increase transdermal absorption for certain drugs. For example, ester prodrugs with increased lipophilicity allow them to accumulate in the skin leading to higher efficacy and lower side effects [37].

Fluocinolone acetonide (R=COCH$_3$)
Fluocinolone (R=H)

Figure 15. Chemical structures of fluocinolone and its prodrug, fluocinolone acetonide.

Topical corticosteroids are widely used as anti-inflammatory and immune-suppressants agents for skin problems. However, they may be absorbed systemically and cause side effects [38]. For example, fluocinolone acetonide ester prodrugs (Figure 15) have high membrane retention (in epidermis) and low permeation which is preferred for local application of corticosteroids [39]. The high lipophilicity of the fluocinolone acetonide prodrug makes it more potent than its less lipophilic parent drug, fluocinolone [40].

Prodrugs to Increase Polarity

Prodrugs are designed to increase aqueous solubility by esterification with amino acids or phosphate group [34].

Phosphate Prodrug for Oral Delivery

For example, fosamprenavir (Figure 16), a protease inhibitor used as antiviral, is converted to amprenavir by alkaline phosphatase in the gut epithelium [41]._The phosphate promoiety is linked to a free hydroxyl group which makes fosamprenavir 10-fold more water soluble than amprinavir. An enhanced patient compliance is achieved by producing this antiviral prodrug, instead of administering the drug 8 times daily, dosage regimen is reduced into 2 times per day [42].

Figure 16. Chemical structure of the oral prodrug fosamprenavir.

Another example is 2-fluoroadenosine (F-ara-A), which has a clinical use as anti-neoplastic agent. However, it is difficult to be formulated because of its lipophilicity. Therefore fludarabine phosphate (2F-ara-AMP), which is a prodrug that is rapidly dephosphorylated to give fludarabine (F-ara-A), was synthesized (Figure 17) [43].

Fludarabine phosphate is available as an oral dosage form and its systemic bioavailability is 85% [44]. Fludarabine enters the cells by a carrier mediated transport and it undergoes phosphorylation to furnish 2-fluoroadenosine (F-ara-ATP, the cytotoxic form of the drug) [43].

Figure 17. Chemical structures of 2-fluoroadenosine and its prodrug, fludarabine phosphate.

Prodrugs for Site Selective Drug Delivery

Prodrugs are applied for targeting drugs to a specific organ or tissue; they are widely used in chemotherapy. Targeted prodrugs are used to increase absorption and decrease toxicity, they are targeted to an enzyme or membrane transporter [32].

Tumor Targeted Drug Delivery

Cancer chemotherapeutics are toxic and nonselective which limits their use for cancer therapy [45]. Their selectivity depends on the rapidly dividing cells that are more prone to toxic effects [46]. Hence, they are toxic for rapidly proliferating normal tissue such as hair follicles, gut epithelia, bone marrow, and red blood cells. Therefore, in order to improve toxicity and efficacy chemotherapy prodrugs were designed to target tumor cells; this targeting is achieved by binding drugs to ligands having high affinity to specific antigens, receptors, or transporters that are over expressed in tumor cells [47].

One of the targeting methods is enzyme activated prodrug therapy where the nontoxic prodrug is converted to the active drug in the tumor tissue [37]. The enzyme should be specifically expressed or over expressed in tumor. Plasmin, prostate specific antigen, matrix metalloproteaes, cathepsin B, D, H and L are examples of tumor associated enzymes that are used for prodrug activation in malignant cells [48].

Monoclonal antibodies (mAbs) have a high affinity, hence they are the first ligands used for tumor targeting [47]. MAbs are designed as drug-antibody conjugate or antibody enzyme conjugate [48].

Drug-Antibody Conjugate

Tumor specific mAbs bind to receptors on tumor cells and the cytotoxic drug is selectively delivered to the tumor. For example, mylotarge consists of anti-CD33 mAbs conjugated to the cytotoxic ozogamicin, which was approved by the FDA for treatment of AML, acute myeloid leukemia [46].

Antibody Enzyme Conjugates

- Antibody-directed enzyme prodrug therapy (ADEPT)

In this approach tumor specific antibody is delivered into tumor cells. Then the prodrug is administered systemically, and converted to the active toxic drug inside the tumor [48].

- Gene-directed enzyme prodrug therapy (GDEPT)

In this method, a gene encoding the activating enzyme is delivered to tumor cells as a first step. The second step is an administration of the inactive prodrug which is converted to the toxic drug by the tumor enzyme [47]. Viral vectors are the most popular vectors used for gene delivery [48].

Membrane Transporter Prodrug Targeting

Membrane transporters selectively transport peptides, amino acids, phosphates, ascorbic acid, bile acids and others. For example, dipeptides and tripeptides are transported in the intestinal epithelial cells by peptide transporters ($PepT_1$) [32].

Targeting specific transporters, which have an important role in drug absorption, distribution, and elimination, via a prodrug is efficient and selective strategy [32)], in which a prodrug is selectively attached to a molecule that targets a specific membrane transporters; $PepT_1$ is the most promising transporter due to its selectivity and high capacity [34].

For example, the antiviral drug acyclovir, used to treat herpes simplex virus, by acting as a competitive substrate for DNA polymerase [49], has low oral bioavailability, because of its hydrophilic nature and poor permeability which limited its efficacy [50].

Figure 18. Chemical structures of acyclovir and its valine prodrug, valacyclovir.

To increase the oral bioavailability of acyclovir, L-valine (valacyclovir) prodrug was developed to target PepT transporters in the G.I (Figure 18). This prodrug has a high affinity for PepT transporter, therefore, it is highly absorbed through small intestine and is converted to acyclovir in the gut lumen [51]. Oral bioavailability of acyclovir is 21.5%, whereas the bioavailability of valacyclovir after oral administration of the prodrug is 70.1%, in addition to the three-fold increase in bioavailability the inter-individual variations are less in the case of valacyclovir [52].

Several valine-valine dipeptide prodrugs of acyclovir were synthesized, in order to protect the prodrug against enzymatic hydrolysis before it reaches the PepT transporter. For example, D-isomers of valine were incorporated, since the hydrolytic enzymes have low affinity for the D-isomer.

It was found that dipeptide prodrug with one D-valine isomer keeps its affinity for the PepT transporter [50].

Another example, is zanamivir, which has poor oral bioavailability because of its polar nature, which limits its use in influenza infection [53]. L-Valyl zanamivir a prodrug of zanamivir was developed (Figure19). The prodrug has a higher uptake through the PepT transporters, which improved its absorption after oral administration [34].

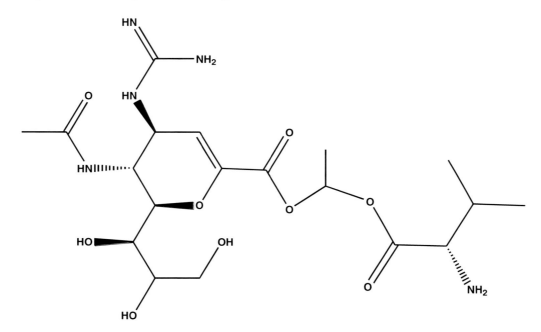

Figure 19. Chemical structure of L-valyl zanamivir.

Prodrugs for Longer Duration of Action

Drugs with short half-life require frequent dosing, to maintain blood concentration, which leads to poor patient compliance and fluctuation in the drug concentration. The development of prodrugs with long duration of action can be used to overcome these problems [11].

Long acting antipsychotic therapy is important to control symptoms and prevent relapse. These long acting agents also improve patient compliance and increase efficacy. For example, fluphenazine decanoate, an ester prodrug of fluphenazine (Figure 20), is used as long acting intramuscular depot injection for the treatment of schizophrenia; this prodrug is administered once every 2 weeks [54].

Fluphenazine decanoate

Figure 20. Chemical structure of fluphenazine decanoate prodrug.

Buprenorphine ester prodrugs are another example of prodrugs used for longer duration of action. Patients with moderate to severe pain like postoperative pain and burn pain may need analgesics for 3 days after a trauma. Therefore, there is a need for depot analgesics. Buprenorphine decanoate, enanthate, and propionate were synthesized and formulated in sesame oil for I.M injection. Pharmacokinetic studies on buprenorphine decanoate (Figure 21) showed that it produced 4.1 day duration of action, which is 14-fold longer than the traditional buprenorphine [55].

Figure 21. Chemical structure of buprenorphine decanoate prodrug.

Reduction of Toxicity

For therapeutically active drugs it is preferred to have minimum or no toxicity, therefore, prodrugs can be used to minimize toxicity of many drugs [11]. For example, doxorubicin, _an anthracycline antibiotic, which is highly used as anticancer drug, but its use, is limited by its cardiotoxicity. Hence, there was a crucial need to design drug targeting system to increase doxorubicin availability in tumor tissue and decrease its accumulation in cardiac tissue [56]. A galactoside prodrug that is linked to doxorubicin via a carbamate spacer was developed (Figure 22). This prodrug is solely activated by β-galactosidase that is highly expressed in tumor tissue; additionally, the hydrophilic nature of galactoside moiety prevents its distribution to other tissues. This prodrug is more effective and less toxic than its parent drug due to low concentration in cardiac tissue [57].

Figure 22. Chemical structure of doxorubicin galactoside prodrug.

Protecting from Rapid Metabolism and Excretion

Presystemic metabolism causes low oral bioavailability of drugs; certain sites or groups in the molecule are subjected to presystemic metabolism therefore prodrugs can be used to block these sites and increase oral bioavailability [45].

Nalbuphine is a potent analgesic used in moderate to severe pain; it has a low oral bioavailability of only 17% due to presystemic metabolism at the 3-hydroxyl position. Nalbuphine acetylsalicylate (Figure 23) an ester prodrug of nalbuphine was synthesized and it has shown an increased oral bioavailability in dogs by 5-folds [58].

Figure 23. Chemical structure of nalbuphine ester prodrug.

Estrogens such as estradiol and ethinyl estradiol have low oral bioavailability due to the conjugation at the phenolic hydroxyl position [45]. Estrogen sulfamate prodrug (Figure 24) was synthesized by replacing the phenolic hydroxyl group with sulfamate; this sulfamate prodrug protects estrogens from the liver first pass effect which leads to higher systemic activity of oral estrogens [59].

Figure 24. Chemical structures of estrogen sulfamate prodrug and the active drug estradiol.

Improvement of Taste

Taste is an important factor in the development of dosage forms, and masking bitter taste of oral drugs is crucial for patient compliance especially in pediatric and geriatric patients.

Drugs interact with taste buds on the tongue to give bitter taste. Many technologies were developed to prevent this interaction, including use of physical barrier, chemical or solubility modification and solid dispersion [60].

Chemical modification to eliminate interaction with taste receptors can be achieved by using prodrug approach. For example, paracetamol, an antipyretic and pain killer drug, has a bitter taste, it is believed that the phenolic hydroxyl group of paracetamol interacts by hydrogen bonding with bitter taste receptors. Therefore, blocking the hydroxyl group with a suitable linker could inhibit the interaction and mask the bitter taste of paracetamol. Karaman's group synthesized some paracetamol prodrugs that were found to lack the bitter taste sensation of paracetamol (Figure 25) [61].

Another example is cefuroxime antibiotic, which has extremely bitter taste. This bitter taste is mostly due to the interaction between the amido group at position 3 and the active site of bitter taste receptors. Some prodrugs with an amide linker were proposed (Figure 26) [62)].

Figure 25. Chemical structures of paracetamol and its bitterless taste prodrugs.

Figure 26. Chemical structures of cefuroxime prodrugs.

Improvement of Odor

Odor is an aesthetic concern for drugs with high vapor pressure or low boiling point, which makes them difficult to be formulated. For example, ethyl mercaptan a tuberculostatic agent used for the treatment of leprosy has unpleasant smell because of low boiling point 25°C. The most attractive derivative prodrugs were its ethyl thiol esters [63]; diethyl dithiolisophthalate prodrug of ethyl mercaptan was developed (Figure 27); this prodrug was found to be highly active and odorless [64].

Ethyl mercaptan

Phthalate ester prodrug

Figure 27. Chemical structures of ethyl mercaptan and its phthalate prodrug.

Minimizing Pain at Injection Site

Pain at the injection site is caused by precipitation of drug that causes cell lyses and tissue injury. This problem may be related to the vehicle composition or vehicle pH needed for formulation purposes.

For example, phenytoin injection, which is approved for the treatment of status epilepticus has poor aqueous solubility, therefore, the pH in the vehicle for injection is adjusted to 12, which leads to soft tissue injury and pain in the site of administration, due to phenytoin precipitation [65].

Fosphenytoin, a phosphate ester prodrug of phenytoin was approved by the FDA in 1996 (Figure 12). This prodrug has high aqueous solubility, no apparent pain was observed upon its use and its intramuscular bioavailability was 100% [66].

Another example is propofol injectable formulations, which are difficult to be developed because propofol is highly lipid soluble. The available formulations are oil in water emulsions that are associated with pain on the site of the injection [67]. Fospropofol, a phosphoester prodrug of propofol was synthesized (Figure 28). The synthesized prodrug is a water soluble form of propofol and upon its use no pain on the site of the injection was detected [68].

Propofol

Fospropofol

Figure 28. Chemical structures of propofol and its prodrug fospropofol.

Summary and Conclusion

Over the past 50 years, considerable attention has been focused on the development of bioreversible derivatives, such as prodrugs, to alter the physicochemical, pharmacokinetic and biopharmaceutical properties of drugs. Prodrugs are pharmacologically inactive form of their active agents, which undergo chemical and/or enzymatic biotransformation to release the corresponding active drug. The conversion product (i.e., parent drug) subsequently elicits the desired pharmacological response. Since the synthesis of new compounds is a time consuming and too costly, designing derivatives of existing clinically used drugs is definitely an interesting and promising area of research.

Pharmacokinetic and pharmaceutical problems are the most important causes of high attrition rates in drug development. Prodrug design is an efficient approach used to overcome these problems. The lipophilicity of poorly permeable drugs can be increased by linking the drug to a lipophilic linker such that it can be used for oral, ocular or local drug delivery [69]. Prodrugs can be also used to increase aqueous solubility by linking the drug to a polar or ionizable groups [69]. Site selectivity can be achieved by targeting a specific enzyme or receptor, such as targeting an enzyme that is over expressed in tumor cells. Additionally, mAbs are also used as ligands to transport prodrugs to tumor cells. They are designed as drug-antibody conjugate or antibody enzyme conjugate [48], targeting membrane transporters_ are used to increase absorption such as in the case of valacyclovir prodrug.

Prodrugs are also have been used for prolongation of action, such as buprenorphine decanoate and fluphenazine decanoate ester prodrugs [55]. Prodrugs also are applied to decrease pain at injection site by making drugs more water soluble. Masking bitter taste and improvement of odor are important applications of prodrugs to increase patient compliance. Taste masking is achieved by blocking chemical groups that are involved in the drug interaction with bitter taste receptors.

References

[1] Stella, V. (2010) Prodrugs: Some thoughts and current issues. *J. Pharm. Sci.* 99(12), 4755-65.

[2] Karaman, R.; Fattash B. & Qtait A. (2013). The future of prodrugs – design by quantum mechanics methods. *Expert Opinion on Drug Delivery10*, 713–729.

[3] Jana, S.; Mandlekar, S. & Marathe, P. (2010) Prodrug design to improve pharmacokinetic and drug delivery properties: challenges to the discovery scientists. *Curr. Med. Chem.* 17(32), 3874-908.

[4] Venkatesh, S. & Lipper, R. A. (2000) Role of the development scientist in compound lead selection and optimization. *J. Pharm. Sci.* 89(2), 145-54.

[5] Albert, A. (1958) Chemical aspects of selective toxicity. *Nature.* 182, 421–2

[6] Stella, V; Borchardt, R.; Hageman, M.; Oliyai, R.; Maag, H. & Tilley, J. Prodrugs: challenges and Rewards Published by AAPS Press and Springer2007. p. 1-2.

[7] Stella, V.J. & Nti-Addae, K. W. (2007) Prodrug strategies to overcome poor water solubility. *Adv. Drug. Deliv. Rev.* 59(7), 677-94.

[8] Rautio, J.; Kumpulainen, H.; Heimbach, T.; Oliyai, R.; Oh, D.; Jarvinen, T. &Savolainen, J. (2008) Prodrugs: design and clinical applications. *Nat. Rev. Drug Discov.* 7(3), 255-70.

[9] Müller, C.E. (2009) Prodrug Approaches for Enhancing the Bioavailability of Drugs with Low Solubility. *Chemistry & Biodiversity.* 6(11), 2071-83.

[10] Chipade, V.; Dewani, A.; Bakal, R. & Chandewar, A. (2012) Prodrugs: adevelopment ofcapping drugs. *PDFARDI*J 4A, 17-34.

[11] Stella, V.J.; Charman, W.N. & Naringrekar, V.H. (1985) Prodrugs. Do they have advantages in clinical practice? Drugs 29(5), 455-73. *Pub. Med. PMID*: 3891303.

[12] Han, H. & Amidon, G. (2000) Targeted prodrug design to optimize drug delivery. *AAPS Pharm. Sci.* 2(1), E6.

[13] del Amo, E.M.; Urtti, A. & Yliperttula, M. (2008) Pharmacokinetic role of L-type amino acid transporters LAT1 and LAT2. *Eur. J. Pharm. Sci.* 35(3), 161-74.

[14] Harper, N,J. (1959) Drug latentiation. *J. Med. Pharm. Chem.* 1, 467-500.

[15] Huttunen, K.M.; Raunio, H. & Rautio, J. (2011) Prodrugs-from serendipity to rational design. *Pharmacol. Rev.* 63(3), 750-71.

[16] Albert, A. Selective Toxicity: *The PhysicoChemical Basis of Therapy.* 7 ed. New York: Chapman and Hall 1985.

[17] Bertolini, A.; Ferrari, A.; Ottani, A.; Guerzoni, S.; Tacchi, R. & Leone, S. (2006) Paracetamol: new vistas of an old drug. *CNS Drug. Rev.* 12(3-4), 250-75.

[18] Burke AS, Emer; FitzGerald, Garret A *Goodman and Gilman's the pharmacological basis of therapeutics.* 11 ed. New York: McGraw-Hill; 2006.

[19] Testa, B. (2009) Prodrugs: bridging pharmacodynamic/pharmacokinetic gaps. *Curr. Opin. Chem. Biol.* 13(3), 338-44.

[20] Glazko, A.J.; Carnes, H.E.; Kazenko, A.; Wolf, L.M. & Reutner, T.F. (1957) Succinic acid esters of chloramphenicol. *Antibiot Annu.* 5, 792-802.

[21] Stella, V. Pro-drugs: An Overview and Definition. Pro-drugs as Novel Drug Delivery Systems. ACS Symposium Series. 14: *American Chemical Society*; 1975. p. 1-115.

[22] Roche, E.B. Design of biopharmaceutical properties through prodrugs and analogs. Washington, DC: *American Pharmaceutical Association*; 1977.

[23] Wu, K-M. (2009) A New Classification of Prodrugs: Regulatory Perspectives. *Pharmaceuticals* 2(3), 77-81. Pub. Med. PMID: doi:10.3390/ph2030077.

[24] Croft, D.N.; Cuddigan, J.H. & Sweetland, C. (1972) Gastric bleeding and benorylate, a new aspirin. *Br. Med. J.* 3(5826), 545-7.

[25] Azadkhan, A.K.; Truelove, S.C. & Aronson, J.K. (1982) The disposition and metabolism of sulphasalazine (salicylazosulphapyridine) in man. *Br. J. Clin. Pharmacol.* 13(4), 523-8.

[26] Peppercorn, M.A. & Goldman, P. (1973) Distribution studies of salicylazosulfapyridine and its metabolites. *Gastroenterology* 64(2), 240-5.

[27] Peppercorn, M. A. & Goldman, P. (1972) The role of intestinal bacteria in the metabolism of salicylazosulfapyridine. *J. Pharmacol. Exp. Ther.* 181(3), 555-62.

[28] Hosokawa, M.; Maki, T. & Satoh, T. (1990) Characterization of molecular species of liver microsomal carboxylesterases of several animal species and humans. *Arch. Biochem. Biophys.* 277(2), 219-27.

[29] Liederer, B.M. & Borchardt, R.T. (2006) Enzymes involved in the bioconversion of ester-based prodrugs. *J. Pharm. Sci.* 95(6), 1177-95.

[30] Yuan, H.; Li, N. & Lai, Y. (2009) Evaluation of in vitro models for screening alkaline phosphatase-mediated bioconversion of phosphate ester prodrugs. *Drug Metab. Dispos.* 37(7), 1443-7.

[31] Kokil, G. R. & Rewatkar, P.V. (2010) Bioprecursor prodrugs: molecular modification of the active principle. *Mini Rev. Med. Chem.* 10(14), 1316-30.

[32] Anand, B. S.; Dey, S. & Mitra, A. K. (2002) Current prodrug strategies via membrane transporters/receptors. *Expert opinion on biological therapy* 2(6), 607-20. Pub. Med. PMID: 12171505.

[33] Gomez-Orellana, I. (2005) Strategies to improve oral drug bioavailability. *Expert opinion on drug delivery* 2(3), 419-33. Pub. Med PMID: 16296764.

[34] Dahan, A.; Khamis, M.; Agbaria, R. & Karaman, R. (2012) Targeted prodrugs in oral drug delivery: the modern molecular biopharmaceutical approach. *Expert opinion on drug delivery* 9(8), 1001-13. Pub. Med. PMID: 22703376.

[35] Eisert, W. G.; Hauel, N.; Stangier, J.; Wienen, W.; Clemens, A. & van Ryn, J. (2010) Dabigatran: an oral novel potent reversible nonpeptide inhibitor of thrombin. *Arteriosclerosis, thrombosis, and vascular biology* 30(10), 1885-9. Pub. Med. PMID: 20671233.

[36] Hankey, G. J. & Eikelboom, J. W. (2011) Dabigatran etexilate: a new oral thrombin inhibitor. *Circulation.* 123(13), 1436-50. Pub. Med PMID: 21464059.

[37] Zawilska, J. B.; Wojcieszak, J. & Olejniczak, A.B. (2013) Prodrugs: a challenge for the drug development. *Pharmacological reports* : PR. 65(1), 1-14. Pub. Med PMID: 23563019.

[38] Sweetman, S. C. MartindaleThe Complete Drug Reference. 36 ed. 1 Lambeth High Street, London SEl 7JN, UK: the Pharmaceutical Press; 2009.

[39] Markovic, B. D.; Vladimirov, S.M.; Cudina, O.A.; Odovic, J.V.& Karljikovic-Rajic. K.D. (2012) A PAMPA assay as fast predictive model of passive human skin permeability of new synthesized corticosteroid C-21 esters. *Molecules.* 17(1), 480-91. PubMed PMID: 22222907.

[40] Markovic, B. D.; Dobricic, V.D.; Vladimirov, S.M.; Cudina, O.A.; Savic, V.M. & Karljikovic-Rajic, K.D. (2011) Investigation of solvolysis kinetics of new synthesized fluocinolone acetonide C-21 esters--an in vitro model for prodrug activation. *Molecules.* 16(3), 2658-71. Pub Med. PMID: 21441868.

[41] Becker, S. & Thornton, L. (2004) Fosamprenavir: advancing HIV protease inhibitor treatment options. *Expert opinion on pharmacotherapy* 5(9), 1995-2005. Pub. Med PMID: 15330736.

[42] Chapman, T. M.; Plosker, G.L. & Perry C.M. (2004) Fosamprenavir: a review of its use in the management of antiretroviral therapy-naive patients with HIV infection. *Drugs.* 64, 2101-24.

[43] Chun, H.G.; Leyland-Jones, B. & Cheson, B.D. (1991) Fludarabine phosphate: a synthetic purine antimetabolite with significant activity against lymphoid malignancies. Journal of clinical oncology : *official journal of the American Society of Clinical Oncology.* 9(1), 175-88. Pub. Med. PMID: 1702143.

[44] Yin, W.; Karyagina, E.V.; Lundberg, A.S.; Greenblatt, D.J. & Lister-James, J. (2010) Pharmacokinetics, bioavailability and effects on electrocardiographic parameters of oral fludarabine phosphate. *Biopharmaceutics & drug disposition.* 31(1), 72-81. Pub. Med. PMID: 19862681.

[45] Stella, V. J.; Borchardt, R.T.; Hageman, M. J.; Oliyai, R.; Maag, H. & Tilley, Jw. editors. *Prodrugs: Challenges and rewards*. 2007 Vol. 5. New York, NY:: Springer.

[46] Schrama, D.; Reisfeld, R. A. & Becker, J. C. (2006) Antibody targeted drugs as cancer therapeutics. Nature reviews Drug discovery. 5(2), 147-59. PubMed PMID: 16424916.

[47] Mahato, R.; Tai, W. & Cheng, K. (2011) Prodrugs for improving tumor targetability and efficiency. *Advanced drug delivery reviews*. 63(8), 659-70. Pub. Med. PMID: 21333700. Pub. Med. Central PMCID: 3132824.

[48] Singh, Y.; Palombo, M. & Sinko, P.J. (2008) Recent trends in targeted anticancer prodrug and conjugate design. *Current medicinal chemistry*. 15(18), 1802-26. Pub. Med. PMID: 18691040. Pub. Med. Central PMCID: 2802226.

[49] Tyring, S. K.; Baker, D. & Snowden, W. (2002) Valacyclovir for herpes simplex virus infection: long-term safety and sustained efficacy after 20 years' experience with acyclovir. *The Journal of infectious diseases*. 186 Suppl 1, S40-6. Pub. Med. PMID: 12353186.

[50] Talluri, R. S.; Samanta, S.K.; Gaudana, R. & Mitra, A.K. (2008) Synthesis, metabolism and cellular permeability of enzymatically stable dipeptide prodrugs of acyclovir. *International journal of pharmaceutics*. 361(1-2), 118-24. Pub. Med. PMID: 18573320. Pubmed Central PMCID: 2556549.

[51] MacDougall, C. & Guglielmo, B.J. (2004) Pharmacokinetics of valaciclovir. The *Journal of antimicrobial chemotherapy*. 53(6), 899-901. Pub. Med. PMID: 15140857.

[52] Steingrimsdottir, H.; Gruber, A.; Palm, C.; Grimfors, G.; Kalin, M. & Eksborg, S. (2000) Bioavailability of aciclovir after oral administration of aciclovir and its prodrug valaciclovir to patients with leukopenia after chemotherapy. *Antimicrobial agents and chemotherapy*. 44(1), 207-9. PubMed PMID: 10602752. Pub. Med. Central PMCID: 89657.

[53] Gupta, S. V.; Gupta, D.; Sun, J.; Dahan, A.; Tsume, Y.; Hilfinger, J.;Lee, K. D. & Amidon, G.L. (2011) Enhancing the intestinal membrane permeability of zanamivir: a carrier mediated prodrug approach. *Mol. Pharm.* 8(6), 2358-67. Pub. Med. PMID: 21905667. Pubmed Central PMCID: 3304100.

[54] Park, E.J.; Amatya, S.; Kim, M.S.; Park, J.H.; Seol, E.; Lee, H.;Shin, Y.H.; Na, D.H.et al. (2013) Long-acting injectable formulations of antipsychotic drugs for the treatment of schizophrenia. *Archives of pharmacal research*. 36(6), 651-9. PubMed PMID: 23543652.

[55] Liu, K.S.; Tzeng, J.I.; Chen, Y.W.; Huang, K.L,.; Kuei, C.H. & Wang, J.J. (2006) Novel depots of buprenorphine prodrugs have a long-acting antinociceptive effect. *Anesthesia and analgesia*. 102(5), 1445-51. Pub. Med. PMID: 16632824.

[56] Platel, D.; Bonoron-Adele, S.; Dix, R. K. & Robert, J. (1999) Preclinical evaluation of the cardiac toxicity of HMR-1826, a novel prodrug of doxorubicin. *British journal of cancer.* 81(1), 24-7. PubMed PMID: 10487608. Pub. Med. Central PMCID: 2374342.

[57] Devalapally, H.; Rajan, K.S.; Akkinepally, R. R. & Devarakonda, R. K. (2008) Safety, pharmacokinetics and biodistribution studies of a beta-galactoside prodrug of doxorubicin for improvement of tumor selective chemotherapy. *Drug development and industrial pharmacy*. 34(8), 789-95. Pub. Med. PMID: 18608462.

[58] Harrelson, J.C. & Wong, Y.(1988) J. Species variation in the disposition of nalbuphine and its acetylsalicylate ester analogue. *Xenobiotica; the fate of foreign compounds in biological systems*. 18(11), 1239-47. Pub. Med. PMID: 3245223.

[59] Elger, W.; Barth, A.; Hedden, A.; Reddersen, G.; Ritter, P.; Schneider, B.;Züchner, J.; Krahl, E.; Müller, K.; Oettel, M. & Schwarz, S. (2001) Estrogen sulfamates: a new approach to oral estrogen therapy. *Reproduction, fertility, and development.* 13(4), 297-305. PubMed PMID: 11800168.

[60] Douroumis, D. (2007). Practical approaches of taste masking technologies in oral solid forms. *Expert opinion on drug delivery* 4(4), 417-26. Pub. Med. PMID: 17683254.

[61] Hejaz, H.; Karaman, R. & Khamis, M. (2012) Computer-assisted design for paracetamol masking bitter taste prodrugs. *Journal of molecular modeling* 18(1), 103-14. PubMed PMID: 21491187.

[62] Karaman, R. (2013) Prodrugs for masking bitter taste of antibacterial drugs-a computational approach. *Journal of molecular modeling* 19(6), 2399-412. Pub. Med. PMID: 23420399.

[63] Davies, G. E.; Driver, G. W.; Hoggarth, E.; Martin, AR.; Paige, M. F.; Rose, F. L. & Wilson, B. R. (1956) Studies in the chemotherapy of tuberculosis: ethyl mercaptan and related compounds. *British journal of pharmacology and chemotherapy.* 11(4), 351-6. PubMed PMID: 13383112. Pub. Med. Central PMCID: 1510553.

[64] Davies, G. E. & Driver, G. W. (1957) The antituberculous activity of ethyl thiolesters with particular reference to diethyl dithiolisophthalate. *British journal of pharmacology and chemotherapy.* 12(4), 434-7. Pub. Med. PMID: 13489170. Pub. Med. Central PMCID: 1510584.

[65] Spengler, R. F.; Arrowsmith, J. B.; Kilarski, D. J.; Buchanan, C.; Von Behren, L. & Graham, D. R. (1988) Severe soft-tissue injury following intravenous infusion of phenytoin. Patient and drug administration risk factors. *Archives of internal medicine.* 148(6), 1329-33. Pub. Med. PMID: 3377616.

[66] Boucher, B. A. Fosphenytoin: a novel phenytoin prodrug. *Pharmacotherapy.* 1996 Sep-Oct;16(5):777-91. Pub. Med. PMID: 8888074.

[67] Wang, H.; Cork, R. & Rao, A. (2007) Development of a new generation of propofol. *Current opinion in anaesthesiology.* 20(4), 311-5. Pub. Med. PMID: 17620837.

[68] Fechner, J.; Ihmsen, H.; Jeleazcov, C. & Schuttler, J. (2009) Fospropofol disodium, a water-soluble prodrug of the intravenous anesthetic propofol (2,6-diisopropylphenol). *Expert opinion on investigational drugs.* 18(10), 1565-71. Pub. Med. PMID: 19758110.

[69] Karaman, R. (2013) Prodrugs design based on inter- and intramolecular processes. *Chem. Biol. Drug. Des. 82*, 643–668.

In: Prodrugs Design – A New Era
Editor: Rafik Karaman

ISBN: 978-1-63117-701-9
© 2014 Nova Science Publishers, Inc.

Chapter III

Chemical Approaches Used in Prodrugs Design

*Beesan Fattash[1] and Rafik Karaman[1,2]**

[1] Pharmaceutical Sciences Department, Faculty of Pharmacy,
Al-Quds University, Jerusalem, Palestine.
[2] Department of Science, University of Basilicata, Potenza, Italy

Abstract

Generally, prodrugs are designed to improve aqueous solubility, to enhance permeability through lipophilicity modification, to achieve site specific delivery and to increase GI absorption through targeting specific transporters and enzymes, and to improve taste, odor and other pharmaceutical and pharmacokinetic properties.

Accordingly, it would be noteworthy to describe the chemistry of prodrugs, in particular various chemical approaches employed to address deficiencies of existing drugs which represent the main focus of this chapter. Moreover, the possibility and suitability of exploiting a number of functional groups like carboxyl, hydroxyl, amine, phosphate/phosphonate and carbonyl groups for undergoing different chemical modifications will be highlighted. In addition, a detailed discussion of the major strategies utilized in prodrug design will be presented along with various prodrug examples that were implemented in clinical practice.

Keywords: Prodrugs, Chemical modifications, Pharmacokinetic and pharmaceutical barriers, Permeability, Lipophilicity.

---

* Corresponding author: Rafik Karaman, e-mail: dr_karaman@yahoo.com; Tel and Fax +972-2-2790413.

List of Abbreviations

ADME	absorption, distribution, excretion, and metabolism.
GIT	Gastro Intestinal Tract.
BBB	Blood Brain Barrier.
POM	Phosphono Oxy Methyl
ACEIs	Angiotensin Converting Enzyme inhibitors.
5-FU	5- Fluorouracil.
HPMPC	(S)-1-(3-Hydroxy-2-phosphonylmethoxypropyl) cytosine.
LPC	Lysophosphatidylcholine
RBCs	Red Blood Cells.
GABA	γ-aminobutyric acid

Introduction

In the past few decades, the pharmaceutical sciences have been subjected to considerable alterations [1-3] in terms of improving drug drawbacks that are related to pharmacokinetic (absorption, distribution, excretion, and metabolism (ADME)) pharmaceutical and biological performance of existing drugs which may hinder drug development process [4].

Overcoming the undesirable physicochemical, biological and organoleptic properties of some existing drugs [1-3], can be achieved through the development of new chemical entities with desirable efficacy and safety. However, this is an expensive and time consuming process that needs a screening of thousands of molecules for biological activity [5]. Therefore, it becomes much more feasible to modify and improve the properties of already existing drugs through exploring the prodrug approach [5]. This is in order to overcome their undesirable properties and increase their commercial life cycle and patentability [4]. The prodrug approach is a promising and well established strategy for the development of new entities that possess superior efficacy, selectivity and reduced toxicity. Hence an optimized therapeutic outcome can be accomplished [5].

Approximately, 10% of all worldwide marketed medicines can be categorized as prodrugs, and in 2008 alone, 33% of all approved small-molecular weight drugs were prodrugs [4]. This data clearly indicates the success of the prodrug approach [4].

To emphasize the significance of this approach, a comprehensive overview of chemical strategies employed to produce a variety of prodrugs that serve to minimize different drawbacks associated with important drugs, is highlighted throughout this chapter.

Prodrugs of Carboxylic Acid and Hydroxyl Functional Groups...Esters

The major direction in prodrug research is toward developing ester prodrugs. This is attributed to their acceptable in vitro chemical stability, consequently lower formulation problems, along with their susceptibility to the action of esterases that are distributed throughout the body, which allows subsequent elaboration of the active drug once it exposes to physiological environments within the body (Figure 1) [7].

Figure 1. Schematic representation for an interconversion of ester prodrug to its parent drug, carboxylic acid.

Ester prodrugs are commonly used to enhance lipophilicity, thus increasing membrane permeation through masking the charge of polar functional groups [8], and the alkyl chain length and configuration (Figure 2) [4].

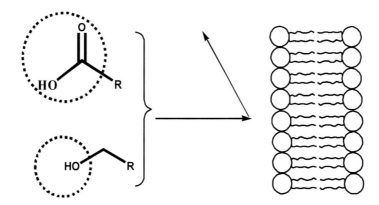

Figure 2. Schematic representation for a membrane barrier that inhibits penetration of carboxylic acid and hydroxyl functional groups.

Carboxylic acids, alcohols and phenols are common functional groups that can be modified into ester based prodrugs. This topic will be covered in the following sections which concentrate on ester based prodrugs of the previously mentioned functional groups.

Ester Prodrugs of Carboxylic Acids - Alkyl Esters

Methyl, ethyl, isopropyl and n-butyl esters are frequently used in the prodrug approach. The usefulness of these moieties arises from their unique characteristics; such that the overall features that will be offered for prodrugs are distinctive and based on the alkyl chain utilized.

Furthermore, each moiety represents an attractive option in addressing certain requirements for certain drugs.

Methyl esters are usually used in drugs that are given in low doses, as being an important group required for activity or needed for slow interconversion to the corresponding carboxylic acid [9].

Prostaglandins like misoprostol (cytotic) represent an example of methyl esters of carboxylic acids (Figure 3). Prostaglandins are commonly derivatized into simple esters due to the fact that their pharmacokinetics is metabolism dependent, and alkyl derivatization is not expected to have any effect upon their exposure to metabolism [9].

Levomet, a methyl ester of L-dopa is another example, which is the only alkyl ester that has reached the market after many attempts to develop other alkyl esters [10].

Figure 3. Chemical structure of misoprostol; a methyl ester derivative of carboxylic acid.

It is worthy to note, that methyl esters are ideal for certain drugs and they are not commonly used as prodrugs promoities due to the toxicity associated with methanol that is released upon cleavage of the prodrug ester bond once the prodrug is exposed to the body esterases (Figure 4). It was shown that methanol toxicity is due to its secondary metabolites; formaldehyde and formic acid that cause acidosis and blindness [11]. Although, it is reported that quite high methanol concentration is needed to reveal to this toxicity [9].

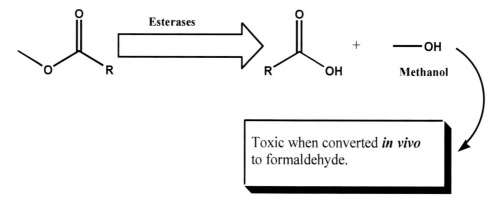

Figure 4. Schematic representation for the conversion of methyl esters into methanol and formaldehyde.

In contrast to methyl esters, ethyl esters are more commonly used as prodrug moieties. This is mainly due to the low levels of ethanol liberated upon cleavage of ester bond and consequently toxicity concerns are not quite significant.

As mentioned before, ester prodrugs are generally exploited in order to offer increased lipophilicity to the parent drug; hence an increased intestinal absorption can be achieved. Ethyl esters are employed to obtain prodrugs with these characteristics. The ethyl ester prodrug, oseltamivir; an anti-influenza (anti-viral) agent has an oral bioavailability of nearly 80%, which represents a significant improvement over the bioavailability of the parent compound which is nearly 5% [12]. In clinical practice this improvement in bioavailability enables oral administration of oseltamivir. This is contrary to the more polar antiviral zanamivir which is administered via the nasal route.

Additional example is ximelagatran, an ethyl ester prodrug of melagatran which acts as thrombin inhibitor (Figure 5). Studies have showed that an 80-fold increase in permeability in caco 2 cells was achieved with this prodrug compared with the active drug melagatran. In addition, the studies revealed that the bioavailability of ximelagatran is 20% in man which represents 2.7 to 5.5-fold increase in bioavailability over its parent drug, melagatran [9].

Oseltamevir

Melgatran

Ximalgatran

Figure 5. Chemical structures of oseltamevir, melgatran and ximalgatran.

Further, utilizing PEPT1 intestinal transport system has been achieved by utilizing ethyl ester prodrugs. Using PEPT1 aids in achieving a higher absorption rate as a result of an increase in lipophilicity and passive absorption process [13]. Angiotensin converting enzymes (ACE) inhibitors are examples of ethyl ester prodrugs that are substrates of PEPT1.

A significant part of ACE inhibitor drugs have two carboxylic acid groups, however, they are derivatized into mono esters and not into diesters. This can mainly be related to the following reasons:

1) To maintain the hydrophilic/lipophilic balance required for optimum absorption [9] and

2) To exploit the PEPT1 transport system through developing substrates suitable for these transporters. Illustrative examples of ACE inhibitors are shown in Figure 6.

It is worth noting, that for the ACE inhibitors mentioned above to be successful in achieving the desired bioavailability, a complete evaluation of their carboxylic acid prodrugs for lipophilicity, solubility and their active transport systems is a mandatory step [9].

Imidapril

Moexipril.

Figure 6. Chemical structures of imidapril and moexipril.

The main idea that is described earlier and is presented afterward is that drug characteristics are modified in a certain way utilizing specific moieties for achieving optimum pharmacokinetic properties. Isopropyl esters offer the best pharmacokinetic characteristics for a number of prostaglandins that are intended for the use in ocular application, especially in animal models [9]. Latanoprost and travoprost (Figure 7) are representatives of isopropyl ester prodrugs. Further, aryl esters such as carbenicillin, carfecillin (phenyl ester) and carindacillin (indanyl ester) exhibit an improved oral bioavailability (Figure 8) [14].

Latanoprost

Travoprost

Figure 7. Chemical structures of latanoprost and travoprost.

Chemical Approaches Used in Prodrugs Design 109

Carbenicillin

Carfecillin

Cardinacillin

Figure 8. Chemical structures of carbenicillin, carfecillin and cardinacillin.

Another class of carboxylic acid ester prodrugs is the acyloxy and alkyl or [(alkoxycarbonyl) oxy] methyl esters. Practically, there is no difference between acyloxy and alkyl [(alkoxycarbonyl) oxy] methyl esters, since both are cleaved in vivo in an efficient manner [9]. Acyloxyalkyl esters of benzyl penicillin undergo rapid enzymatic transformation into their antibacterial active drugs due to the spacing provided by the acyloxycarbonyl linker [15]. In contrast, alkyl ester prodrugs of other β-lactams are slowly interconverted into their active drugs due to the crowding surroundings the carbonyl group in these compounds (Figure 9) [9].

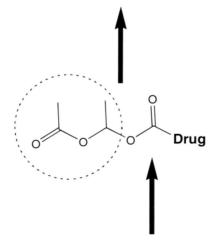

Figure 9. Schematic representation illustrating the minimized steric hindrance around the carbonyl group provided by the acyloxymethyl ester moiety.

Figure 10. Sultamicillin; a mutual prodrug of ampicillin and sulbactam.

Sultamicillin is another example of this class in which the irreversible β-lactamase inhibitor, sulbactam, has joined chemically via ester linkage with an ampicillin molecule to obtain a mutual prodrug. This mutual prodrug possesses a synergistic effect [16] and upon oral administration, sultamicillin is completely hydrolyzed to equimolar proportions of sulbactam and ampicillin, thereby acting as an efficient mutual prodrug (Figure 10) [17].

Oxodioxolyl methyl esters group is another example of ester prodrug, a representative example for this group is lenampicillin [18] and the ACE inhibitor olmesartan medoxomil (Benicar) [19].

It was demonstrated that this class of prodrugs exhibit chemical and enzymatic instability; ester hydrolysis takes place upon addition of water or a base, as well it was observed that in vivo hydrolysis of lenampicilline in plasma is mainly performed via the action of paraoxonase [9].

As mentioned before, carboxylic acid group can be modified into several ester derivatives. However, these modifications are not only restricted to drugs that bear carboxylic acid group. Hydroxyl group is also amenable to be manipulated in order to circumvent pharmaceutical and pharmacokinetic barriers; nevertheless carboxylic acid esters are more clinically successful. This can be as a result of masking the more polar carboxylic acid group which by its own serve to solve problems associated with parent drugs. Despite this fact, a group of esters by which the alkoxide is aliphatic or aromatic are clinically applied.

Increasing lipophilicity and thus permeation as well as tumor targeting are the main objectives of hydroxyl group modifications [20].

Dipivefrine, dipivalyl acid diester of epinephrine, intended for the treatment of high ocular pressure, is 600 times more lipophilic than epinephrine because it incorporates a substituted acyl group; the tri methyl ester pivallic acid, which offers higher lipophilicity and enzymatic stability than epinephrine [21]. Thus, systemic levels of epinephrine are reduced since lower doses of dipiverfine are administered due to enhanced penetration achieved by this strategy. However, the application of pivallic acid as an ester promoiety in other prodrug strategies seems to be not preferable. For instance, the O-pivaloyl ester of the ß-blocker oxprenolol is not suitable for ocular application due to its high stability (t $_{1/2}$ 700 minutes) [22]. Furthermore, long chain acyl esters can be utilized to increase lipophilicity of certain drugs as in the case of the antipsychotic agents, haloperidol and fluphenazine (Figure 11). A deaconate ester of haloperidol is prepared and dissolved in sesame oil to produce a prodrug intended for sustained release of haloperidol [23]; hence, aiding to overcome the low patient compliance associated with the use of haloperidol for long periods in psychiatric patients, the apparent t $_{1/2}$ of this pro drug is 3 weeks [20]. On the other hand, sesame oil solutions of the enthanate and deconate fluphenazine ester prodrugs intended to be used for the same purposes as haloperidol decanoate were synthesized and studied. The enthanate ester has an apparent t $_{1/2}$ of 3-4 days while for decanoate ester the t $_{1/2}$ value was in the range 6 -10 days [24].

haloperidol

Figure 11. Chemical structure of haloperidol.

It should be noted, that the prolonged elimination half-life is associated with increased plasma and tissue protein binding which is a direct consequence of the increased lipophilicity, which reduces enzymatic elimination and thus increasing the $t_{1/2}$ value [20].

Enhancement of aqueous solubility is a main requirement for a group of drugs as enhancing lipophilicity is an obligation for others. For instance, ionizable acyl ester promoieties are exploited to increase aqueous solubility of chloramphenicol, hydrocortisone and propranolol [25, 26]. Furthermore, increasing water solubility of poorly soluble drugs is not restricted to conjugating ionizable acyl group to a hydroxyl group but also this can be achieved by joining ionizable amino groups and phosphate group to generate amino acid esters and phosphate esters, respectively. These aspects will be discussed briefly in the following sections.

Amino Acid Esters of Hydroxyl Group

Eighteen amino acid esters of acyclovir were synthesized as potential prodrugs intended for oral administration and the hydrolytic activation of these prodrugs was shown to be catalyzed by biphenyl hydrolase; an enzyme exists in epithelial cells [27]. Valacyclovir hydrochloride is the L-valyl amino acid ester of the anti-viral agent acyclovir [28]. The L-valine promoiety severs two purposes: (i) enhanced chemical stability at physiological pH of the prodrug, which is vital to allow for long term storage and (ii) provides an acceptable hydrophilic lipophilicity balance that is essential to achieve a desirable blood levels of acyclovir after oral administration, this is actually attained by valacyclovir [18]. An enhancement of 3-10 fold in oral bioavailability is achieved utilizing this promoiety compared to that of the parent drug, acyclovir. This is corresponding to 54% of absolute acyclovir [29], after its liberation by an extensive enzymatic hydrolysis in the blood [30].

Valganciclovir is the l-valyl ester of gancyclovir [31] offers an increased oral bioavailability of gancyclovir up to 60% [32]. Actually, it produces gancyclovir levels equivalent to the IV administered dose. This improvement is also achieved by valacyclovir (Figure 12) [29].

It was reported that PEPT 1 transport system plays an important role in increasing bioavailability of both acyclovir and gancyclovir. The prodrugs act as substrates for these transporters and as a result of the interaction between the prodrugs and the PEPT 1 transport system, high systemic levels of the parent drugs are achieved after biotransformation [33].

Phosphate Ester Prodrugs of Hydroxyl Group

In phosphate ester prodrugs, the phosphate group is either directly connected to the hydroxyl group to produce phospho-monoester or indirectly via a linker (Figure 13). Phosphate ester prodrugs strategy is a beneficial approach in terms of circumventing poor aqueous solubility of poorly soluble drugs. In addition, phosphate prodrugs are relatively stable when are formulated, however, upon being subjected they undergo extensive in vivo conversion into their parent drugs through the action of alkaline phosphatases; an abundant enzymes in human body (Figure 13) [34].

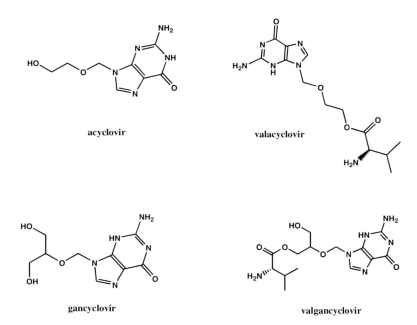

Figure 12. Chemical structures of acyclovir, valacyclovir, gancyclovir and valganciclovir.

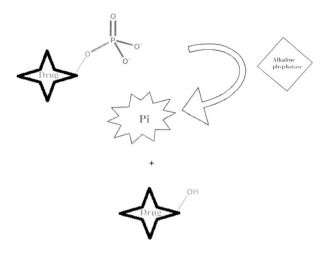

Figure 13. Interconversion of phosphate prodrugs into their hydroxyl active drugs and inorganic phosphate.

Upon parenteral administration of clindamycin, an extremely irritating sensation at the injection site takes place [35]. However, administration of clindamycin phosphate ester prodrug overcomes this concern due to improved aqueous solubility with subsequent in vivo efficient release of clindamycin (Figure 14) [36]. Consequently, clindamycin phosphate was approved for parenteral and topical application [37].

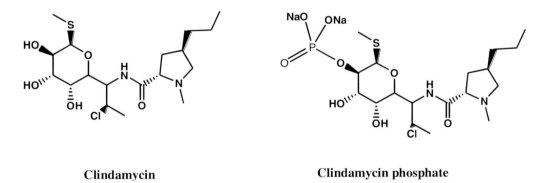

Figure 14. Chemical structures of clindamycin and clindamycin phosphate.

Another example of such approach is the broad spectrum antifungal agent fluconazole (Figure 15) [38]. The phosphate ester derivative, fosfluconazole, allows the administration of small volume, concentrated infusions to the patients, thus the required steady-state concentration can be reached within a short time (Figure 15) [20].

fluconazole   **fosfluconazole**

Figure 15. Chemical structures of fluconazole and fosfluconazole.

Another commonly used phosphate prodrug is fosamprenavir, a phosphate ester prodrug of the HIV protease inhibitor, amprinavir. The phosphate promoiety is linked to a free hydroxyl group and is 10-fold more water soluble than amprinavir. An enhanced patient compliance is achieved by the use of this antiviral prodrug since dosage regimen is reduced to only twice daily [39] compared to its parent drug which is given 8 times daily. Once reaches the gut and via the action of alkaline phosphatases, this prodrug is cleaved back to the corresponding active drug and then absorbed into the systemic circulation [4].

Another application of this approach is fosphnytoin a prodrug of the anticonvulsant agent phenytoin. Fosphenytoin has an enhanced solubility over the corresponding drug. The utility of this strategy can be exploited to drugs that don't contain hydroxyl groups [40].

It should be indicated that phosphomonoester prodrug approach is applicable to aromatic alcohols (phenols) as well as aliphatic alcohols [41]. For instance, etoposide (Figure 16) a podophyllotoxin antineoplastic agent [42] suffers from low chemical stability and insufficient aqueous solubility [43] which results in drug precipitation upon dilution and injection. Therefore, the phosphorylation of the phenolic hydroxyl was a practical solution to enhance water solubility and thus minimizing the probability of precipitation upon injection. Then in the systemic circulation a rapid cleavage of etoposide phosphate into etoposide takes place [44].

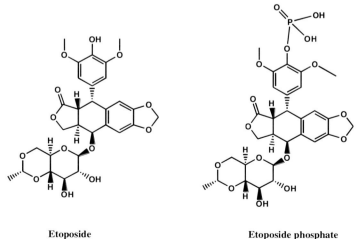

Etoposide   Etoposide phosphate

Figure 16. Chemical structures of etoposide and etoposide phosphate.

As was previously mentioned in this section a rapid hydrolysis of the phosphate ester linkage is required to liberate the hydroxyl-parent drug and an inorganic phosphate group. However, phosphomonoesters of secondary and tertiary alcohols undergo a slow conversion rate which is due to the existence of steric hindrance at the cleavage site which in turn impedes the catalytic efficiency of the enzyme [45]. This obstacle was eliminated by attaching the phosphate group to the hydroxyl group via a chemical linker thus separating the phosphate group away from the crowding site and hence facilitating the enzyme catalytic action. Such examples include phosphonooxymethyl (POM) prodrugs containing a methylene linker. These prodrugs undergo an initial dephosphorylation followed by cleavage of the hemiester intermediate to liberate the parent drug [20].

The benefits of phosphate prodrugs stem from improved aqueous solubility of the parent drugs via linking the phosphate moiety to a hydroxyl group in order to yield a phosphate ester prodrug with high chemical stability and rapid in vivo hydrolysis [46].

Carbamates Ester Prodrugs

Carbamate esters (Figure 17) are esters of carbamic acid and are usually designed to enhance metabolic stability of alcohols and phenols. In general, carbamate prodrugs are converted back to their parent drugs by chemical or enzymatic hydrolysis.

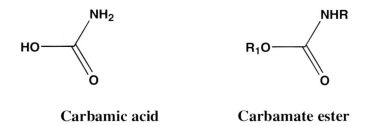

Figure 17. Chemical structures of carbamic acid and carbamate ester.

Carbamate esters of alcohols and phenols are available. However, the carbamate esters of alcohols offer very high stability and a few examples for such class are in clinical use [20], while phenolic carbamates are more clinically applicable. This can be attributed to the fact that the degree of substitution on the carbamate ester nitrogen can be controlled and this offers a different degree of stability to phenolic carbamate prodrugs. For example, prodrugs of two dopaminergic 7-hydroxy [5] benzazepines, exhibit different stability depending on N-substitution. The N-monosubstituted carbamate shows extremely low enzymatic and chemical stability [47] while the N, N-disubstitueted exhibits high enzymatic and chemical stability which is desirable in the case of dopaminergic 7-hydroxy benzazepines to provide the required protection against first pass metabolism upon oral administration [20].

An example that illustrates the benefit of using carbamate esters to enhance metabolic stability which then can be translated into prolonged pharmacologic action of the parent drug is bambuterol, a bis-dimethyl carbamate prodrug of the β2-adrenoreceptor agonist, terbutaline, used in asthma control. Bambuterol is slowly hydrolyzed by buteryl cholinesterase, an enzyme present in human plasma, to yield monocarbamate which further undergoes hydrolytic cleavage to furnish terbutaline (Figure 18) [48].

The catalytic activity of buteryl cholinesterase has shown to be slowed down once the binding of carbamate group to the serine residue in the enzyme's active site is taking place [49]. This drop in catalysis is attributed to a slow recovery of the enzyme's activity which happens after 2 days, consequently a slow release of terbutaline occurs, and hence a sustained release and reduced dosing frequency of the active drug are achieved [50].

Bambuterol   **terbutaline**

Figure 18. Enzymatic cleavage of bambuterol to terbuline.

Sulfamate Ester Prodrugs

The metabolic instability of natural or synthetic estrogens is worth considering because the conjugation of sulfamic acid to the metabolically labile hydroxyl group of estrogens to yield estrogenic prodrugs has the potential to achieve a superior efficiency for these contraceptive agents. An improved systemic levels is attained which leads to improved estrogenic activity [51].

The conversion of estrogen prodrugs into their parent estrogen takes place at the membrane of the red blood cells (RBCs). This is because a preferential uptake of these prodrugs into RBCs due to the high affinity to carbonic anhydrase an enzyme presents in RBCs [52].

Aryl Esters

Aromatic esters or aryl esters are among the preferred promoieties in prodrug approaches because the hydrolysis rate is controlled by the substitution on the aromatic ring [20]. For instance, a number of substituted and unsubstituted benzoate esters of timolol were assessed for ocular application [53]. A great variation in both enzymatic and chemical stability among different prodrugs was reported, and this can be related to electronic and steric effects arise from different substituents. It was concluded from different studies that electron withdrawing or electron donating substituents affect the hydrolysis rate of ester bond and these variations found to be practically beneficial in clinical applications, in terms of generating prodrugs with particular hydrolytic rate to meet specific clinical needs [20].

N-acyl derivatives, Carbamates, N-Oxides and Others Prodrugs of Amines

Another common functional group amenable to chemical alteration is the amine group.

The Amine group is differentiated by two main properties; basicity and nucleophilicity. Basicity is a physicochemical property related to the ability of amines to accept protons according to Bronsted-Lowrey definition of acids and bases [54], while nucleophilicity is a property related to chemical reactivity of amines and hence chemical stability of amine containing drugs. The former is directly related to the ability of amines to cross biological membranes at physiological pH due to the fact that amines can exist in ionized and non-ionized forms corresponding to protonated and non-protonated forms, respectively. Accordingly, amine prodrugs are intended either to improve membrane permeation through enhancing lipophilicity, or enhancing water solubility. Obviously the intended goal can be achieved through proper selection of the promoiety. Additionally, amine prodrugs are also considered to improve chemical and metabolic stability of their corresponding drugs [55] in particular those that undergo intramolecular aminolysis. Further, site targeted delivery is one of the intended goals of developing amine prodrugs [54].

To ensure the importance of selecting a suitable promoiety that aids in alteration of the undesirable physicochemical properties of amines, and hence overcoming barriers associated with the use of these therapeutically active drugs, a number of amine prodrugs examples are introduced in the following sections.

Amides

Amides are derivatives (Figure 19) that result from simple acylation of amines, thus they are classified as N- acyl derivatives. Amides are characterized by their high chemical and enzymatic stability. This feature can be exploited to acquire a sustained release system of drugs from their prodrugs. This concept was applicable for phenylethylamine and dopamine [56].

Amide Group

Figure 19. Chemical structure for amides.

It is believed that amine containing drugs experience inadequate penetration into the blood brain barrier (BBB) due to their ionization at physiological pH. Therefore, efforts were made in an attempt to solve permeability for these concerned drugs. It was found that linking amine drugs to dihydropyridine generates prodrugs containing an amide linkage which possess the following characteristics:

1) Enhanced BBB permeability.
2) Targeted delivery to the CNS, since the prodrugs are entrapped inside the BBB after their oxidation via CNS specific enzymes such that their redistribution out of CNS is not allowed (Figure 20).
3) Sustained release of the active parent amines due to the slow hydrolytic rate of their amide prodrugs [56].

On the other hand, in most situations the slow hydrolysis is not required. Instead, a fast conversion into the parent drug is needed. Two main strategies are utilized to accelerate hydrolytic rate. The first is the exploitation of peptidases and the second is utilizing intramolecular cyclization strategy.

Amide prodrugs can be converted back to the parent drugs either by non-specific amidases or specific enzymatic activation such as renal γ-glutamyl transpeptidase [57]. The dopamine double prodrug; γ-glutamyl-L-dopa (gludopa) undergoes specific activation by renal γ-glutamyl transpeptidase. It achieves relatively 5-fold increase in dopamine level in the kidney compared to L-dopa prodrug. However, because gludopa has low oral bioavailability [57], docarpamine, [N-(N-acetyl-L-methionyl)-O, O-bis (ethoxycarbonyl) dopamine), a pseudopeptide prodrug of dopamine (Figure 21) was developed and showed improved oral absorption, thus it is given by the oral route and is used in the treatment of renal and cardiovascular diseases. Basically, dopamine prodrugs are developed to overcome inactivation by COMT and MAO enzymes when they are administered orally [58].

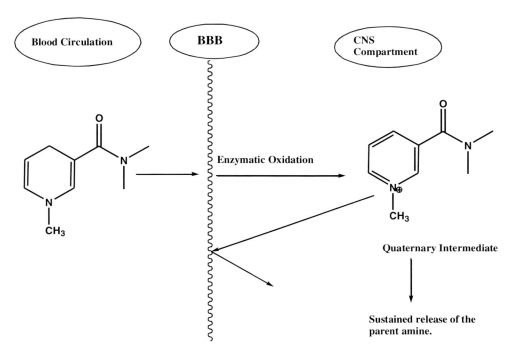

Figure 20. Targeted delivery of amide containing prodrugs to the CNS.

Dopamine

Docarpamine

Figure 21. Chemical structures of dopamine and docarpamine, respectively.

Several amine conjugates with amino acids via amide bonds that are subjected to peptidase catalyzed hydrolysis have been remarkably considered especially due to their high solubility like dapsone [59].

Amine conjugation with L- or D-amino acid exhibits different stability. D-amino acid has a half-life of 30-60 minutes, while that of the L-isomer is less than 2 minutes. This data suggest that the peptidase responsible for the amide hydrolysis is stereo-selective. Another explanation of this observation is that multiple enzymes are responsible for catalyzing the cleavage of the different prodrug isoforms [59].

The second approach used to accelerate hydrolysis involves the design of promoieties capable for undergoing intramolecular cyclization, as depicted in Figure 22.

Figure 22. Intramolecular cyclization reaction of amide prodrugs.

Carbamate Derivatives of Amines

Carbamates are prodrugs of carboxylic acids and amines [60]. Carbamates has no specific enzymes for their hydrolysis, however they are degraded by esterases to generate their parent drugs [45]. Co-carboxy methyl phenyl ester of amphetamine is an example of carbamate prodrug of amphetamine that can be hydrolyzed by esterases [45]. Generally carbamates are more stable than esters but less stable than amides [60]. Although simple carbamic acid derivatives show high instability, their esters are much more stable and consequently they are clinically used [54].

Carbamates are considered to be double prodrugs (pro-prodrug) since they are first being enzymatically activated followed by spontaneous cleavage of the resulted carbamic acid, as shown in the case of capecitabine, an anticancer prodrug of 5-FU that undergoes a multistep activation (Figure 23). The first activation is accomplished by liver carboxyl esterase then followed by subsequent transformation into 5-FU which is catalyzed by cytidine deaminase and thymidine phosphorylase (Figure 23). The former enzyme is present in plasma while the latter is highly expressed in tumor cells and allows for selective production of 5-FU in tumor cells. Capecitabine is less toxic than 5-FU, more selective and is widely used in clinical practice [61].

N-acyloxy Derivatives

Acyloxyalkyl carbamates (Figure 24) are known to be appropriate as promoities for drugs containing an acidic amino group with the aim of enhancing their delivery [54].

For example, acyloxyalkyl carbamates such as the hydrophilic ß-blockers show an increase in skin and corneal permeability [62]. Furthermore, acyloxyalkyl carbamate prodrugs were used to mask the bitter sensation of the antibacterial agent, norfloxacin [63].

It is well known that amines are classified as primary, secondary or tertiary amines. Studies demonstrated that derivatizing primary and secondary amines using acyloxyalkyl promoiety yields highly unstable prodrugs, while prodrugs of tertiary amines have a relatively high enzymatic stability. This can be related to the fact that derivatizing tertiary amines using acyloxyalkyl moiety actually generates quaternary ammonium compounds that are known to exhibit stability and at the same time undergo *in vivo* hydrolysis.

Figure 23. Schematic representation of the conversion of capecitabine into 5-FU.

Figure 24. A chemical structure of N-acyloxyalkyl carbamates.

An additional advantage offered by the resultant quaternary ammonium compounds (as a result of tertiary amines modifications) is that these compounds are ionized at all pH values; therefore, the main goal that is accomplished here is to increase water solubility of tertiary amines (Figure 25) [54], such as the N- acyl oxyalkyl derivatives, antagonists of the platelet activating factor, that were developed for enhancing water solubility of the corresponding parent amines [64].

Figure 25. Chemical structure of quaternary ammonium acyloxyalkyl amines.

N- Oxides

N- Oxides are among the bio-reductive prodrug strategies that explore a low oxygen environment linked with tumor cells (hypoxia). Tirapazamine (Figure 26) is an anti-cancer prodrug that undergoes tumor specific activation where NADPH cytochrome P450 reductase enzyme catalyzes the formation of the cytotoxic nitroxide through one electron reduction process [65] which in turn results in the formation of high levels of radicals around the DNA area to cause DNA strands destruction [66].

Figure 26. Chemical structure of tirapazamine.

Another anticancer agent is AQ4N, an aliphatic N-Oxide that undergoes tumor specific reduction to yield its parent active drug, a tertiary amine which inhibits DNA topoisomerase II resulting in strong DNA binding (cancer cells killer) [67].

N-Mannich Bases

N- Mannich base formation is another approach used to manipulate amine group containing drugs. N-Mannich bases (Figure 27) are prepared by Mannich reaction that includes NH-acidic compound, an aldehyde and an amine in ethanol [68]. This approach can be utilized to enhance solubility and to improve membrane permeation.

Figure 27. Chemical structure of N-Mannich base.

Rolitetracycline is a Mannich derivative of tetracycline, and it is the only prodrug available for intravenous administration (Figure 28) [69]. Another example is the N-Mannich base of dipyrone (metamizole) the methane sulfonic acid of the analgesic 4-(methylamino) antipyrine, is more water soluble than its active drug, antipyrine, and is suitable for parenteral and oral use. When it is given orally it undergoes hydrolysis in the stomach to provide its active form [10].

Figure 28. Chemical structure of rolitetracyclin.

Moreover, N-Mannich bases are developed in order to enhance permeability through membranes. This is believed to be due to a drop in the pK_a value caused by the amine derivatization in general and by N- Mannich bases in particular [70]. Hence, the ionization of N-Mannich prodrugs at physiological pH will be much lower than that of their corresponding amines.

In addition, the advantages of N-Mannich bases over their corresponding amines are their ability to minimize the N acylation of their parent active amines that can take place pre-systemically. On the other hand, N-Mannich bases suffer from stability/formulation problems that arise from poor in vitro stability [69]; this is in addition to the undesired formation of formaldehyde upon their cleavage [68].

On the other hand, a study conducted by Cogan and coworkers [71] on anthracycline N-Mannich prodrugs has showed that formaldehyde has a clinical advantage when it is released near DNA encouraging covalent binding of chemotherapeutic agents with DNA in cancer cells [72].

Schiff Bases

Schiff bases, imines (Figure 29) are considered to be more lipophilic than their parent drugs.

Figure 29. Chemical structure for Schiff base.

Progabide (Figure 30), an anticonvulsant agent, is a prodrug of γ-aminobutyric acid (GABA). Progabide is developed to improve the poor BBB permeability associated with GABA. The prodrug is converted back to GABA after crossing BBB due to its improved lipophilic character. Nevertheless, progabide can't be considered as a prodrug because it possesses intrinsic activity [60]. Another example of Schiff prodrugs is the histamine derivative (R)-α–methylhistamine, an H3-receptor agonist, which has poor CNS penetration ability. The diaryl and benzaryl imines prodrugs show satisfactory stability and improved CNS delivery [73].

Figure 30. Chemical structure of progabide.

Enamines and Enaminones

Enamines (α, β-unsaturated amines) [74], are unstable at low pH, therefore, they are unsuitable for oral administration [68]. Nonetheless, an ampicillin prodrug was prepared for rectal use and it exhibits an increased absorption [75].

Enaminones (Figure 31) are enamines of β-dicarbonyl compounds that undergo keto-enol and imine-enamine tautomeric equilibriums which may offer stability to these compounds [10].

Figure 31. Chemical structure for enaminone.

Enaminones are generally more lipophilic than their parent drugs; hence they have an improved oral absorption. Typically, enaminones have high chemical stability which results in a limitation for their use as potential prodrugs. It is expected that enaminones derived from ketoesters and lactone may be subjected to enzymatic degradation hence a better conversion rate to the active drug can be obtained [76].

Furthermore, the usefulness of enaminones in reducing the nucleophilicity of amines is exemplified by acetyl acetone, a prodrug of cycloserine, in which a nucleophilic dimerization that occurs in solid and concentrated solutions of cycloserine is prevented in the case of the acetyl acetone prodrug [77].

Azo Compounds

Colonic bacteria have been exploited in the prodrug approach as means of prodrugs activation through the action of azo reductases (Figure 32). This approach is particularly applied in targeted drug release [69].

Generally, this approach is usually limited to aromatic amines, since azo compounds of aliphatic amines exhibit instability [68].

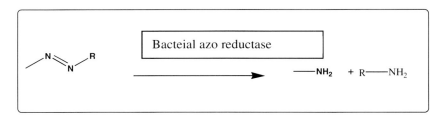

Figure 32. Conversion of an azo bond via the action of bacterial reductases.

Sulfasalazine (Figure 33) used in the treatment of ulcerative colitis [78] is a prodrug of 5-aminosalycilic acid and sulfapyridine. Upon reaching the colon, sulfasalazine undergoes a cleavage of the azo bond to release the two active moieties [16].

Figure 33. Chemical structure of sulfasalazine.

In addition, illustrative examples of prodrugs that are activated by azo reductases are osalazine, a dimer of 5-aminosalycilic acid, balsalazide and ipsalazide, in which 5-aminosalicylic acid moiety is conjugated to 4-aminobenzoyl-β-alanine and 4-aminobenzoylglycine, respectively [79].

Oxazolidines and 4- Imidazolidinones

The clinical advantage of oxazolidines prodrugs is to enhance membrane permeability. This strategy is adequate for primary and secondary amines that have beta hydroxyl group [54]. The synthesis of prodrugs is based on cyclic condensation of the ß-aminoalochol with an aldehyde or ketone (Figure 34).

Figure 34. Chemical structure of oxazolidines.

Hetacillin is produced from condensation of ampicillin with acetone [80], an example of 4- imidazolidinones (Figure 35) prodrugs.

Figure 35. Chemical structure of imidazolidinone.

Hetacillin was developed in order to overcome the polymerization phenomenon [81], observed with ampicillin molecules at elevated concentrations and it happens as a result of the intermolecular nucleophilic attack by the free NH terminal present in the peptide, like ampicillin, on the beta lactam ring of an adjacent molecule. So attempts were directed toward creating a prodrug of ampicillin in order to enhance stability. By conjugating 1, 4-imidazolidinone into NH (Figure 36) the resulted prodrug exhibits a six-fold increase in stability which is achieved by the equilibrium obtained between the drug and the prodrug. In a later stage, the prodrug converts back to ampicillin within 11 minutes. Using this approach the oral bioavailability of ampicillin was slightly increased [82].

Another application of this strategy is to obtain a sustained release drug delivery from an oily vehicle as in the case of prilocaine condensation with formaldehyde or acetaldehyde [83].

Figure 36. Chemical structures of ampicillin and hetacillin.

Simple Alkyl, Benzyl, Aryl Halo Alkyl Esters and Others-Prodrugs of Phosphonates

Phosphonates (Figure 37) is a category of drugs having two negative charges at physiological pH; accordingly they possess high polarity and suffer from extremely low bioavailability which results from poor membrane penetration [84]. Therefore, masking both charged groups has the potential to increase membrane permeation due to an increase in lipophilicity.

Figure 37. Chemical structure of phosphonate.

Phosphonates exhibit sufficient chemical and enzymatic stability due to the chemical nature of P---C bond. This is in contrary to phosphates that show low stability as being substrates to phosphatases. Consequently only few phosphate prodrug derivatives are available, while a significant number of phosphonate prodrugs have successfully reached the market.

It should be indicated that the prodrug rules applied to carboxylic acid functional group are the same for phosphonate functional group. However, phosphonate prodrug strategy is much more problematic due to structural aspects related to the phosphonate group [84]. One of these concerns is the incomplete conversion of phosphonate prodrugs into their corresponding phosphonic acid derivatives, such in the case of simple alkyl diesters of 9-[2-(phosphonomethoxy) ethoxy] adenine which were developed by Serafinowska and co-workers in an attempt to increase 9-[2-(phosphonomethoxy) ethoxy] adenine poor bioavailability [85].

It was mentioned earlier that phosphonates are highly polar and this results in low membrane permeability. In certain situations this aspect can be explored in such a way that allows the entrapment of the parent drug inside a target cell, hence a targeted drug delivery can be achieved. This issue can be accomplished if:

1) The prodrug is chemically and enzymatically stable in the GIT and blood circulation.
2) The drug has an intracellular target.
3) The prodrug can be converted into the parent drug in the intracellular compartment by certain enzymes (Figure 38).

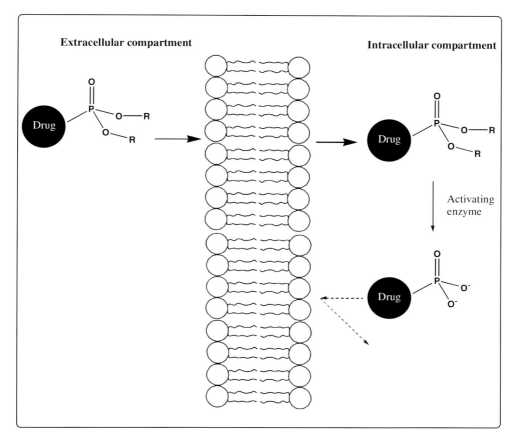

Figure 38. Schematic representation of the utilization of phosphonates having high polarity and low membrane permeability in targeted drug delivery.

An illustrative example is (S)-1-(3-Hydroxy-2-phosphonylmethoxypropyl) cytosine, cidofovir or HPMPC (Figure 39), an antiviral agent intended for the treatment of cytomegalovirus retinitis in AIDS patients by IV infusion [86].

Figure 39. Chemical structure of cidofovir.

Cidofovir causes nephrotoxicity when administered by IV infusion. In order to circumvent this drawback, cyclic HPMPC [(S)-1-(2-hydroxy-2-oxo-1, 4, 2-dioxaphosphorinan- 5-yl) methyl) cytosine], a cyclic analogue of cidofovir, was developed. This analogue exhibits an identical in vitro and in vivo activity to cidofovir but it shows a 10-40 fold reduction in nephrotoxicity in rats, guinea pig, and monkeys [87]. This improvement in pharmacokinetic profile of cidofovir can be explained as follows:

In vitro studies have demonstrated that cyclic HPMPC is stable in liver, plasma and intestinal homogenates [88]. Once it penetrates the cells it is transformed into cidofovir by cCMP phosphodiesterase which stays inside the cell due to cidofovir high polarity and low membrane permeation, thus minimizing systemic exposure and toxicity. In this situation cidofovir is called intracellular prodrug [89].

Acyloxyalkyl prodrugs represent neutral lipophilic compounds having the ability to cross membranes, and to break down intracellularly through the action of esterases into their parent drugs and spacers. The most commonly used bridge herein is a methylene group that is converted into an acetaldehyde without containing any chiral center, hence chirality concern that was associated with the previously mentioned prodrugs is eliminated [84].

Niemi and coworkers [90] studied some alkyl ester and acyloxymethyl ester prodrugs of etidronic acid (Figure 40) in an attempt to enhance membrane permeation and oral bioavailability of the corresponding active drugs.

Figure 40. Chemical structure of etidronic acid.

Etidronic and acetyletidronic acids are members of the bisphosphonates family used for the treatment of osteoporosis that are characterized by their high polarity that limits their oral absorption [91]. Among the prepared prodrugs; the tri substituted pivaloyloxymethyl ester of acetyletidronate. In vitro evaluation showed satisfactory water solubility and desirable lipophilicity [90].

This approach was utilized by a group of researchers for the antiviral agent adefovir (Figure 41) in an effort to promote its antiviral activity and enhance its oral bioavailability.

A group of adefovir bis (pivaloyloxymethyl) prodrugs were synthesized. *In vitro* evaluation showed that these prodrugs exhibit an improved antiviral activity in comparison with adefovir [91]. This can be attributed to an increase in the permeability of these prodrugs. The study also showed a rapid intracellular transformation of the prodrugs into their active drugs.

Figure 41. Chemical structure of adefovir.

Furthermore, pivaloyloxymethyl and 1-pivaloyloxyethyl prodrugs of adenofovir showed the highest bioavailability among all studied prodrugs. However, the break-down products of these prodrugs affect carnitine homeostasis; this represents a toxicological concern, which arises from pivalic acid; one of the breakdown products [84].

An alternative approach to facilitate conversion of phosphonate prodrugs is phosphonamidates. This strategy has been applied because the P----N bond has the tendency to be cleaved chemically and enzymatically.

More and more attempts to improve lipophilicity, oral bioavailability and specific cellular uptake of drugs continued and were relatively achieved by using long-chain alkyloxy alkyl monoesters. By employing this approach a considerable improvement of drug accumulation in the target cells is accomplished. Long-chain alkyloxy alkyl cidofovir monoester prodrugs were prepared and tested for their ability to cross membranes. It was proposed that these prodrugs permeate cell membranes through the following mechanisms:

1) Phospholipids uptake pathway.
2) Passive diffusion.
3) Membrane flippase activity.

The activity of phospholipase c enzyme on P-O alkyl bond is explored to cleave the prodrug and release cidofovir once it is inside the cell. Furthermore, exploiting lysophosphatidylcholine (LPC) uptake pathway in the intestine to increase oral bioavailability of cidofovir is possible because of the resemblance of long-chain alkyloxyalkyl monoester to lysophosphatidylcholine (LPC) [84].

Phosphinate Prodrugs

Phosphinate drugs contain one ionizable group which needs to be masked in order to meet pharmacokinetic requirement. Owing to its high polarity, phospinates suffer from low membrane penetration and hence low oral bioavailability. Masking the negative charge using a lipophilic linker aids in achieving enhanced penetration through intestinal wall. Acyloxyalkyl group that is used for carboxylic acids is also employed in this case. Fosinoprilat, an antihypertensive agent, has a very low bioavailability (<5%) due to the presence of a negative charged phosphinate group which inhibits its development as antihypertensive agent [82]. However, extensive efforts were made to develop the acyloxyalkyl prodrug fosinopril which is hydrolyzed by intestinal and liver esterases prior or during absorption [92], which then is converted to fosinoprilate, the parent active drug. The latter inhibits ACE enzyme through binding of its phosphinic acid to the zinc present in ACE binding site.

Phosphate Prodrugs

Nucleosides have been found to be widely applied in the treatment of cancer and viral infections [93]. Phosphorylation of nucleoside by cellular kinases (viral or host) is a crucial step for their biological activity. However, the emergence of kinases resistance over time of these kinases to activate the corresponding nucleoside limits their utility as effective medications [94]. Consequently, the idea of administering these agents as monophosphates to overcome the resistance issue was theoretically applicable but practically not feasible because of several pharmacokinetic barriers. Firstly, the presence of the phosphate group imparts high polarity to these agents; therefore low membrane permeability and thus low oral bioavailability will be the end result. Secondly, in vivo dephosphorylation of these monophosphates was found to be relatively fast [95].

Accordingly, masking the phosphate group by an appropriate moiety will be beneficial in terms of generating prodrugs with increased lipophilicity and hence improved permeability. Additionally, prodrug approaches can be employed to overcome the instability problem associated with this class of drugs.

Hence, simple alkyl, benzyl, aryl and halo alkyl esters were developed in an attempt to achieve superior pharmacokinetic characteristics.

As investigated by Rosowsky group [96] various mono-5'-(alkyl phosphate) esters of ara C were examined in order to improve ara CMP delivery to cancer cells. It was demonstrated that as the alkyl chain length increased the activity is decreased.

Summary and Conclusion

In summary, it has become apparent that pharmacokinetic and physiological barriers represent an obstacle for proper utilization of therapeutically active drugs. Hence, attention was paid towards exploring many approaches to solve these problems. The prodrug approach has captured the greatest attention because it aids in overcoming various negative aspects associated with drugs in a short and a relatively low cost way. A number of these aspects were already discussed previously in this chapter; including increasing lipophilicity, improving water solubility, and achieving targeted drug delivery through the development of carboxylic acid, hydroxyl, amino phosphonate, phosphonite and phosphate prodrugs.

References

[1]   Dahan, A.; Khamis, M.; Agbaria, R. & Karaman, R. (2012) Targeted prodrugs in oral delivery: the modern molecular biopharmaceutical approach. *Expert Opinion on Drug Delivery9*, 1001–1013.

[2]   Karaman, R.; Fattash B. & Qtait A. (2013) The future of prodrugs – design by quantum mechanics methods. *Expert Opinion on Drug Delivery10*, 713–729.

[3]   Karaman, R. (2013) Prodrugs design based on inter- and intramolecular processes. *Chem. Biol. Drug. Des* 82, 643–668.

[4]   Huttunen, K. M.; Raunio, H.; Rautio, J. (2011) Prodrugs--from serendipity to rational design. *Pharmacological reviews*63(3), 750-71.

[5]   Jana, S.; Mandlekar, S.; Marathe, P. (2010) Prodrug design to improve pharmacokinetic and drug delivery properties: challenges to the discovery scientists. *Current medicinal chemistry*. 17(32), 3874-908.

[6]   Stella, V. J. (2010) Prodrugs: Some thoughts and current issues. *Journal of pharmaceutical sciences* 99(12), 4755-65.

[7]   Bundgaard, H. (1989) The Double Prodrug Concept and its Applications. *Advanced drug delivery reviews* 3, 39-65.

[8]   Li, F.; Maag, H.; Alfredson, T. (2008) Prodrugs of nucleoside analogues for improved oral absorption and tissue targeting. *Journal of pharmaceutical sciences* 97(3), 1109-34. Epub 2007/08/19.

[9]   Stella, V. J.; Borchardt, R. T.; Hageman, M. J.; Oliyai, R.; Maag, H.; Tilley, J. W., editors. (2007) prodrugs, challenges and rewards part I: Prodrugs of Carboxylic Acids 2000/07/13 ed. New York, NY 10013, USA),: Springer Science+Business Media, LLC.

[10]   Testa, B.; Mayer, J. M. (2003) Hydrolysis in Drug and Prodrug metabolism, Chemistry, biochemistry and enzymology, 690-5 p.

[11]   Kostic, M. A.; Dart, R.C. (2003) Rethinking the toxic methanol level. *Journal of toxicology Clinical toxicology* 41(6), 793-800.

[12]   He, G.; Massarella, J.; Ward, P. (1999) Clinical pharmacokinetics of the prodrug oseltamivir and its active metabolite Ro 64-0802. *Clinical pharmacokinetics* 37(6), 471-84.

[13]   Moore, V.A.; Irwin, W. J.; Timmins, P.; Chong, S.; Dando, S. A.; Morrison, R. A. (2000) A rapid screening system to determine drug affinities for the intestinal dipeptide transporter 1: system characterisation. *International journal of pharmaceutics* 210(1-2), 15-27.

[14]   Modr, Z.; Dvovacek, K.; Janku, I.; Krebs, V. (1997) Pharmacokinetics of carfecillin and carindacillin. *International journal of clinical pharmacology and biopharmacy* 15(2), 81-3. Epub 1977/02/01.

[15]   Jansen, A. B.; Russell, T.J. (1965) Some Novel Penicillin Derivatives. *Journal of the Chemical Society* 65, 2127-32.

[16]   Bhosle, D.; Bharambe, S. D.; Gairola, N.; Dhaneshwar, S. (2006) Mutual prodrug concept: Fundamentals and applications. *Indian journal of pharmaceutical sciences* 68(3), 286-94..

[17]   English, A. R.; Girard, D.; Haskell, S. L. (1984) Pharmacokinetics of sultamicillin in mice, rats, and dogs. *Antimicrobial agents and chemotherapy* 25(5), 599-602.

[18]   Saito, A.; Kato, Y.; Ishikawa, K.; Odagaki, E.; Shinohara, M.; Fukuhara, I.; Tomizawa, M.; Nakayama, I.; Morita, K.; Sato, K. (1984) Lenampicillin (KBT-1585): Pharmacokinetics and Clinical Evaluation . *Chemotherapy-Tokyo* 32 (Suppl.8), 209-21.

[19]   Warner G. T., Jarvis B. (2002) Olmesartan medoxomil. *Drugs* 62(9), 1345-53; discussion 54-6.

[20] Stella, V. J., Ronald, T. B.; Michael, J. H.; Reza, O.; Hans, M.; Jefferson, w.T., editors. (2007) Prodrugs: Challenges and Rewards part I: Prodrugs of Alcohols and Phenols.

[21] Wei, C. P.; Anderson, J. A.; Leopold, I. (1978) Ocular absorption and metabolism of topically applied epinephrine and a dipivalyl ester of epinephrine. *Investigative ophthalmology & visual science* 17(4), 315-21.

[22] Jordan, C. G. (1998) How an increase in the carbon chain length of the ester moiety affects the stability of a homologous series of oxprenolol esters in the presence of biological enzymes. *Journal of pharmaceutical sciences* 87(7), 880-5. Epub 1998/07/02.

[23] Beresford, R.; Ward, A. (1987) Haloperidol decanoate. A preliminary review of its pharmacodynamic and pharmacokinetic properties and therapeutic use in psychosis. *Drugs* 33(1), 31-49. Epub 1987/01/01.

[24] Jann, M. W.; Ereshefsky, L.; Saklad, S. R. (1985) Clinical pharmacokinetics of the depot antipsychotics. *Clinical pharmacokinetics* 10(4), 315-33. Epub 1985/07/01.

[25] Brent, D. A.; Chandrasurin, P.; Ragouzeos, A.; Hurlbert, B. S; Burke, J. T. (1980) Rearrangement of chloramphenicol-3-monosuccinate. *Journal of pharmaceutical sciences.* 69(8), 906-8. Epub 1980/08/01.

[26] Garceau, Y.; Davis, I.; Hasegawa, J. (1967) Plasma propranolol levels in beagle dogs after administration of propranolol hemisuccinate ester. *Journal of pharmaceutical sciences* 10, 1360-3. Epub 1978/10/01.

[27] Kim, I.; Chu, X. Y.; Kim, S.; Provoda, C. J.; Lee, K. D.; Amidon, G. L. (2003) Identification of a human valacyclovirase: biphenyl hydrolase-like protein as valacyclovir hydrolase. *The Journal of biological chemistry* 278(28), 25348-56. Epub 2003/05/07.

[28] Beutner, K. R. (1995) Valacyclovir: a review of its antiviral activity, pharmacokinetic properties, and clinical efficacy. *Antiviral research* 28(4), 281-90. Epub 1995/12/01.

[29] Soul-Lawton, J.; Seaber, E.; On, N.; Wootton, R.; Rolan, P.; Posner, J. (1995) Absolute bioavailability and metabolic disposition of valaciclovir, the L-valyl ester of acyclovir, following oral administration to humans. *Antimicrobial agents and chemotherapy* 39(12), 2759-64. Epub 1995/12/01.

[30] de Miranda, P.; Krasny, H. C.; Page, D. A.; Elion, G. B. (1981) The disposition of acyclovir in different species. *The Journal of pharmacology and experimental therapeutics* 219(2), 309-15. Epub 1981/11/01.

[31] Martin, D. F.; Sierra-Madero, J.; Walmsley, S.; Wolitz, R.A.; Macey, K.; Georgiou, P.; Robinson, C.; and Stempien, M. (2002) A controlled trial of valganciclovir as induction therapy for cytomegalovirus retinitis. *The New England journal of medicine* 346(15), 1119-26. Epub 2002/04/12.

[32] Jung, D.; Dorr, A. (1999) Single-dose pharmacokinetics of valganciclovir in HIV- and CMV-seropositive subjects. *Journal of clinical pharmacology* 39(8), 800-4. Epub 1999/08/06.

[33] Sugawara, M.; Huang, W.; Fei, Y. J.; Leibach, F. H.; Ganapathy, V.; Ganapathy, M. E. (2000) Transport of valganciclovir, a ganciclovir prodrug, via peptide transporters PEPT1 and PEPT2. Journal of pharmaceutical sciences 89(6), 781-9. Epub 2000/05/29.

[34] Gani, D; Wilkie, J. (1995) Stereochemical, Mechanistic, and Structural Features of Enzyme-catalyzed Phosphate Monoester Hydrolyses. *Chemical Society reviews* 24, 55-63.

[35] Novak, E.; Wagner, J.G.; Lamb, D. J. (1970) Local and systemic tolerance, absorption and excretion of clindamycin hydrochloride after intramuscular administration. *International journal of clinical pharmacology, therapy, and toxicology* 3(3), 201-8. Epub 1970/07/01.

[36] Riebe, K.W.; Oesterling, T.O.(1972) Parenteral development of clindamycin-2-phosphate. Bulletin of the Parenteral Drug Association 26(3), 139-46. Epub 1972/05/01.

[37] Cambazard, F. (1998) Clinical efficacy of Velac, a new tretinoin and clindamycin phosphate gel in acne vulgaris. *Journal of the European Academy of Dermatology and Venereology : JEADV*. 11 Suppl 1, S20-7; discussion S8-9. Epub 1999/01/19.

[38] Richardson, K.; Cooper, K.; Marriott, M. S.; Tarbit, M. H.; Troke, P. F.; Whittle, P. J. (1990) Discovery of fluconazole, a novel antifungal agent. *Reviews of infectious diseases* 12 Suppl, 3:S267-71. Epub 1990/03/01.

[39] Chapman, T. M.; Plosker, G. L.; Perry, C.M. (2004) Fosamprenavir: a review of its use in the management of antiretroviral therapy-naive patients with HIV infection. *Drugs* 64, 2101-24. Epub 2005/02/01.

[40] Varia, S.A.; Schuller, S.; Sloan, K. B.; Stella, V. J. (1984) Phenytoin prodrugs III: water-soluble prodrugs for oral and/or parenteral use. *Journal of pharmaceutical sciences* 73(8), 1068-73. Epub 1984/08/01.

[41] Pettit, G. R.; Lippert, J.W. (2000) 3rd. Antineoplastic agents 429. Syntheses of the combretastatin A-1 and combretastatin B-1 prodrugs. *Anti-cancer drug design* 15(3), 203-16. Epub 2000/10/26.

[42] Saulnier, M. G.; Langley, D. R.; Kadow, J. F.; Senter, P. D.; Knipe, J. O.; Tun, M. M.; Vyas, D.; Doyle, T. (1994) Synthesis of Etoposide Phosphate, BMY-40481: A Water-soluble Clinically Active Prodrug of Etoposide. *Bioorganic & medicinal chemistry letters* 4, 2567-72.

[43] Shah, J. C.; Chen, J. R.; Chow, D. (1989) Preformulation Study of Etoposide: Identification of Physicochemical Characteristics Responsible for the Low and Erratic Oral Bioavailability of Etoposide. *Pharmaceutical research* 6, 408-12.

[44] Budman, D,R.; Igwemezie, L. N.; Kaul, S; Behr, J.; Lichtman, S.; Schulman, P.; Vinciguerra, P.; Allen, S.; Kolitz, J.; Hock, K.; O'Neill, K.; Schacter, L.; Barbhaiya, R. (1994) Phase I evaluation of a water-soluble etoposide prodrug, etoposide phosphate, given as a 5-minute infusion on days 1, 3, and 5 in patients with solid tumors. *Journal of clinical oncology : official journal of the American Society of Clinical Oncology* 12(9), 1902-9. Epub 1994/09/01.

[45] Safadi, M.; Oliyai, R.; Stella, V. J. (1993) Phosphoryloxymethyl carbamates and carbonates--novel water-soluble prodrugs for amines and hindered alcohols. *Pharmaceutical research*. 10(9), 1350-5. Epub 1993/09/01.

[46] Bentley, A.; Butters, M.; Green, S. P.; Learmonth, W. J.; MacRae, J. A.; Morland, M.C.; O'Conno, R.G.; Skuse,J. (2002) The Discovery and Process Development of a Commercial Route to a Water Soluble Prodrug, Fosfluconazole. *Org Process Res Dev* 6, 109-12.

[47] Hansen, K. T.; Faarup, P.; Bundgaard, H. (1991) Carbamate ester prodrugs of dopaminergic compounds: synthesis, stability, and bioconversion. *Journal of pharmaceutical sciences* 80(8), 793-8. Epub 1991/08/01.

[48] Svensson, L. A.; Tunek, A. (1988) The design and bioactivation of presystemically stable prodrugs. *Drug metabolism reviews* 19(2), 165-94. Epub 1988/01/01.

[49] Olsson, O.; Svensson, L. A. (1984) New Lipophilic Terbutalin Ester Prodrugs with Long Effect Duration. *Pharmaceutical research* 1, 19-23. Epub 1993/01/01.

[50] Fugleholm, A. M. ; Ibsen, T. B.; Laxmyr, L.; Svendsen, U. G. (1993) Therapeutic Equivalence between Bambuterol, 10 mg Once Daily, and Terbutaline Controlled Release, 5mg Twice Daily, in Mild to Moderate Asthma. *Eur Respir J* 6, 1474-8. Epub 1979/01/01.

[51] Elger, W.; Schwarz, S.; Hedden, A.; Reddersen, G.; Schneider, B. (1995) Sulfamates of various estrogens are prodrugs with increased systemic and reduced hepatic estrogenicity at oral application. *The Journal of steroid biochemistry and molecular biology* 55(3-4), 395-403. Epub 1995/12/01.

[52] Bauer, K.; Elger, W; Schneider, B.; Krahl, E; Bauer, R. (2003) Effect of EstradiolSulfamate (ES-J995) on Affinity of Hemoglobin for Oxygen, CardiovascularFunction and Acid-Base Balance in Ovariectomized Rats. *Exp Toxicol Pathology* 55, 301-7. Epub 1971/08/01.

[53] Bundgaard, H.; Buur, A.; Chang, S. C.; Lee, V. H. L. (1988a) Timolol Prodrugs: Synthesis,Stability and Lipophilicity of Various Alkyl, Cycloalkyl and Aromatic Esters ofTimolol. *International journal of pharmaceutics* 46, 77-88. Epub 1973/08/24.

[54] Stella, V. J.; Ronald, T. B.; Michael, J. H.; Reza, O.; Hans, M.; Jefferson,W. T.N, editors. (2007) Prodrugs: Challenges and Rewards part I: Prodrugs of Amines.

[55] Kalgutkar, A. S.; Marnett, A. B.; Crews, B. C.; Remmel, R. P.; Marnett, L. J. (2000) Ester and amide derivatives of the nonsteroidal antiinflammatory drug, indomethacin, as selective cyclooxygenase-2 inhibitors. *Journal of medicinal chemistry* 43(15), 2860-70. Epub 2000/08/24.

[56] Bodor, N.; Simpkins, J. W. (1983) Redox delivery system for brain-specific, sustained release of dopamine. *Science* 221(4605), 65-7. Epub 1983/07/01.

[57] Lee, M. R. (1990) Five years' experience with gamma-L-glutamyl-L-dopa: a relatively renally specific dopaminergic prodrug in man. *Journal of autonomic pharmacology* 10 Suppl 1:s103-8. Epub 1990/01/01.

[58] Casagrande, C.; Merlo, L.; Ferrini, R.; Miragoli, G.; Semeraro, C. (1989) Cardiovascular and renal action of dopaminergic prodrugs. *Journal of cardiovascular pharmacology.* 14 Suppl 8:S40-59. Epub 1989/01/01.

[59] Pochopin, N. L.; Charman, W. N.; Stella, V. J. (1994) Pharmacokinetics of dapsone and amino acid prodrugs of dapsone. Drug metabolism and disposition: *the biological fate of chemicals* 22(5), 770-5. Epub 1994/09/01.

[60] Bundgaard, H. (1985) Design of Prodrug p. 3-79.

[61] Ajani, J. (2006) Review of capecitabine as oral treatment of gastric, gastroesophageal, and esophageal cancers. *Cancer* 107(2), 221-31. Epub 2006/06/14.

[62] Alexander, J.; Cargill, R.; Michelson, S. R.; Schwam, H. (1988) (Acyloxy)alkyl carbamates as novel bioreversible prodrugs for amines: increased permeation through biological membranes. *Journal of medicinal chemistry* 31(2), 318-22. Epub 1988/02/01.

[63] Alexander, J.; Fromtling, R. A.; Bland, J. A.; Pelak, B. A.; Gilfillan, E. C. (1991) (Acyloxy)alkyl carbamate prodrugs of norfloxacin. *Journal of medicinal chemistry* 34(1), 78-81. Epub 1991/01/01.

[64] Davidsen, S. K,; Summers, J. B.; Albert, D. H.; Holms, J. H.; Heyman, H. R.; Magoc, T. J.; Conway, R .; Rhein, D .; Carter, G. (1994) N-(acyloxyalkyl)pyridinium Salts as Soluble Prodrugs of a Potent Platelet Activating Factor Antagonist. *Journal of medicinal chemistry* 37, 4423–9. Epub 1974/09/29.

[65] Riley, R. J.; Workman, P. (1992) Enzymology of the reduction of the potent benzotriazine-di-N-oxide hypoxic cell cytotoxin SR 4233 (WIN 59075) by NAD(P)H: (quinone acceptor) oxidoreductase (EC 1.6.99.2) purified from Walker 256 rat tumour cells. *Biochemical pharmacology* 43(2), 167-74. Epub 1992/01/22.

[66] Brown, J. M. (1999) The hypoxic cell: a target for selective cancer therapy--eighteenth Bruce F. Cain Memorial Award lecture. *Cancer research* 59(23), 5863-70. Epub 1999/12/22.

[67] Smith, P. J.; Blunt, N. J.; Desnoyers, R.; Giles, Y.; Patterson, L. H. (1997) DNA topoisomerase II-dependent cytotoxicity of alkylaminoanthraquinones and their N-oxides. *Cancer chemotherapy and pharmacology* 39(5), 455-61. Epub 1997/01/01.

[68] Simplicio, A. L.; Clancy, J. M.; Gilmer, J. F. (2008) Prodrugs for amines. *Molecules* 13(3), 519-47. Epub 2008/05/09.

[69] Krogsgaard, L. P.; Liljefors, T.; Madsen, U., editors. (2002) A textbook of drug design and discovery. 3rd ed.

[70] Bundgaard, H.; Johansen, M. (1980) Prodrugs as drug delivery systems IV: N-Mannich bases as potential novel prodrugs for amides, ureides, amines, and other NH-acidic compounds. *Journal of pharmaceutical sciences* 69(1), 44-6. Epub 1980/01/01.

[71] Cogan, P. S.; Koch, T. H. (2004) Studies of targeting and intracellular trafficking of an anti-androgen doxorubicin-formaldehyde conjugate in PC-3 prostate cancer cells bearing androgen receptor-GFP chimera. *Journal of medicinal chemistry* 47(23), 5690-9. Epub 2004/10/29.

[72] Taatjes, D. J.; Gaudiano, G.; Resing, K.; Koch, T. H. (1996) Alkylation of DNA by the anthracycline, antitumor drugs adriamycin and daunomycin. *Journal of medicinal chemistry* 39(21), 4135-8. Epub 1996/10/11.

[73] Krause, M.; Rouleau, A.; Stark, H.; Garbarg, M.; Schwartz, J. C.; Schunack, W. (1996) Structure-activity relationships of novel azomethine prodrugs of the histamine H3-receptor agonist (R)-alpha-methylhistamine: from alkylaryl to substituted diaryl derivatives. *Die Pharmazie* 51(10), 720-6. Epub 1996/10/01.

[74] Caldwell, H. C.; Adams, H. J.; Jones, R. G.; Mann, W. A.; Dittert, L. W.; Chong, C. W.; Swintosky, J.V. (1971) Enamine prodrugs. *Journal of pharmaceutical sciences* 60(12), 1810-2. Epub 1971/12/01.

[75] Murakami, T.; Tamauchi, H.; Yamazaki, M.; Kubo, K.; Kamada, A.; Yata, N. (1981) Biopharmaceutical study on the oral and rectal administrations of enamine prodrugs of amino acid-like beta-lactam antibiotics in rabbits. *Chemical & pharmaceutical bulletin* 29(7), 1986-97. Epub 1981/07/01.

[76] Naringrekar, V. H.; Stella, V. J. (1990) Mechanism of hydrolysis and structure-stability relationship of enaminones as potential prodrugs of model primary amines. *Journal of pharmaceutical sciences* 79(2), 138-46. Epub 1990/02/01.

[77] Jensen, N. P.; Friedman, J. J.; Kropp, H.; Kahan, F. M. (1980) Use of acetylacetone to prepare a prodrug of cycloserine. *Journal of medicinal chemistry* 23(1), 6-8. Epub 1980/01/01.

[78] Azadkhan, A. K.; Truelove, S. C.; Aronson, J. K. (1982) The disposition and metabolism of sulphasalazine (salicylazosulphapyridine) in man. *British journal of clinical pharmacology* 13(4), 523-8. Epub 1982/04/01.

[79] Sandborn, W. J. (2002) Rational selection of oral 5-aminosalicylate formulations and prodrugs for the treatment of ulcerative colitis. *The American journal of gastroenterology* 97(12), 2939-41. Epub 2002/12/21.

[80] Tsuji, A.; Yamana, T. (1974) Kinetic approach to the development in beta-lactam antibiotics. II. Prodrug. (I). Simultaneous determination of hetacillin and ampicillin, and its application to the stability of hetacillin in aqueous solutions. *Chemical & pharmaceutical bulletin* 22(10), 2434-43. Epub 1974/10/01.

[81] Schwartz, M. A.; Hayton, W. L. (1972) Relative stability of hetacillin and ampicillin in solution. *Journal of pharmaceutical sciences* 61(6), 906-9. Epub 1972/06/01.

[82] Jusko, W. J.; Lewis, G. P. (1973) Comparison of Ampicillin and HetacillinPharmacokinetics in Man. *J Pharm Sci* 62, 69-76. Epub 1983/01/01.

[83] Larsen, S. W.; Sidenius, M.; Ankersen, M.; Larsen, C. (2003) Kinetics of degradation of 4-imidazolidinone prodrug types obtained from reacting prilocaine with formaldehyde and acetaldehyde. *European journal of pharmaceutical sciences : official journal of the European Federation for Pharmaceutical Sciences* 20(2), 233-40. Epub 2003/10/11.

[84] Stella, V. J.; Borchardt, R. T.; Hageman, M.J.; Oliyai, R.; Maag, H.; Tilley, J. W., editors. (2007) Prodrugs: Challenges and Rewards part I: Prodrugs of Phosphonates, Phosphinates, and Phosphates

[85] Serafinowska, H. T; Ashton, R. J; Bailey, S; Harnden, M. R; Jackson, S. M; Sutton, D. (1995) Synthesis and In Vivo Evaluation of Prodrugs of 9-[2-(Phosphonomethoxy)ethoxy]adenine. *J Med Chem* 38, 1372–9.

[86] Hitchcock, M. J. M.; Jaffe, H. S.; Martin, J. C.; Stagg, R. J. (1996) Cidofovir, A New Agent with Potent Anti-Herpesvirus Activity.1996; 7:115–127. *Antiviral chemistry & chemotherapy* 7, 115-27. Epub 1985/11/01.

[87] Bischofberger, N.; Hitchcock, M. J. M.; Chen, M. S.; Barkhimer, D. B.; Cundy, K. C.; Kent, K. M.; Lacy, S. A.; Lee, W. A.; Li, Z. H.; Mendel, D. B. (1994) 1-[((S)-2-Hydroxy-2-oxo-1,4,2-dioxaphosphorinan-5-yl)methyl] Cytosine, anIntracellular Prodrug for (S)-1-(3-Hydroxy-2-Phosphonylmethoxypropyl)cytosine with Improved Therapeutic Index In Vivo. *Antimicrobial Agents and Chemotherapy* 38, 2387–91. Epub 2009/04/29.

[88] Mendel, D. B.; Cihlar, T.; Moon, K.; Chen, M.S. (1997) Conversion of 1-[((S)-2-hydroxy-2-oxo-1,4,2-dioxaphosphorinan-5-yl)methyl]cytosine to cidofovir by an intracellular cyclic CMP phosphodiesterase. *Antimicrobial agents and chemotherapy* 41(3), 641-6. Epub 1997/03/01.

[89] Hitchcock, M. J. M.; Lacy, S.; Lindsey, J.; Kern, E. (1995) The Cyclic Congener of Cidofovir Has Reduced Nephrotoxicity in Three Species. *Antiviral research* 26, A358.

[90] Niemi, R.; Turhanen, P.; Vepsalainen, J.; Taipale, H.; Jarvinen, T. (2000) Bisphosphonate prodrugs: synthesis and in vitro evaluation of alkyl and acyloxymethyl esters of etidronic acid as bioreversible prodrugs of etidronate. *European journal of pharmaceutical sciences : official journal of the European Federation for Pharmaceutical Sciences* 11(2), 173-80. Epub 2000/08/01.

[91] Starrett, J. E.; Tortolani, D. R.; Hitchcock, M. J.; Martin, J.C.; Mansuri, M.M. (1992) Synthesis and in vitro evaluation of a phosphonate prodrug: bis(pivaloyloxymethyl) 9-(2- phosphonylmethoxyethyl)adenine. *Antiviral research* 19(3), 267-73. Epub 1992/09/11.

[92] Morrison, R. A. ; Singhvi, S. M. ; Peterson, A. E. ; Pocetti, D. A.; Migdalof, B. H. (1990) Relative contribution of the gut, liver, and lung to the first-pass hydrolysis (bioactivation) of orally administered 14C-fosinopril sodium in dogs. In vivo and in vitro studies. *Drug metabolism and disposition: the biological fate of chemicals* 18(2), 253-7. Epub 1990/03/01.

[93] Cooney, D. A.; Dalal, M.; Mitsuya, H.; McMahon, J.B.; Nadkarni, M.; Balzarini, J.; Broder, S.; Johns, D. G.. (1986) Initial studies on the cellular pharmacology of 2',3-dideoxycytidine, an inhibitor of HTLV-III infectivity. *Biochemical pharmacology* 35(13), 2065-8. Epub 1986/07/01.

[94] Reichard, P.; Skold, O.; Klein, G.; Revesz, L.; Magnusson, P. H. (1962) Studies on resistance against 5-fluorouracil. I. Enzymes of the uracil pathway during development of resistance. *Cancer research* 22, 235-43. Epub 1962/02/01.

[95] Schrecker, A. W.; Goldin, A. (1968) Antitumor effect and mode of action of 1-beta-D-arabinofuranosylcytosine 5'-phosphate in leukemia L1210. *Cancer research* 28(4), 802-3. Epub 1968/04/01.

[96] Rosowsky, A.; Kim, S. H.; Ross, J.; Wick, M. M. (1982) Lipophilic 5'-(alkyl phosphate) esters of 1-beta-D-arabinofuranosylcytosine and its N4-acyl and 2,2'-anhydro-3'-O-acyl derivatives as potential prodrugs. *Journal of medicinal chemistry* 25(2), 171-8. Epub 1982/02/01.

In: Prodrugs Design – A New Era
Editor: Rafik Karaman

ISBN: 978-1-63117-701-9
© 2014 Nova Science Publishers, Inc.

Chapter IV

Targeted Prodrugs

Maryam Bader[1], Ameen Thawabteh[1] and Rafik Karaman[1,2,] *

[1]Pharmaceutical Sciences Department, Faculty of Pharmacy
Al-Quds University, Jerusalem, Palestine;
[2]Department of Science, University of Basilicata, Potenza, Italy

Abstract

Generally, prodrugs are obtained to overcome certain problems associated with their parent drugs. The old classical/ traditional prodrugs suffer from decreased bioavailability and a high profile of side effects due to activation at sites other than the desired site. Recently, they have been replaced by the new targeted prodrugs which have more therapeutic efficiency and less associated side effects.

Targeted prodrugs are synthesized to deliver the desired drugs to a certain organ/cell in the body, thus, overcoming problems associated with traditional prodrugs. This type of prodrugs achieves its aim depending on the presence of unique cellular conditions at the desired target, especially the availability of certain enzymes and transporters at these target sites.

In this chapter, the majority of the discussion is devoted to cover and address many methods for targeting different organs and cells. Some of these methods have proved their success while others are still under investigation.

Due to an increase in the number of detected cancers and lack of effective treatments, targeting methodology was given a high priority and greatest devotion in this chapter. Several methods including active and passive targeting and many others are discussed in details. Targeting the central nervous system by studying the physiological nature of the blood brain barrier; taking advantage of the presence of certain transporters has been addressed. Another respected part of this chapter was devoted to colon targeting by the prodrug approach which covers some of prodrugs based on linkers that can be solely cleaved by the colonic microflora. This chapter documents in details the human immune deficiency virus and kidney targeting methods as well.

---

* Corresponding author: Rafik Karaman, e-mail: dr_karaman@yahoo.com; Tel and Fax +972-2-2790413.

Keywords: Targeted prodrugs, prodrugs, GDEPT, bystander effect, cancer, chemotherapy, metabolic enzymes

List of Abbreviations

GIT	Gastro-intestinal tract
ADME	Absorption, distribution, metabolism and excretion
mAbs	Monoclonal antibodies
P-GP	P-glycoprotein
FDA	Food and drug administration
AML	Acute myeloid leukemia
CPT	Camptothecin
ABC	ATP-binding cassette
SLC	Solute carrier
EPR	Enhanced permeability and retention
PEG	Polyethylene glycol
PGA	Polyglutamate
HPMA	Hydroxypropylmethacrylamide
PDEPT	Polymer directed enzyme prodrug therapy
ADEPT	Antibody-directed enzyme prodrug therapy
GDEPT	Gene-directed enzyme prodrug therapy
PELT	Polymer directed enzyme liposome therapy
PSA	Prostate specific antigen
SERCA	Sarcoplasmic/endoplasmic reticulum calcium ATPase
CYP	Cytochrome P450
CPA	Cyclophosphamide
IFA	Ifosfamide
NMP	Nucleoside monophosphate
BBB	Blood brain barrier
CES	Carboxyl esterase
Doxaz	Doxazolidine
PABA	Para-aminobenzyl alcohol
5-FU	5-*Fluorouracil*
LEAPT	Lectin-directed enzyme activated prodrug therapy
ASGPRs	Asialoglycoprotein receptors
HIV	Human immunodeficiency virus
CNS	Central nervous system
BTCDS	Brain-targeting chemical delivery system
DADLE	Tyr-D-Ala-Gly-Phe-D-Leu
POP	Prolyloligopeptidase
SASP	Salicylazosulphapyridine
OSZ	Osalazine
5-ASA	5-Aminosalicylic acid
PSI	Proximal small intestine

DSI	Distal small intestine
IBD	Inflammatory bowel disease
BPAA	Biphenylacetic acid
CyDs	Cyclodextrins
RT	Reverse transcriptase
HAART	Highly active antiretroviral therapy
NRTIs	Nucleoside reverse-transcriptase inhibitors
TDP	Tenofovir diphosphate
SQV	Saquinavir
fMLF	Formyl-methionine-leucine-phenylalanine
EPO	Erythropoietin

Introduction

Classical/traditional prodrug approach aims to make better properties of drugs such as solubility and absorption by linking them covalently to a chemical moiety. This moiety is intended to be cleaved inside the body non-specifically or specifically by certain enzymes to give rise to the active drug. The moiety can be hydrophilic aiming to increase solubility in gastro-intestinal tract (GIT) or hydrophobic aiming to increase membrane permeability. Such prodrugs suffer from non-specific activation at sites other than the active site resulting in related toxicities and low bioavailability [1-3].

The molecular revolution in recent years and the increasing knowledge of the structure and functions of enzymes and transporters have created a new era of prodrugs which are termed 'targeted prodrugs'. Scientists have now replaced their way of synthesizing classical prodrugs into designing prodrugs for specific targeting of certain enzymes and transporters, thus increasing bioavailability and reducing toxicity that lead to the goal of achieving a better therapeutic efficiency.

Now it is no longer the old absorption, distribution, metabolism and excretion (ADME) barriers what we care about but the modern ADME which takes into consideration the presence of influx/efflux proteins and the distribution and expression of cellular proteins [4-7].

Targeted prodrugs in which a chemical moiety is attached to a parent drug to selectively target an activating enzyme or transporter is considered the main cornerstone for making efficient clinical profiles.

A successful prodrug targeting must fulfill the following requirements: the drug must be transported to its site rapidly, cleaved there selectively and retained at its site of action for a reliable time [8].

Targeting using both enzymes and transporters requires a great knowledge of the molecular structure and functionalities of those transporters/enzymes. When synthesizing a prodrug to target a specific site in the body, the prodrug must contain a chemical moiety that is specifically recognized by the aimed enzyme/transporter which is usually present exclusively or overexpressed at the desired site of action [4-7].

Targeting Cancer Cells

Cancer is defined as an uncontrolled cell division of abnormal cells [9, 10]. It can affect any type of cells of the body organs such as lung, liver and colon. Because the cells dividing are normal cells, cancer drugs are not selective and results in many side effects [11].

In the recent years cancer diagnosed patients have been gradually increasing, the most common treatments used are surgery, radiation and chemotherapy which can be used alone or in combination [11]. With the absence of an ultimate cure and due to the limited efficiency of currently available chemotherapeutics, it is a supreme goal for scientists to develop an effective anticancer treatment. Researchers often focus on the development of available drugs into more effective regiments with better properties by making prodrugs, especially targeted prodrugs; which produce their effect at the desired site of action, increasing efficiency and reducing toxic side effects that are well known to be caused with by these cytotoxic agents.

Drugs used in cancer treatment fall into one of the following classes: DNA complexing agents, alkylating agents, antimetabolites, mitosis inhibitors and hormones. They all act by interfering with normal DNA processes necessary to cell division [12].

Tumor cell targeting can be active or passive taking advantage from specific conditions available at these cancerous cells such as: hypoxia, existence and/or over expression of certain enzymes, tumor specific antigens and low extracellular pH [12].

Tumor Active Targeting

Tumor Specific Antigens and Receptors

Tumor active targeting is targeting tumor cells through a specific interaction with antigens or receptors that are present at the tumor cell surface. A prodrug conjugate linked to a moiety that has the potential to achieve the required interaction is to be used. This moiety can be monoclonal antibodies (mAbs) or any other ligand [13-16]. These systems can be activated inside or outside the cell gaining the names internalizing and non-internalizing, respectively [12]. Drugs that gain entrance to the cell by receptor-mediated endocytosis are expected to have a significant low resistance as a result of efflux by P-glycoprotein (P-GP). Once inside the cells the active drug is released by endosomes or lysosomes activation.

Besides its usefulness, such a technique in tumor targeting suffers from some drawbacks including some off-targets that occur as a result of a presence of the same receptors or ligands at sites in the body other than tumor cells, producing undesired side effects [17]. In addition, the expression of these receptors on cancer cells is variable and the preclinical models used which are mouse and human transplanted tumors do not reflect the real image of a drug bio-distribution [12].

Conjugating a drug to mAb was one of the first methods to be tested because of its high binding affinity with certain antigens. When drugs bind to antigens they act by blocking signal transduction or they may activate the complementary system which activates natural killer cells resulting in cytotoxicity. A number of studies have been conducted on linking chemotherapeutic agents with mAbs. These studies have shown that the mAb-drug conjugates were capable of entering the cell by receptor-mediated endocytosis and have shown better selectivity towards cancerous cells. However, a major drawback was developing immunogenicity that resulted from the use of murine mAbs [16].

At the start of this approach murine mAbs were used and have caused immunogenic reactions. To avoid such immune reactions, the murine derived mAbs were replaced with newer chimeric and humanized ones. Some of these FDA approved chimeric and humanized mAbs that were used to treat some types of tumors are: trastuzumab (Herceptin), rituximab (Rituxan), alemtuzumab (campath), cetuximab (Erbitux) and bevacizumab (Avastin) [18-20].

Mylotarg (gemtuzumab, Wyeth) [21] is an FDA approved immunoconjugate for the treatment of acute myeloid leukemia (AML) for elderly patients that cannot tolerate other chemotherapeutic agents or for those suffer from relapse. It consists of humanized anti-CD33 mAb linked to the cytotoxic antibiotic ozogamicin, N-acetyl-γ calicheamicin (Figure 1).

Figure 1. Antibody conjugate of maytansinoid (huC242-DM1).

Another immunoconjugate which is currently in phase three clinical trials is cantuzumab-mertansine conjugate of DM1 [22]. This agent kills cancer cells by inhibiting microtubules assembly thus preventing mitosis [23]. It consists of DM1 coupled to ε-amino group of lysine residues on humanized antibody C242 through a disulfide bond. Once inside the cell it is activated via reductive cleavage in the lysosomal/endosomal compartments (Figure 2).

Differently from mAbs, some ligands show high affinity for receptors on the surface of tumor cells. Such ligands are used for tumor specific targeting by linking the desired drug/prodrug to them [12]. Most of such research had focused on using folic acid drug conjugates. The reason behind that is that even when conjugated to drug folic acid still shows high affinity to its receptor which is overexpressed on some kinds of tumor cells.

Patrick and coworkers have developed several camptothecin (CPT) conjugates and tested them for folate receptor targeting [24]. One conjugate was CPT-Gly-PEG-Folate; it was prepared by linking CPT to one end of PEG through glycine peptide and the other end was linked directly to folic acid (Figure 3).

Figure 2. Auristatins (cAC10-vcMMAE) - an antibody conjugate.

Results from in vitro tests on KB cells have shown specificity towards folate receptor with less associated cytotoxicity. The same group has also prepared the following CPT conjugates: glycine (gly), alanine (ala), proline (pro), prolineglycine (pro), proline-alanine (pro-ala), glycine-glycine-glycine (gly-gly-gly) and glycineglycine- phenylalanine-glycine (gly-gly-phe-gly). The aim of the mono and dipeptides was to investigate the effect of the steric hindrance on the release of the drug, whereas the tri- and tetra-peptides were used to target the enzyme cathepsin B, thus achieving dual targeting. In the terms of effectiveness and safety the conjugate PEG-Gly-Gly-Phe-Gly-folate was the most promising for further development.

Figure 3. Camptothecin folate conjugate.

Cancer Targeting via Membrane Transporters

The knowledge of the existence of a certain membrane transporter on the surface of a certain type of cell allows specific targeting.

Transporters are protein structures which are present on the cell surface and their work depends on the presence of a secondary substrate. Two major families of transporters are known: the ATP-binding cassette (ABC) family which is responsible for resistance through efflux mechanism and the solute carrier (SLC) transporters which is responsible for influx [25]. The idea of drug targeting through membrane transporters have been advocated after the study on the prodrug valcyclovir which is a prodrug of L-valyl ester of the antiviral acyclovir; the addition of the peptide into the drug have efficiently increased the drug's bioavailability after oral administration through the targeting of the peptidic membrane transporter PEPT1 which is highly expressed on the walls of the small intestine [26-29]. After uptake into the blood the prodrug is rapidly converted to the active drug acyclovir by the action of blood esterases.

Many cancer cells overexpress certain membrane transporters thus making them vulnerable to specific drug targeting. Zhao et al. have synthesized a prodrug of the anticancer agent β-arboline by linking it to several amino acids via an ester bond. From the in vitro results it was shown that the permeability was the highest utilizing the amino acids lysine and arginine. The receptor PEPT1 is thought to be responsible for the increased influx [12].

Of the disadvantages of such a method is that the transporters are not exclusive to specific cell type but they are also expressed on other cells to a lesser extent resulting in toxic effects. However, there are some advantages which include among other, increasing oral absorption, especially for hydrophilic drugs. Further, it is usual to target these receptors with an addition of a nutrient to the parent drug to ensure a minimum toxicity of the resulting by product [12].

Passive Targeting of Tumor

Passive Targeting Taking Advantage of the Enhanced Permeability and Retention Effect

Not only receptors or antigens may allow for targeting cancer cells. Taking advantages of other properties of these cells is another possibility for targeting. One of the most important characteristics of tumor cells is angiogenesis. To grow at high rates cancer cells require a continuous supply of nutrients and oxygen. These needs are coped by biosynthesis of new blood vessels. These newly formed blood vessels are different from the normal ones; they have large pores (in the size range 100-1200 nm) [30] as a result of the disorganized alignment of endothelial cells and absence or existence of abnormal perivascular cells and smooth muscles.

Due to this fenestrated structure of vessels and referring to the fact that tumor tissues suffers from poor lymphatic drainage the phenomena of enhanced permeability and retention (EPR) effect was elucidated [31].

Taking benefit of this phenomena tumor cell targeting is achieved by linking a drug/prodrug molecule into a macro/nanomolecular carrier or to a polymeric structure. Such structures are kept away from targeting normal cells having normally structured blood vessels. Although smaller molecules can gain access into these tumor cells but they usually leave through the lymphatic drainage, while the larger molecules tend to get retained.

Of the polymers that are used in such targeting are polyethylene glycol (PEG), polyglutamate (PGA) and hydroxypropylmethacrylamide (HPMA). Recently, new polymeric architectures are being developed and are used in this field such as star-like polymers, dendronized linear polymers and graft copolymers. It is important to make sure that the polymers used are safe, non-toxic and non-irritant [12].

Polymer Directed Enzyme Prodrug Therapy (PDEPT)

Another method of passive targeting is called polymer directed enzyme prodrug therapy (PDEPT). This method of passive targeting relies on delivering a prodrug-polymer conjugate followed by an enzyme-polymer conjugate to achieve specific site activation. Both the enzyme and prodrug take advantage of EPR effect to reach tumor cells [32, 33]. When compared to antibody-directed enzyme prodrug therapy (ADEPT) or gene-directed enzyme prodrug therapy (GDEPT) PDEPT is found to be less toxic, and with easier synthesis and purification steps [912].

When the same method is applied using a liposome-prodrug conjugate instead of a polymer-prodrug it is called polymer directed enzyme liposome therapy (PELT) [32].

Duncan et al. have studied this concept with PK1 prodrug which consists of doxorubicin conjugated to HPMA copolymer through the linker Gly-Phe-Leu-Gly which is found to be sensitive to the enzyme cysteine protease. From in vivo testing study that was conducted on B16F10 melanoma-bearing mice it was shown that an increase of 3-4 fold in free doxorubicin AUC was achieved after administrating HPMA-cathepsin when compared to an administration of doxorubicin-polymer conjugate alone.

Tumor Targeting Using Acid Sensitive Linkers

Tumor tissues extracellular environment has an acidic pH which is lower than normal tissues by 0.5-1 pH units. This pH difference can be used in tumor targeting by incorporating acid sensitive linkages into the prodrug design such as: imine, ketal, acetal and hydrazonebonds [34].

Tumor Targeting by Enzymatic Cleavage

Enzymatic cleavage via the advantageous of enzymes expressed intra/extracellular at the tumor cell represents a major method for targeting cancerous cells. Usually a peptide linker which is a substrate for a specific tumor enzyme is conjugated to the desired drug/prodrug. When acted upon by the enzyme there are two possibilities: one is that the drug is released after the peptide cleavage by the enzyme and the other is that a peptide-drug derivative is released and subjected to further hydrolysis releasing the active moiety [34].

The most important enzymes in cancer targeting are:

1)   Cathepsin B,D,H and L

They represent a large family of lysosomal cysteine proteases that exist in all mammalian cells. Some of their subtypes are considered a prognostic factor for the presence of some tumors such as cathepsin D which indicates a presence of metastatic breast cancer. Cathepsin enzymes are present at the surface of cancer cells or they are secreted at extracellular space.

Prodrugs with these peptide sequences Arg-Arg-X, Ala-Leu-X, Gly-Leu-Phe-Gly-X, Gly-Phe-Leu-Gly-X and Ala-Leu-Ala-Leu-X are considered as substrates for cathepsin B, H and L which are responsible for lysosomal degradation processes. While prodrugs with the following structures: Phe-Ala-Ala-Phe (NO2)-Phe-Val-Leu-OM4P-X and Bz-Arg-Gly-Phe-Phe-Pro-4mβNA are considered substrates for cathepsin D which is responsible for the degradation of extracellular matrix.

2)   γ-Glutamyl transpeptidase

High levels of this enzyme are associated with several types of liver cancer. Substrates for this enzyme include the γ-Glutamyl derivatives of many drugs such as phenylenediamine mustard, cytosine arabinoside and adriamycin.

3)   Acid phosphatase

High levels of this enzyme are associated with prostate cancer. Substrates are prodrug derivatives containing an acid phosphatase cleavable bond.

Other enzymes that can be used in tumor specific targeting include: matrix metalloproteases and beta-glucoronidases [35, 36].

Hypoxia

Some cancer cells are known to be hypoxic resulting from a poor vasculature; such cells overexpress angiogenic factors and have low levels of oxygen and nutrients. Because of decreased blood flow these cells are resistant to treatment by radiation and chemotherapy [37]. Also, they were found to have more resistance patterns including up-regulation of genes responsible for P-glycoproteins.

The principle of targeting hypoxic cancer cells relies on using inactive prodrug that becomes activated by reductases, such as NADPH: cytochrome P450 reductase (P450R), DT-diaphorase, xanthine oxidase and xanthine dehydrogenase. After being reduced to produce a free radical the drug is oxidized by molecular oxygen forming the initial prodrug.

Prodrugs produced by this way are transformed into electrophiles or free radicals so they locked in hypoxic cells. Hypoxic anticancer prodrugs are classified into three categories: N-oxides, nitro compounds and quinones [9].

Two prodrugs in clinical trials based on this principle are tirapamazine [38] and anthraquinone [39].Such a process suffers from the lack of reductive enzymes required for activation because these hypoxic cells are nercotic. So an alternative method was developed and is being tested on some drugs such as nitrobenzyl quaternary ammonium salts [40] and oxypropyl-substituted 5-fluoruracilderivatives [41].This method depends on the use of ionizing radiation which is commonly used for cancer treatment. When water is exposed to these radiation an electron is formed which have a high reductive potential, leading to the formation of a superoxide when scavenged by O2 [42].

Targeting Prostate Cancer

Prostate cancer is of the most common cancer in old men but also can affect the young [43]. Cancer cells in metastatic colon cancer are divided into androgen dependent and androgen independent cells [44]. When given androgen deprivation therapy androgen dependent cells undergo apoptosis showing an initial clinical response [45]. After repeated administration the clinical effect subsides due to the presence of androgen independent cells [46].The need for drugs that will cause selective apoptosis in androgen independent cells without affecting normal cells is crucial.

The main idea of prostate cancer targeting relies on the presence of prostate specific antigen (PSA) in the extracellular fluid of prostate cells. PSA is secreted both from normal and cancerous cells, it also exists in serum but in an inactive state. A major characteristic of the presence of prostate cancer is high levels of PSA which is used as diagnostic measurement [47-49].

A prodrug containing a moiety that is cleaved specifically by PSA near the prostate represents the main idea of prostate cancer targeting [50].

Samuel et al. have synthesized and studied a targeted prodrug of thapsigargin for prostate cancer. Thapsigargin (Figure 4) which is naturally extracted from the plant *Thapsia garganica* is a potent inhibitor of sarcoplasmic/endoplasmic reticulum calcium ATPase (SERCA) pump in both proliferating and quiescent cells. It causes an increase in intracellular free calcium levels, leading to an elevation of the intracellular calcium levels resulting from the depletion of the ER calcium pools which further creates a signal that affects cellular membrane permeability leading to the opening of calcium channels causing more calcium influx which has resulted in cell death [51-53]. The drawback of this cytotoxic drug is not selective in its action between cancerous and normal cells leading to toxic effects which had led the researchers to develop a targeted prodrug of the drug thapsigargin.

Thapsigargin prodrug was synthesized by incorporating the drug into a primary amine which was linked to a specific peptide sequence that was found to be highly cleaved specifically by prostate not serum PSA. This specific sequence is His-Ser-Ser-Lys-Leu-Gln (HSSKLQ) by which the primary amine is linked to the terminal carboxyl group of glutamine [50].

From in vitro studies it was found that the prodrug was stable in human plasma and not cleaved by serum PSA and it was selectively toxic to PSA producing cancerous prostate cells.

Attempts using the same principle were made on doxorubicin but have not succeeded because the prodrug for doxorubicin have shown a nearly 30% cleavage of the specific peptide has occurred by serum PSA which was associated with systemic toxicity. Another drawback was that doxorubicin was not found to be active in low proliferative prostate cancer cells [54]. This is in contrast to thapsigargin which was found to have activity against this specific population of cells and to other cancerous cells regardless of their proliferative state [55].

Figure 4. Thapsigargin and thapsigargin prodrug. The arrow shows the point of recognition by PSA.

Targeting Liver Cancer

The liver which is made of hepatocytes is considered the main organ responsible for metabolism in the body also it is involved in the synthesis of many essential compounds. The surface of the hepatocytes is full with receptors and carriers and many enzymes are available inside providing several targets for specific liver drug delivery [56, 57].

The vital liver functions can be affected with a wide variety of acute or chronic diseases resulting from many reasons such as toxicity by an overdose of alcohol or drugs, viral infections, metabolic disorders such as diabetes as well as chronic congenital disorders such as Wilson disease and Gilbert syndrome. If left untreated they will lead to mortality resulting from liver cancer and failure [58].

The most successful strategy followed in liver targeting is through the cytochrome P450 liver enzyme family (CYPs) [59]. These are a group of more than fifty enzymes upon which six of them are responsible for metabolizing about ninety percent of drugs. They are crucial for the production of certain substances such as cholesterol and prostacyclins [60].

CYP families 1, 2 and 3 are responsible for the metabolism of xenobiotics and are found to have wide substrate specificity, while CYP families 4, 5, 7, 8, 11, 17, 19, 21, 24, 27, and 51 are responsible for the metabolism of endogenous compounds and are found to have very strict substrate specificity [61-63]. When targeting CYPs, polymorphism and possible drug-drug interactions should be taken in consideration [64].

The knowledge of the mechanism of activation of cancer agents CPA, IFA, and trofosfamideby CYPs has led to the development of HepDirect prodrugs; a class of phosphates and phosphonates including in their structures cyclic 1,3-propanyl esters containing a ring substituent that has the tendency to undergo an oxidative cleavage reaction catalyzed by a cytochrome P450 [65].

The isoenzyme family CYP3A is highly expressed in the parenchymal cells of liver. Among substrates for this family are prodrugs containing 4-aryl substituent [66]. Upon exposure to CYP oxidative reaction, the ring opens irreversibly creating anionic intermediate which becomes locked inside the hepatocyte. An elimination reaction follows creating the phosphate/phosphonate drug with an aryl vinyl ketone as a byproduct [67, 68]. This byproduct becomes rapidly conjugated by the glutathione (GSH) which is normally present inside hepatocytes as a protective mechanism against oxidative damage (Figure 5).

Figure 5. Mechanism of activation of HepDirect prodrugs via CYP3A4 oxidation forming the corresponding active phosphate/phosphonate and the side product aryl vinyl ketone.

In vivo testing of HepDirect prodrugs for liver-targeted drug delivery in rats and mice using two structurally different nucleoside monophosphate (NMP) analogs, namely adefovir(PMEA) and cytarabine (araC) 5-monophosphate have shown an improved safety profile and no byproduct-related toxicities. These results suggest that HepDirect prodrugs have the potential to be used in achieving targeted liver delivery with less associated side effects for liver chronic diseases such as liver cancer and hepatitis B and C [69].

Targeting the enzymes carboxyl estrase-1(CES-1) and carboxyl estrase-2(CES-2) which are over expressed in liver cancer have made a new approach for specific liver targeting. Carboxyl esterases are serine esterases that cause hydrolysis of various esters and carbamates.

Carbamate prodrugs were synthesized to target these carboxylases. The enzyme carboxyl esterase has two pockets one is small; which accommodates small alcohols or esters and the other is large which is flexible and have the capability to accommodate many molecules [70].

Doxazolidine (Doxaz) is oxazolidine derivative of doxorubicin. Several doxazolidine prodrugs were synthesized Doxaz ethyl carbamate, Doxaz butyl carbamate and PentylDoxaz ethyl carbamate (Figure 6).

After in vivo testing it was found that most inhibition has occurred with butyl and pentyl carbamates, while the prodrug with the simplest structure ethyl carbamate resulted in the least inhibition indicating the necessity of the existence of a lipophilic moiety for the interaction to occur with the enzyme. Cardiotoxic effects were found due to the final formation of doxorubicin [71].

New carbamate prodrugs were synthesized by using a self-eliminating linker, p-aminobenzyl alcohol (PABA), between the doxazolidine and alkyl carbamate. These compounds were found to inhibit cancer cells with less cardio-toxicity than the simple carbamates (Figure 7).

Capecitabine is carbamate prodrug of 5-FU.Capcitabine is the pentyl carbamate of 5-Flurocytidine derivative that functions as a prodrug of the antitumor compound 5-FU (Figure 8).

Another prodrug to be mentioned is Irinotecan which is a carbamate prodrug of a water soluble camptothecin that is hydrolyzed primarily by CES2 [72].Capecitabine and irinotecan can be hydrolyzed by both esterases CES1 and CES2.

Another approach utilized in liver targeting is platinum compounds that have been conjugated with galactose taking benefit of galactose receptors expressed on the level of hepatocytes [73].

While in another method platinum was attached to bile acid to be taken into hepatocytes by sodium independent transport carriers [74].

Figure 6. Doxazolidine carbamate prodrug.

Figure 7. The newer less toxic doxazolidine carbamate prodrug with the PABA linker.

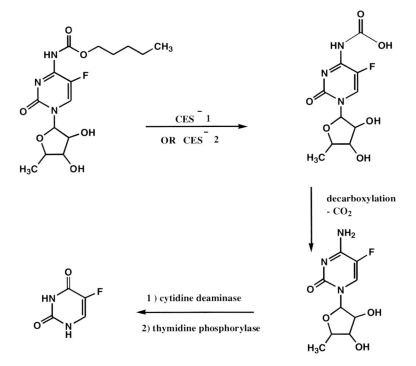

Figure 8. Activation of capecitabine by human CES.

One conjugate-based strategy capable of delivering drugs to an extravascular site uses glycoprotein and glycolipid-containing drug carriers that recognize the Asialoglycoprotein receptor expressed on hepatocytes [75]. This method relies on delivering a glycoslated enzyme into the body. This glycosylation process will ensure a specific organ/tissue targeting through an interaction between the sugar unit on the enzyme and a specific receptor. Then anon-mammalian sugar capped prodrug is administered; using non-mammalian sugar to ensure that the drug will be intact until it reaches its active site. When it reaches the enzyme site, the enzyme acts to break down the prodrug releasing the active drug specifically to its site of action, thus decreasing associated toxicities and unwanted side effects [76].

A method with this principle was applied in targeting liver cancer, it is called lectin-directed enzyme activated prodrug therapy (LEAPT) [77]. An example using this method was demonstrated in a study that utilizes the enzyme rhamnosidase which was specifically bioengineered to form d-galactosylatedrhamnosidase, d-galactosylatedrhamnosidase ensures its way to the liver through specific internalization into hepatocytes by receptor mediated endocytosis which occurs as a result of binding to Asialoglycoprotein receptors (ASGPRs) which are highly expressed on hepatocytes. Prodrugs of both doxorubicin and 5-fluorouracil were capped with the non-mammalian sugar l-rhamnosyl [78].

The results of bio-distribution of the enzyme have shown that strong localization in the liver was achieved with a minimum amount localized in the kidney and bladder. The results have shown stability in blood and a halving decrease in tumor burden after 42 days of treatment compared to control in a disease model of rats [78].

Despite some success in preclinical models, advancement of these and other drug conjugates remains slow due to concerns over manufacturing costs, conjugate-induced immunogenic reactions, and limitations in drug loading and the route of administration [69].

Targeting the Central Nervous System

As the health care system in the developed world is improving an increase in the elderly population is observed. Making CNS diseases like Parkinson's disease and Alzheimer's a critical public problem. An inefficient treatment for these neurodegenerative diseases is caused partly by the physiological nature of the CNS which is secured from the entry of any foreign substances including drugs to the brain by the blood brain barrier (BBB).

The BBB contains tight-junctions which only permit the transport of lipophilic compounds to traverse it by diffusion or if the compound is a substrate for DBB carrier mediated transporters, also transcytosis takes place which can be absorptive mediated or receptor mediated transcytosis [79].

Many recent advances have been made in the last decades for better CNS delivery. Of these used methods are nanoparticles, liposomes, and some invasive strategies such as BBB disruption and intracerebral implants [80].

CNS targeting via prodrugs is considered a pharmacological strategy. Classical prodrugs are inactive chemical entities usually prepared for improving physicochemical properties. Prodrugs become activated spontaneously or enzymatically giving rise to the active parent compound. When talking about prodrugs to target CNS the first thing to come in mind is to link the drug to a lipophilic moiety such as fatty acid, glyceride or phospholipids which will permit BBB transmission. Regardless of the achievement of successful entry of the drug into the CNS via this method many disadvantages are to be faced including poor selectivity, poor retention and the creation of toxic/reactive metabolites [81].

Vector mediated delivery is also used for CNS specific targeting. The principle of this method relies on using a non-transportable drug conjugated to BBB transport vector. The vector can be a modified protein or receptor specific antibody. The vector gains access to the brain via BBB transporters (for modified proteins) or via receptor mediated transcytosis (for monoclonal antibodies) [82]. The drug can be conjugated to the vector through several methods such as chemical linkers, avidin-biotin technology, polyethylene glycol linkers and liposomes [83].

Chemical delivery systems are also used in which at least one bond needs to be broken to release the active drug. Redox chemical delivery systems have shown efficiency in CNS targeting. It is composed of two parts target promoting moiety; responsible for site specificity and modifier functions which increase hydrophobicity, these modifier functions are designed to prevent the conversion to unwanted metabolites mentioned before. Of these chemical delivery systems are the ones that depend on an enzymatic oxidation reaction to covert the lipophilic dihydropyridine to the ionic pyridinium salt, thus retaining the drug in the brain for a longer time [80].

Based on the principle of redox chemical delivery one system was applied for enkephalin delivery to the brain. Enkephalins are naturally occurring opioids used as analgesics which can replace the currently used morphine derivatives and alkaloids minimizing their associated side effects [84]. The problem of such compounds is that they are proteins which make them vulnerable to degradation by peptidases, also being hydrophilic limits their blood brain barrier (BBB) permeability [85].

A way for resolving this problem was utilizing the prodrug approach. A prodrug was made with improved in vivo stability. This prodrug is δ opioid receptor-selective enkephalin analogue Tyr-D-Ala-Gly-Phe-D-Leu (DADLE), even it is stable it cannot cross the BBB because of its hydrophilic nature [86].

Brain-targeting chemical delivery system (BTCDS) for DADLE was made. This system is inactive on its own but is enzymatically activated in the brain by the act of peptidases. This system consists of lipophilic 1,4-dihydrotrigonellyl moiety which is attached to the N terminus of the drug via peptidic spacer. In the brain, oxidoreductases act to oxidize the dihydropyridine into the positively charged N-methylpyridinium thus retaining the drug in the brain for a longer time [87]. Then the drug is released by the action of several peptidases specially the enzyme prolyloligopeptidase (POP) which acts to remove the spacer from the oxidized BTCDS (Figure 9) [88]. In vitro studies on rats brain homogenates have shown increased half-lives which were correlated with in vivo analgesic effects using tail-flick model [89].

Targeting Colon

The aim of colon drug targeting is to increase the efficiency of treating colon diseases with less side effects and higher bioavailability.

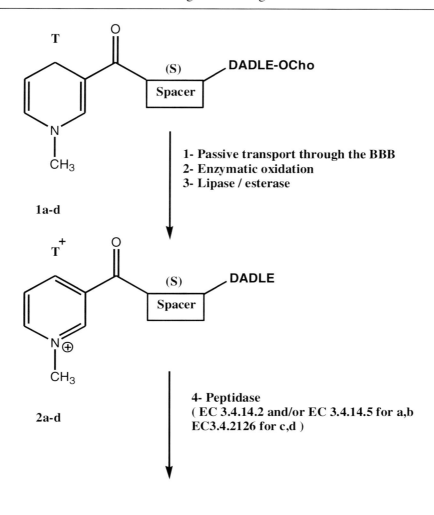

Figure 9. DADLE brain targeting delivery system. (a) DADLE (b) peptidic spacer (c) lipophilic 1, 4-dihydrotrigonellyl moiety (d) N-methylpyridine moiety.

Due to the relatively hostile environment of the stomach it remains hard to transport intact drugs to the colon. Colonic drug targeting is not only very important for treating several colonic diseases such as Chron's disease, ulcerative colitis, colon cancer, irritable bowel disease and many others but also the colon was found to be an appropriate site for the absorption of many therapeutic peptides [90].

One of the successful ways to deliver intact chemical entities to the colon is via using the prodrug approach. Using prodrugs with linkers that are selectively cleaved at colon by the enzymatic activity, colonic microflora is a very common approach in colon specific targeting [91]. The linker used must be covalently attached to the drug in order to prevent early degradation in the stomach and small intestine [90].

Advantages of colonic targeting include increasing the efficiency of treating colon diseases with less side effects and higher bioavailability. The lymphoid tissue present at the colon facilitates the uptake of antigens into mast cells which leads to antibodies production and thus more efficient vaccination [92]. A drawback of colon targeting is due to colonic microflora which may cause some unwanted reactions [90].

Azo bond prodrugs, glycosidic prodrugs and natural polysaccharides are of the most common compounds used in colon-specific targeting.

Azo Bond Conjugates

The microflora in the colon is a complex, relatively stable microorganisms which are involved in many metabolic processes including the reduction of many chemical functionalities such as azo and nitro groups. In addition, the microflora serves as defender against invasion of pathogenic microorganisms [93-95].

Of the prodrugs that were synthesized on the basis of azo bond conjugates is sulfasalazine which is also chemically called salicylazosulphapyridine (SASP). It is widely used for anti-inflammatory diseases [96]. This drug is acted upon the azoreductase enzyme secreted by the colonic microflora causing azo bond cleavage producing one molecule of sulfapyridine and 5-aminosalicylic acid (Figure 10). Because of the production of sulfapyridine the prodrug has been associated with side effects, so a safer prodrug with less toxic moiety was made which is called osalazine (OSZ). OSZ is a dimer connecting two molecules of 5-ASA through an azo bond (Figure 11).

The prodrug was found to cause watery diarrhea in 15% of patients administered the prodrug [97]. Balsalazine was also synthesized by linking one molecule of 5-ASA and 4-aminobenzoyl-b-alanine (Figure 11) which has shown good efficiency with fewer side effects than SASP (Figure 11) [98].

Figure 10. Cleavage of sulfasalazine by the colonic azoreductases.

Figure 11. Another azo bond containing prodrugs OSZ (2 units of 5-ASA linked together) and balsalazine (5-ASA linked to 4-aminobenzoyl-b-alanine).

Drugs based on high molecular weight azo polymer coating have been also developed and tested with the same principle of getting activated by microflora enzymes. Such drugs are prevented from absorption from upper GIT because of their large size [99].

Amino Acid Conjugation

Amino acid conjugation is used in colon targeting by linking the drug to amino acids. The hydrophilic nature of amino acids due to the presence of COOH and NH2 functions results in a limited absorption in the upper GIT. A trial contained salicylic acid conjugated to a non-essential amino acid such as glycine and tyrosine was tested in dogs and rabbits. Salicylic acid was released by the action of microflora (Figure 12). The results also have shown that a small amount of the prodrug was detected in the systemic circulation of the tested dogs and rabbits which was unwanted. This had led to a synthesis of a new prodrug containing a more hydrophilic and higher chain length amino acid, glutamine. After testing the new prodrug has shown satisfactory results with minimal GIT absorption [100-103].

Glycoside Conjugates

Glycoside conjugates are used for colon targeting based on the existence of several glycosidase enzymes in the colon and on the brush border of small intestine. Several subtypes were detected from human feces; they are β-D-galactosidase, β-D-glucosidase, β-D-xylopyranosidaseandα-L- arabinofuranosidase [104]. Glycosides are prevented from an absorption in the upper GIT parts because of their bulkiness and polarity.

Figure 12. Amino acid conjugated prodrugs of salicylic acid. (a) salicyluric acid. (b) salicyl-glutamic acid.

Dexamethasone-21-β-glucoside and prednisolone-21-β-glucoside were prepared by Friend and Chang to be tested for colon targeting. The drugs were administered to rats, intagastrically, using a negative control of the free steroid dexamethasone and prednisolone, respectively. The results have shown that both drugs needed nearly 5 hours to reach the colon where the free steroids were released. When studied after oral administration 60% of dexamethasone-21-β-glucoside and 15% of prednisolone-21-β-glucoside have reached the colon compared to only 1% of the dose was reached when the corresponding steroids were administered in the same manner [105].

The effect of the structure of the prodrug on the specificity of glycoside/glycosidase was studied by synthesizing nine steroidal glycoside prodrugs. The reaction used was a modified method of Koenigs-Knorr. The prodrugs were 21-ylB-D-glucosides and galactosides of dexamethasone, prednisolone, hydrocortisone, fludrocortisones and 21-ylB-D-cellobioside of prednisolone. The prodrugs were subjected to hydrolysis by the contents of a rat stomach, proximal small intestine (PSI), distal small intestine (DSI) and caecum. The results have shown that the hydrolysis in caecum had the highest rate followed by the DSI then the stomach and PSI. All of the prodrugs were hydrolyzed fast in the caecum except hydrocortisone-21-ylB-D-glucoside and fludrocortisones-21-ylB-D-glucoside. These results indicate that the activity of glucosidase in the colon is more heterogeneous than the activity of galactosidase as was suggested by Eadie-Hofstee [106].

In an experimental model of inflammatory bowel disease (IBD) conducted in guinea pig it was found that 0.65 mol/kg of dexamethasone-B-D-glucoside gave the same effect in reducing the total number of ulcers as 1.3 mol/kg of dexamethasone [107].

Glucoronide Conjugates

It is widely known that glucoronidation is naturally occurring metabolic pathway which leads to the production of hydrophilic metabolites limiting their membrane permeability. Glucoronidases which are secreted by the colonic microflora enables the release of the active drug in the colon in an absorbable form to exert its activity [108].

Two narcotic antagonists, nalmefene and naloxone, and their glucoronide conjugates were tested on morphine dependent rats. When nalmefene hydrochloride and nalmefene glucoronide were given subcutaneously the latter had shown no efficacy as was indicated by tail skin temperature responses. When the glucoronide conjugates for nalmefene and naloxone were given orally only 0.2-0.5% of the administered dose had reached the circulation indicating a successful colon delivery of the drugs [109].

A more efficient treatment of ulcerative colitis with lower steroid side effects was observed by Haeberlin et al. after testing two glucoronide prodrugs of dexamethasone and budesonide [110].

Cyclodextrin Conjugates

Cyclodextrins (CyDs) are cyclic oligosaccharides consisting of six to eight units linked together by α -1,4glycosidic bonds. They are hydrophilic from outside while their interior part is relatively hydrophobic thus allowing the drug to be captured in forming an inclusion body which allows an improvement in some unwanted properties of the drug such as low solubility and bioavailability. Their large size limits their permeability and absorption from upper GIT [111,112]. After reaching the colon they get fermented by the act of the colonic microflora releasing small sugar units and the drug to be ready for absorption [113]. One can control the rate of drug release depending on the nature of cyclodextrin. For example, ionizable cyclodextrins allow for delayed release whereas hydrophilic ones allow for an immediate release.

It was shown from a study on healthy human volunteers that there was a minimum digestion of β-cyds in small intestine, whereas it was completely fermented in the large intestine [90].

A study was conducted on the release of the anti-inflammatory biphenylacetic acid (BPAA) from different cyd conjugates in a rat gastrointestinal tract after oral administration. The drug was linked through an ester or an amide bond to the primary OH of α, β or γ cyds. Results have shown that both α- andγ-cyds with an amide bond were hydrolyzed to maltose in the colon while no absorption of the drug had occurred. Whereas when the same cyds were linked through an ester linkage a drug absorption and release had occurred as it was indicated by measuring the drug concentration from the systemic circulation. β -cyds linked through an ester or an amide had led to a minimum hydrolysis to maltose and negligible drug release. This is attributed to the low solubility of β -cyds in the physiological media. Another study on the same drug, BPAA, was conducted using a model of carrageenan induced acute-edema in rat paw. The drug was administered alone and in combination with β-and γ-cyds. From the results it was shown that β-cyd resulted in immediate effect indicating that intestinal absorption that had taken its part. Whereas, γ-cyd resulted in a delayed effect indicating that absorption had occurred mainly in the colon [114,115].

Prednisolone which is widely used for the treatments of IBD suffers from associated side effects due to absorption at upper GIT. To reduce these effects conjugating the drug to α-cyd through an ester linkage was made and the new entity was tested in a rat IBD model and compared to prednisolone succinate. The results have shown reduced toxicity of the conjugate using cyd because the drug conjugate was only degraded in the colon [116]. Yano et al. also studied the anti-inflammatory and side effects of prednisolone conjugated to secondary hydroxyl of α, β and γ-cyds in a 2,4,6-trinitrobenzeneusulfonic acid induced rat colitis model. From the ones tested α-cyd has shown decreased side effects and good efficacy when administered intracolonically [117].

α - and β-cyds are widely known for causing nephrotoxicity which is either attributed to their uptake by kidney tubule cells or extraction of lipid membrane components [118]. This had led the scientists to develop new modified cyds which would not cause such an effect. Of these modified cyds that have shown successful colon targeting in rats dogs and humans are: DM- β -cyds and HP- β –cyd [119].

Dextran Conjugates

Dextrans—hydrophilic polysaccharides synthesized by *Leuconostoc* bacteria—are characterized by their high molecular weight, good water solubility, low toxicity, and relative inertness.

These properties make dextrans effective water-soluble carriers for dyes, indicators, and reactive groups in a wide variety of applications. Moreover, their biologically uncommon α-1, 6-polyglucose linkages are resistant to cleavage by most of endogenous cellular glycosidases. Therefore dextran conjugates make ideal long-term tracers for live cells.

Harboeand coworkers have determined the bioavailability of naproxen after oral administration of the conjugated dextran ester prodrug T-70-naproxen compared to an oral solution containing the same dose of naproxen. The absorption fraction of T-70-naproxen was 91% when compared to the oral solution [120].

Meclodet et al. have synthesized dextran ester prodrugs of dexamethasone and methylprednisolone. Succinic acid wad linked to each of them and another prodrug of dexamethasone was prepared using glutaric acid as a linker. This step was to determine the effect of the linker on the release of the active drug. Kinetic studies were measured as a function of time and pH. Intermolecular migration of the linker from 21- to 17- position was noticed in the three prodrug conjugates. To study their half-lives the dextran conjugates where incubated at 37°C and pH 6.8. The longest half-life was recorded for dexamethasone-glutarate-dextran (103 hours) followed by methylprednisolone-succinate-dextran (82 hours) and it was 73 hours for dexamethasone-21-hemisuccinate [121-123].

Targeting Human Immunodeficiency Virus (HIV)

Human immunodeficiency virus (HIV) is a retrovirus that attacks the immune cells of the body making the person vulnerable to much disease causing what is known under the name of acquired immunodeficiency syndrome. Two types of HIV are defined HIV1 and HIV2 until not specified the term HIV refers to HIV 1.

HIV2 was discovered in 1986 it starts slower and with milder symptoms but finally leads to AIDS and it has the same opportunistic infections caused by HIV 1 [124].

The virus is first adsorbed on the cell surface as a result of electrostatic interaction between the positively charged viral glycolprotein and the negatively charged heparin sulfate on the cell wall then it interacts with the receptor CD4 and the chemokine co-receptor CXCR4 or CCR5[125]. The interaction with CXCR4 or CCR5 depends on the V3 loop of glycoprotein 120. Therefore, the virus is classified as R5 or X4 tropic, or it can be X4R5 dual tropic [126].

Resulting from this binding is a conformational change is a fusion of the viral coat with the cell membrane followed by viral uncoating and releasing of two RNA strands and other viral enzymes including reverse transcriptase (RT) and integrase [127]. The viral RNA is then translocated into the nucleus and the enzyme RT creates a cDNA strand that is translocated into the nucleus and becomes incorporated into the host DNA by the aid of the enzyme integrase [128,129]. After the transcription the viral RNA travels to the cytoplasm, some is reserved to another replication cycles and others are translated to produce new viral proteins which are assembled to make new capsids and envelops; the new virus bud off the plasma membrane and is ready to infect other cells.

Prodrugs and Drug Conjugates for HIV Delivery

From the first report of HIV case in 1981 the numbers of patients are increasing reaching more than 67 million worldwide [130,131]. The disease mostly affects the younger population with an age of 15-24 years [132]. The most affected area is the sub-Saharan Africa [133].

HIV remains a great challenge for scientists due to the development of resistant strains, the cost and tolerability of treatment, the lack of an efficient prophylactic agent and an agent that would eradicate the virus [134].

Currently there are twenty four FDA approved drugs which are called highly active antiretroviral therapy (HAART) for HIV treatment which are often used in combinations. These agents are effective in suppressing the virus but remain insufficient for total eradication and cure. This insufficiency is caused by the physicochemical properties of such drugs which render them with poor solubility and bioavailability, and poor patient compliance due to the associated adverse effects and the need of frequent administration of these drugs [134,135].

Dr. Paul Janssen had described the characteristics that an ideal HIV drug should have. These characteristics include: potency even against resistant strains of the virus, low toxicity, high bioavailability, long half-life and easy synthesis which will be reflected in the cost of the therapy [136].

The number of drugs that meet this criteria is limited, which have led the scientists to focus on modifying the current drugs via prodrug and drug conjugates instead of discovering new chemical entities (Figure 13). Of the successfully made traditional prodrugs for HIV are fosamprenavir and tenofovir disoproxil fumarate (Figure 14) [137].

Fosamprenavir is a water soluble phosphor-ester of the protease inhibitor drug amprinavir [138-140]. It was approved by the FDA in 2003. Two dosage forms are available: tablet or suspension, with a dose equal to 1400 mg twice daily or 700 mg when combined with 100 mg ritonavir [139,140]. The aim of this prodrug was to increase water solubility of the parent drug (amprinavir) which has water solubility of~ 0.04mg/ml; this low solubility leads to poor bioavailability which varies from 35-90%. Administration of the phosphor-ester produg has led to 10 fold increase in water solubility [139].

Fosamprenavir on its own has no in vitro antiviral activity. Activity is noticed after in vivo administration due to its interconversion into amprinavir by alkaline phosphatase enzyme which is located at or near the intestinal epithelium [141]. From animal studies it was shown that less than 1% of fosamprenavir has reached the systemic circulation indicating that nearly all the administered prodrug has complete presystemic conversion. This result was reconfirmed by clinical studies [142].

The drug appeared to be absorbed immediately after administration of the prodrug as was demonstrated by plasma concentrations of the drug which was detected after 15 minutes and reaches its maximum concentration after 1.5-2.5 hours [142].

The drug had also shown to undergo biphasic absorption; the first occurs immediately after administration of the prodrug. This result was demonstrated by plasma concentrations of the drug which was detected after 15 minutes and reaches its maximum concentration after 1.5-2.5 hours. The second slow absorption phase was indicated from the appearance of a second peak in the plasma concentration curve at 10-12 hours but with concentration less than C_{max} [143]. The volume of distribution is ~ 430 liters more than the total body fluids also it is taken by lymphocytes 2-3 times more than plasma. The drug bioavailability was shown not to be affected with the presence or absence of food [144].

Tenofovir disoproxil fumarate is available as once daily tablet [145].It is the first nucleoside approved for AIDS treatment; it belongs to the acyclic nucleoside phosphonates [146,147]. The drug produces its effect after being phosphorylated inside the cell to produce tenofovir diphosphate which causes chain termination when the enzyme reverse transcriptase utilizes it to synthesize the viral DNA [148].

Unlike fosamprenavir which has a phosphor-ester linkage, tenofovir has a phosphonate linkage which is stable in the physiological media. An advantage of tenofovir over other nucleoside reverse-transcriptase inhibitors (NRTIs) is that the presence of the phosphonate group eliminates the need for the initial phosphorylation activation by virus induced kinases which is considered the rate limiting step for NRTIs activation [149-151]. The drug becomes active after two phosphorylations; the first by the enzyme adenylate kinase and the second by the enzyme nucleoside diphosphate kinase which leads to the formation of the active metabolite tenofovir diphosphate (TDP) [148,152,153].

Even that prodrugs have improved the efficiency of HIV treatment, the side effects resulting from unwanted activation remains a major disadvantage which had led for considering targeted prodrugs that are expected to lack associated side effects by releasing the drug at the site of action [154,155].

Protease inhibitors are widely used for HIV treatment. Of the most commonly known limitations of this class of drugs are low solubility, poor absorption, and conversion into inactive metabolites. The first drug that was approved of this class is saquinavir (SQV) which suffers from significant variability in bioavailability ranging from 4- 16% [156-158]. Sinko et al. have developed SQV prodrug by linking the drug covalently to polyethylene glycol (PEG) which was chosen due to its safety profile.

The PEG prodrugs were further attached to biotin or retro-inverso-cysteine-lysine-Tat9 (R.I.C.K-Tat9) or R.I.C.K-Tat9 (stearate); R.I.C.K-Tat9 permits drug penetration and also it has anti HIV properties [159]. Four prodrugs were tested: SQV-Cys (control), SQV-Cys-PEG, SQV-Cys-PEG-biotin, SQV-Cys (R.I.C.K-Tat9)-PEG, SQV-Cys (R.I.C.K (stearate)-Tat9)-PEG. Each prodrug was attached through breakable ester bond while PEG was attached to cysteine residue through stable amide bond. The results revealed that all of the conjugates except the one attached to PEG were active, SQV-Cys (R.I.C.K-Tat9)-PEG was found to be with the highest activity.

Targeting Macrophages

Macrophages are considered a primary target for HIV infection. Macrophages were found to be infected with HIV not only in untreated patients but also in patients receiving highly active antiretroviral therapy HAART. Due to their natural phagocytic ability, targeting an intact drug to macrophages is a major challenge [160].

Macrophage cell activity is controlled by several receptors. Many receptors are available on the macrophage surface [161,162]. Scientists in the field have moved their thought into delivering the required drugs to macrophages through these receptors using Nano carriers or conjugates which can be internalized inside the macrophage via receptor mediated endocytosis.

Of the receptors that were studied is the formyl peptide receptor. A nano carrier based on PEG was synthesized. A PEG-based linear copolymer, poly [poly (ethylene glycol) - alt-poly (aspartic acid)] was developed. The multifunctional PEG nano carriers were made by using four copies of N-formyl-methionine-leucine-phenylalanine (fMLF) peptide (PEG-fMLF4) and/or four and eight copies of digoxigenin (DIG4-PEG-fMLF4 and PEG-DIG8) [163].

Testing these delivery systems on macrophages has revealed the following: (i) the uptake was by active transport mediated by fMLF receptor and (ii) the fMLF copy number and the molecular weight of the PEG polymer have affected the rate of the uptake. It was found that the best rates of uptake were associated with one or two copies of fMLF and PEG molecular weight from 5 to 20 kDa [164-167].

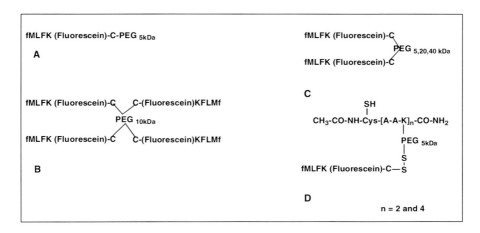

Figure 13. PEG containing nano carriers for targeting macrophages. (A-C) Different number of fMLF copies were used and PEG with different molecular weight to optimize the binding (D) PEG peptide. Fluorescein linked to elucidate uptake and binding.

This system represents a potential to be tested in association with HIV therapies.

Figure 14. Classical HIV prodrugs. (a) activation of fosamprenavir (b) tenofovir disoproxil fumarate.

Targeting the Kidneys

The kidney is the major organ responsible for waste excretion and maintaining electrolyte balance in the body. Also it produces renin and erythropoietin (EPO) which is responsible for regulating blood pressure and manufacture of red blood cells from bone marrow respectively [168,169].

The most common treatments for kidney failure are transplantation or dialysis. Most drugs reach the kidney in an inactive form. Very few drugs were made to specifically target the kidneys. No such drug has reached the clinic.

Proximal tubular cells in the nephron contain many enzymes such as γ- glutamyl transpeptidase at their basolateral side and β-lyase, N-acetyl transferase, or L-amino acid decarboxylase in their cytosolic side [170].

One of the drugs that was made to target the proximal tubular cells is L-γ-Glutamyl-L-dopa; a double prodrug of dopamine. It is intended to be transformed at the proximal tubules by γ--glutamyl transpeptidase to L-dopa then the active dopamine is formed by L-amino acid decarboxylase (Figure 15). Dopamine is used as a renal vasodilator but this double prodrug was found to have low bioavailability [171-173].

Compounds having the moiety N-acyl-L-γ- glutamyl seem to get selective activation in the proximal tubules by the sequential action of kidney-specific acylase and γ-glutamyl transpeptidase. This result was proved from the studies on N-acyl-L-γ- glutamyl derivatives of sulfamethoxazole and the vasodilative drug CGP 18137 (2-hydrazine-5-n-butyl pyridine [174-176]. Nevertheless, it is good to keep in mind that not every compound having this moiety is selectively transported and activated at the proximal tubules; this conclusion was revealed from studies on the drugN-acyl-L-γ-glutamyl-4'-aminowarfarin [177, 178].

L -γ-glutamyl-L- dopa   L-dopa   Dopamine

Figure 15. Specific activation of the dopamine prodrug in the kidney.

Summary and Conclusion

In the past few years, scientists have directed their attention towards developing targeted prodrugs to replace the classical ones. This approach has been accelerated after the encouraging results emerged from several studies on targeted prodrugs that demonstrated better efficiency and safety profiles.

In this chapter many areas of targeted drugs delivery using prodrugs were covered. Methods for targeting organ/disease were reported in details in separate sections. Many of the listed prodrugs in this chapter are still in clinical studies hoping to see the light soon.

Active targeting of cancer cells can be achieved by targeting transporters present at these cells or by using chimeric/humanized mAbs. While passive targeting can be achieved by taking advantage of the EPR effect which is characteristic for tumor cells. Some conditions associated with tumors such as hypoxia and low pH are also considered as good methods for targeting. For prostate cancer specific linkers that can be cleaved by the highly expressed PSA were linked to a number of tested prodrugs. For targeting liver cancer HepDirect prodrugs and carbamate prodrugs were made, tested and are in use.

In colon targeting all the developed prodrugs contain a breakable bond that can be broken by the enzymes secreted by the colonic microflora, such as azo bond containing prodrugs or they are linked to specific conjugates that can be degraded only in the colon.

Redox chemical delivery systems that contain pyridine have shown a good efficacy for CNS targeting.

In targeting HIV, researchers have developed prodrugs to target macrophages by linking them to moieties that make the prodrug-conjugate capable of being internalized by receptor mediated endocytosis.

References

[1] Testa, B. (2009). Prodrugs: bridging pharmacodynamic/pharmacokinetic gaps. *Current opinion in chemical biology*, *13*(3), 338-344.

[2] Ettmayer, P., Amidon, G. L., Clement, B., & Testa, B. (2004). Lessons learned from marketed and investigational prodrugs. *Journal of medicinal chemistry 47*(10), 2393-2404.

[3] Rautio, J., Kumpulainen, H., Heimbach, T., Oliyai, R., Oh, D., Järvinen, T., & Savolainen, J. (2008). Prodrugs: design and clinical applications. *Nature Reviews Drug Discovery*, *7*(3), 255-270.

[4] Dahan, A., Khamis, M., Agbaria, R., & Karaman, R. (2012). Targeted prodrugs in oral drug delivery: the modern molecular biopharmaceutical approach. *Expert Opinion on Drug Delivery*, *9*(8), 1001-1013.

[5] Karaman, R.; Fattash B. & Qtait A. (2013) The future of prodrugs – design by quantum mechanics methods. *Expert Opinion on Drug Delivery10*, 713–729.

[6] Karaman, R. (2013) Prodrugs design based on inter- and intramolecular processes. *Chem. Biol. Drug.Des. 82*, 643–668.

[7] Karaman, R. (2013) Prodrugs Design by Computation Methods- A New Era. Journal of Drug Designing 2: e113. doi:10.4172/2169-0138.1000e113.

[8] Stella, V. J., & Himmelstein, K. J. (1985). Prodrugs: a chemical approach to targeted drug delivery. In *Directed Drug Delivery* (pp. 247-267). Humana Press.

[9] Hanahan, D., & Weinberg, R. A. (2000). The hallmarks of cancer. *cell*, *100*(1), 57-70.

[10] Finkel, T., Serrano, M., & Blasco, M. A. (2007). The common biology of cancer and ageing. *Nature*, *448*(7155), 767-774.

[11] M Huttunen, K., & Rautio, J. (2011). Prodrugs-an efficient way to breach delivery and targeting barriers. *Current Topics in Medicinal Chemistry*, *11*(18), 2265-2287.

[12] Singh, Y., Palombo, M., &Sinko, P. J. (2008). Recent trends in targeted anticancer prodrug and conjugate design. *Current medicinal chemistry*, *15*(18), 1802.

[13] Carter, P. (2001). Improving the efficacy of antibody-based cancer therapies. *Nature Reviews Cancer*, *1*(2), 118-129.

[14] Schrama, D., Reisfeld, R. A., & Becker, J. C. (2006). Antibody targeted drugs as cancer therapeutics. *Nature Reviews Drug Discovery*, *5*(2), 147-159.

[15] King, H. D., Dubowchik, G. M., & Walker, M. A. (2002). Facile synthesis of maleimide bifunctional linkers. *Tetrahedron letters*, *43*(11), 1987-1990.

[16] Allen, T. M., & Cullis, P. R. (2004). Drug delivery systems: entering the mainstream. *Science*, *303*(5665), 1818-1822.

[17] Kratz, F., Müller, I. A., Ryppa, C., & Warnecke, A. (2008). Prodrug strategies in anticancer chemotherapy. *Chem Med Chem*, *3*(1), 20-53.

[18] Adams, G. P., & Weiner, L. M. (2005). Monoclonal antibody therapy of cancer. *Nature biotechnology*, *23*(9), 1147-1157.

[19] Henson, E. S., Johnston, J. B., & Gibson, S. B. (2008). The role of TRAIL death receptors in the treatment of hematological malignancies. *Leukemia & lymphoma*, *49*(1), 27-35.

[20] Zhang, Q., Chen, G., Liu, X., & Qian, Q. (2007). Monoclonal antibodies as therapeutic agents in oncology and antibody gene therapy. *Cell research*, *17*(2), 89-99.

[21] Singh, Y., Palombo, M., &Sinko, P. J. (2008). Recent trends in targeted anticancer prodrug and conjugate design. *Current medicinal chemistry*, *15*(18), 1802.

[22] http://obroncology.com/obrgreen/article/the-promising-outlook-with-immunoconjugate-therapy.

[23] Jordan, M. A., & Wilson, L. (2004). Microtubules as a target for anticancer drugs. *Nature Reviews Cancer*, *4*(4), 253-265.

[24] Paranjpe, P. V., Chen, Y., Kholodovych, V., Welsh, W., Stein, S., &Sinko, P. J. (2004). Tumor-targeted bioconjugate based delivery of camptothecin: design, synthesis and in vitro evaluation. *Journal of controlled release*, *100*(2), 275-292.

[25] Liu, F. S. (2009). Mechanisms of chemotherapeutic drug resistance in cancer therapy— a quick review. *Taiwanese Journal of Obstetrics and Gynecology 48*(3), 239-244.

Targeted Prodrugs

[26] Jacobson, M. A. (1993). Valaciclovir (BW256U87): The L-valyl ester of acyclovir. *Journal of medical virology*, *41*(S1), 150-153.

[27] Beauchamp, L. M., & Krenitsky, T. A. (1993). Acyclovir prodrugs: the road to valaciclovir. *Drugs of the Future*, *18*, 619-619.

[28] Han, H. K., de Vrueh, R. L., Rhie, J. K., Covitz, K. M. Y., Smith, P. L., Lee, C. P., ... & Amidon, G. L. (1998). 5'-Amino acid esters of antiviral nucleosides, acyclovir, and AZT are absorbed by the intestinal PEPT1 peptide transporter. *Pharmaceutical research*, *15*(8), 1154-1159.

[29] Smith, C., Klein, A., & Zimmerman, T. (1993). Influx of valacyclovir into cynomologous monkey intestinal brush border membranes is transporter mediated and enhanced over acyclovir. In *33rd Interscience Conference on Antimicrobial Agents and Chemotherapy, abstract* (No. 1750).

[30] Fang, J., Deng, D., Nakamura, H., Akuta, T., Qin, H., Iyer, A. K. & Maeda, H. (2008). Oxystress inducing antitumor therapeutics via tumor-targeted delivery of PEG-conjugated D-amino acid oxidase. *International Journal of Cancer*, *122*(5), 1135-1144.

[31] Greish, K., Fang, J., Inutsuka, T., Nagamitsu, A., & Maeda, H. (2003). Macromolecular Therapeutics. *Clinical pharmacokinetics*, *42*(13), 1089-1105.

[32] Duncan, R. (2003). The dawning era of polymer therapeutics. *Nature Reviews Drug Discovery*, *2*(5), 347-360.

[33] Satchi-Fainaro, R., Duncan, R., & Barnes, C. M. (2006). Polymer therapeutics for cancer: current status and future challenges. In *Polymer Therapeutics II* (pp. 1-65). Springer Berlin Heidelberg.

[34] Kratz, F., Müller, I. A., Ryppa, C., & Warnecke, A. (2008). Prodrug strategies in anticancer chemotherapy. *Chem Med Chem*, *3*(1), 20-53.

[35] King, H. D., Dubowchik, G. M., & Walker, M. A. (2002). Facile synthesis of maleimide bifunctional linkers. *Tetrahedron letters*, *43*(11), 1987-1990.

[36] Commandeur, J. N., Andreadou, I., Rooseboom, M., Out, M., Laurens, J., Groot, E., & Vermeulen, N. P. (2000). Bioactivation of selenocysteine Se-conjugates by a highly purified rat renal cysteine conjugate β-lyase/glutamine transaminase K. *Journal of Pharmacology and Experimental Therapeutics*, *294*(2), 753-761.

[37] Brown, J. M., & Wilson, W. R. (2004). Exploiting tumour hypoxia in cancer treatment. *Nature Reviews Cancer*, *4*(6), 437-447.

[38] Daniels, J. S., Gates, K. S., Tronche, C., & Greenberg, M. M. (1998). Direct evidence for bimodal DNA damage induced by tirapazamine. *Chemical research in toxicology*, *11*(11), 1254-1257.

[39] Patterson, L. H. (2002). Bioreductively activated antitumor N-oxides: the case of AQ4N, a unique approach to hypoxia-activated cancer chemotherapy. *Drug metabolism reviews*, *34*(3), 581-592.

[40] Kriste, A. G., Tercel, M., Anderson, R. F., Ferry, D. M., & Wilson, W. R. (2009). Pathways of reductive fragmentation of heterocyclic nitroarylmethyl quaternary ammonium prodrugs of mechlorethamine.

[41] Shibamoto, Y., Zhou, L., Hatta, H., Mori, M. & Nishimoto, S. I. (2000). A Novel Class of Antitumor Prodrug, 1-(2'-Oxopropyl)-5-fluorouracil (OFU001), That Releases 5-Fluorouracil upon Hypoxic Irradiation. *Cancer Science*, *91*(4), 433-438.

[42] Denny, W. A., Wilson, W. R., & Hay, M. P. (1996). Recent developments in the design of bioreductive drugs. *The British journal of cancer. Supplement*, *27*, S32.

[43] http://www.nice.org.uk/nicemedia/pdf/CG58NICEGuideline.pdf

[44] Isaacs, J. T. (1999). The biology of hormone refractory prostate cancer: why does it develop? *Urologic Clinics of North America*, *26*(2), 263-273.

[45] Kyprianou, N., English, H. F., & Isaacs, J. T. (1990). Programmed cell death during regression of PC-82 human prostate cancer following androgen ablation. *Cancer research*, *50*(12), 3748-3753.

[46] Samson, D. J., Seidenfeld, J., Schmitt, B., Hasselblad, V., Albertsen, P. C., Bennett, C. L. & Aronson, N. (2002). Systematic review and meta-analysis of monotherapy compared with combined androgen blockade for patients with advanced prostate carcinoma. *Cancer*, *95*(2), 361-376.

[47] Akiyama, K., Nakamura, T., Iwanaga, S., & Hara, M. (1987). The chymotrypsin-like activity of human prostate-specific antigen, γ-seminoprotein. *FEBS letters*, *225*(1), 168-172.

[48] Christensson, A., Laurell, C. B., & Lilja, H. (1990). Enzymatic activity of prostate-specific antigen and its reactions with extracellular serine proteinase inhibitors. *European journal of biochemistry*, *194*(3), 755-763.

[49] Lilja, H., Christensson, A., Dahlén, U., Matikainen, M. T., Nilsson, O., Pettersson, K., & Lövgren, T. (1991). Prostate-specific antigen in serum occurs predominantly in complex with alpha 1-antichymotrypsin. *Clinical Chemistry*, *37*(9), 1618-1625.

[50] Denmeade, S. R., Lou, W., Lövgren, J., Malm, J., Lilja, H., & Isaacs, J. T. (1997). Specific and efficient peptide substrates for assaying the proteolytic activity of prostate-specific antigen. *Cancer research*, *57*(21), 4924-4930.

[51] Furuya, Y., Lundmo, P., Short, A. D., Gill, D. L., & Isaacs, J. T. (1994). The role of calcium, pH, and cell proliferation in the programmed (apoptotic) death of androgen-independent prostatic cancer cells induced by thapsigargin. *Cancer research*, *54*(23), 6167-6175.

[52] Thastrup, O. (1990). Role of Ca2+-ATPases in regulation of cellular Ca2+ signalling, as studied with the selective microsomal Ca2+-ATPase inhibitor, thapsigargin. *Agents and actions*, *29*(1-2), 8-15.

[53] Davidson, G. A., & Varhol, R. J. (1995). Kinetics of Thapsigargin-Ca-ATPase (Sarcoplasmic Reticulum) Interaction Reveals a Two-step Binding Mechanism and Picomolar Inhibition. *Journal of Biological Chemistry*, *270*(20), 11731-11734.

[54] DiPaola, R. S., Rinehart, J., Nemunaitis, J., Ebbinghaus, S., Rubin, E., Capanna, T. & Yao, S. L. (2002). Characterization of a Novel Prostate-Specific Antigen–Activated Peptide-Doxorubicin Conjugate in Patients With Prostate Cancer. *Journal of clinical oncology*, *20*(7), 1874-1879.

[55] Denmeade, S. R., Jakobsen, C. M., Janssen, S., Khan, S. R., Garrett, E. S., Lilja, H. & Isaacs, J. T. (2003). Prostate-specific antigen-activated thapsigargin prodrug as targeted therapy for prostate cancer. *Journal of the National Cancer Institute*, *95*(13), 990-1000.

[56] Hakim, D. (2011). *Zakim and Boyer's Hepatology: A Textbook of Liver Disease; [searchable Full Text Online]*. T. D. Boyer, M. P. Manns, & A. J. Sanyal (Eds.). Elsevier Health Sciences.

[57] Worman, H. J. (2006). *The Liver Disorders and Hepatitis Sourcebook*. McGraw Hill Professional.

[58] M Huttunen, K., & Rautio, J. (2011). Prodrugs-an efficient way to breach delivery and targeting barriers. *Current Topics in Medicinal Chemistry*, *11*(18), 2265-2287.

[59] Stella, V. J. (Ed.). (2007). *Prodrugs: challenges and rewards. P. 1* (Vol. 5). Springer.

[60] http://www.aafp.org/afp/2007/0801/p391.html

[61] Smith, D. A., Ackland, M. J., & Jones, B. C. (1997). Properties of cytochrome P450 isoenzymes and their substrates part 2: properties of cytochrome P450 substrates. *Drug Discovery Today*, *2*(11), 479-486.

[62] Lewis, D. F., & Dickins, M. (2002). Substrate SARs in human P450s. *Drug Discovery Today*, *7*(17), 918-925.

[63] Nebert, D. W., & Russell, D. W. (2002). Clinical importance of the cytochromes P450. *The Lancet*, *360*(9340), 1155-1162.

[64] Ettmayer, P., Amidon, G. L., Clement, B., & Testa, B. (2004). Lessons learned from marketed and investigational prodrugs. *Journal of medicinal chemistry*, *47*(10), 2393-2404.

[65] Erion, M. D., Reddy, K. R., Boyer, S. H., Matelich, M. C., Gomez-Galeno, J., Lemus, R. H., ... & van Poelje, P. D. (2004). Design, Synthesis, and Characterization of a Series of Cytochrome P450 3A-Activated Prodrugs (HepDirect Prodrugs) Useful for Targeting Phosphonate-Based Drugs to the liver. *Journal of the American Chemical Society*, *126*(16), 5154-5163.

[66] De Waziers, I., Cugnenc, P. H., Yang, C. S., Leroux, J. P., & Beaune, P. H. (1990). Cytochrome P 450 isoenzymes, epoxide hydrolase and glutathione transferases in rat and human hepatic and extrahepatic tissues. *Journal of Pharmacology and Experimental Therapeutics*, *253*(1), 387-394.

[67] Curley, S. A., & Izzo, F. (2002). Radiofrequency ablation of primary and metastatic hepatic malignancies. *International Journal of Clinical Oncology*, *7*(2), 72-81.

[68] Rees, A. (Ed.). (1997). *Consumer health USA* (Vol. 2). Greenwood Publishing Group.

[69] Erion, M. D., Van Poelje, P. D., MacKenna, D. A., Colby, T. J., Montag, A. C., Fujitaki, J. M., ... & Bullough, D. A. (2005). Liver-targeted drug delivery using HepDirect prodrugs. *Journal of Pharmacology and Experimental Therapeutics*, *312*(2), 554-560.

[70] Hosokawa, M. (2008). Structure and catalytic properties of carboxylesterase isozymes involved in metabolic activation of prodrugs. *Molecules*, *13*(2), 412-431.

[71] Burkhart, D. J., Barthel, B. L., Post, G. C., Kalet, B. T., Nafie, J. W., Shoemaker, R. K., & Koch, T. H. (2006). Design, synthesis, and preliminary evaluation of doxazolidine carbamates as prodrugs activated by carboxylesterases. *Journal of medicinal chemistry*, *49*(24), 7002-7012.

[72] Li, Q. Y., Zu, Y. G., Shi, R. Z., & Yao, L. P. (2006). Review camptothecin: current perspectives. *Current medicinal chemistry*, *13*(17), 2021-2039.

[73] Ohya, Y., Nagatomi, K., & Ouchi, T. (2001). Synthesis and cytotoxic activity of macromolecular prodrug of cisplatin using poly (ethylene glycol) with galactose residues or antennary galactose units. *Macromolecular Bioscience*, *1*(8), 355-363.

[74] Briz, O., Serrano, M. A., Rebollo, N., Hagenbuch, B., Meier, P. J., Koepsell, H., & Marin, J. J. (2002). Carriers Involved in Targeting the Cytostatic Bile Acid-CisplatinDerivativescis-Diammine-chloro-cholylglycinate-platinum (II) and cis-Diammine-bisursodeoxycholate-platinum (II) toward Liver Cells. *Molecular pharmacology*, *61*(4), 853-860.

[75] Fiume, L., Bonino, F., Mattioli, A., Chiaberge, E., TorraniCerenzia, M., Busi, C. & Verme, G. (1988). Inhibition of hepatitis B virus replication by vidarabine

monophosphate conjugated with lactosaminated serum albumin. *The Lancet, 332*(8601), 13-15.

[76] Davis, B. G., & Robinson, M. A. (2002). Drug delivery systems based on sugar-macromolecule conjugates. *Current Opinion in Drug Discovery and Development, 5*(2), 279-288.

[77] Garnier, P., Wang, X. T., Robinson, M. A., van Kasteren, S., Perkins, A. C., Frier, M. & Davis, B. G. (2010). Lectin-directed enzyme activated prodrug therapy (LEAPT): Synthesis and evaluation of rhamnose-capped prodrugs. *Journal of Drug Targeting, 18*(10), 794-802.

[78] Robinson, M. A., Charlton, S. T., Garnier, P., Wang, X. T., Davis, S. S., Perkins, A. C. & Davis, B. G. (2004). LEAPT: lectin-directed enzyme-activated prodrug therapy. *Proceedings of the National Academy of Sciences of the United States of America, 101*(40), 14527-14532.

[79] van de Waterbeemd, H., Camenisch, G., Folkers, G., Chretien, J. R., & Raevsky, O. A. (1998). Estimation of blood-brain barrier crossing of drugs using molecular size and shape, and H-bonding descriptors. *Journal of drug targeting, 6*(2), 151-165.

[80] Rasheed, A., Theja, I., Silparani, G., Lavanya, Y., & Kumar, C. A. (2010). CNS targeted drug delivery: current perspectives. *JITPS, 1*(1), 9-18.

[81] Belliotti, T. R., Capiris, T., Ekhato, I. V., Kinsora, J. J., Field, M. J., Heffner, T. G. & Wustrow, D. J. (2005). Structure-activity relationships of pregabalin and analogues that target the α2-δ protein. *Journal of medicinal chemistry, 48*(7), 2294-2307.

[82] Wu, J., Yoon, S. H., Wu, W. M., & Bodor, N. (2002). Synthesis and biological evaluations of brain-targeted chemical delivery systems of [Nva2]-TRH. *Journal of pharmacy and pharmacology, 54*(7), 945-950.

[83] Lee, H.J., Pardridge, W.M. (2000). Drug targeting to the brain using avidin-biotin technology in the mouse (blood-brain barrier, monoclonal antibody, transferrin receptor, Alzheimer's disease).*Journal of drug targeting,* 8(6), 413-424.

[84] Gentilucci, L., Tolomelli, A., & Squassabia, F. (2006). Peptides and peptidomimetics in medicine, surgery and biotechnology. *Current medicinal chemistry, 13*(20), 2449-2466.

[85] Prokai-Tatrai, K., Kim, H. S., & Prokai, L. (2008). The utility of oligopeptidase in brain-targeting delivery of an enkephalin analogue by prodrug design. *The open medicinal chemistry journal, 2,* 97.

[86] Prokai, L., & Prokai-Tatrai, K. (Eds.). (2003). *Peptide transport and delivery into the central nervous system* (Vol. 61). Springer.

[87] Prokai, L., Prokai-Tatrai, K., & Bodor, N. (2000). Targeting drugs to the brain by redox chemical delivery systems. *Medicinal research reviews, 20*(5), 367-416.

[88] Chen, P., Bodor, N., Wu, W. M., & Prokai, L. (1998). Strategies to target kyotorphin analogues to the brain. *Journal of medicinal chemistry, 41*(20), 3773-3781.

[89] Prokai-Tatrai, K., Prokai, L., & Bodor, N. (1996). Brain-targeted delivery of a leucine-enkephalin analogue by retrometabolic design. *Journal of medicinal chemistry, 39*(24), 4775-4782.

[90] Chourasia, M. K., & Jain, S. K. (2003). Pharmaceutical approaches to colon targeted drug delivery systems. *J Pharm Pharm Sci, 6*(1), 33-66.

[91] Scheline, R. R. (1973). Metabolism of foreign compounds by gastrointestinal microorganisms. *Pharmacological reviews, 25*(4), 451.

[92] Sarasija, S., & Hota, A. (2000). Colon-specific drug delivery systems. *Indian journal of pharmaceutical sciences, 62*(1), 1.

[93] Rafii, F. A. T. E. M. E. H., Franklin, W. I. R. T., & Cerniglia, C. E. (1990). Azoreductase activity of anaerobic bacteria isolated from human intestinal microflora. *Applied and environmental microbiology, 56*(7), 2146-2151.

[94] Rafil, F., Franklin, W. I. R. T., Heflich, R. H., & Cerniglia, C. E. (1991). Reduction of nitroaromatic compounds by anaerobic bacteria isolated from the human gastrointestinal tract. *Applied and environmental microbiology, 57*(4), 962-968.

[95] Walker, R., & Ryan, A. J. (1971). Some molecular parameters influencing rate of reduction of azo compounds by intestinal microflora. *Xenobiotica, 1*(4-5), 483-486.

[96] Azadkhan, A. K., Truelove, S. C., & Aronson, J. K. (1982). The disposition and metabolism of sulphasalazine (salicylazosulphapyridine) in man. *British journal of clinical pharmacology, 13*(4), 523-528.

[97] Rao, S. S., Read, N. W., &Holdsworth, C. D. (1987). Influence of olsalazine on gastrointestinal transit in ulcerative colitis. *Gut, 28*(11), 1474-1477.

[98] McIntyre, P. B., Rodrigues, C. A., Lennard-Jones, J. E., Barrison, I. G., Walker, J. G., Baron, J. H., & Thornton, P. C. (1988). Balsalazide in the maintenance treatment of patients with ulcerative colitis, a double-blind comparison with sulphasalazine. *Alimentary pharmacology & therapeutics, 2*(3), 237-243.

[99] Sakuma, S., Lu, Z. R., Kopečková, P., & Kopeček, J. (2001). Biorecognizable HPMA copolymer–drug conjugates for colon-specific delivery of 9-aminocamptothecin. *Journal of controlled release, 75*(3), 365-379.

[100] Nakamura, J., Asai, K., Nishida, K., & Sasaki, H. (1992). A novel prodrug of salicylic acid, salicylic acid-glutamic acid conjugate utilizing hydrolysis in rabbit intestinal microorganisms. *Chemical & pharmaceutical bulletin, 40*(8), 2164-2168.

[101] Nakamura, J., Kido, M., Nishida, K., & Sasaki, H. (1992). Hydrolysis of salicylic acid-tyrosine and salicylic acid-methionine prodrugs in the rabbit. *International journal of pharmaceutics, 87*(1), 59-66.

[102] Nakamura, J., Kido, M., Nishida, K., & Sasaki, H. (1992). Effect of oral pretreatment with antibiotics on the hydrolysis of salicylic acid-tyrosine and salicylic acid-methionine prodrugs in rabbit intestinal microorganisms. *Chemical & pharmaceutical bulletin, 40*(9), 2572.

[103] Nakamura, J., Tagami, C., Nishida, K., & Sasaki, H. (1992). Unequal hydrolysis of salicylic acid-D-alanine and salicylic acid-L-alanine conjugate in rabbit intestinal microorganisms. *Chemical & pharmaceutical bulletin, 40*(2), 547.

[104] Friend, D. R. (1992). Glycosides in colonic drug delivery. *Oral colon specific drug delivery. CRC Press, Boca Raton*, 153-187.

[105] Friend, D. R., & Chang, G. W. (1984). A colon-specific drug-delivery system based on drug glycosides and the glycosidases of colonic bacteria. *Journal of medicinal chemistry, 27*(3), 261-266.

[106] Friend, D. R., & Chang, G. W. (1985). Drug glycosides: potential prodrugs for colon-specific drug delivery. *Journal of medicinal chemistry, 28*(1), 51-57.

[107] Friend, D. R., Phillips, S., McLeod, A., & Tozer, T. N. (1991). Relative anti-inflammatory effect of oral dexamethasone-β-D-glucoside and dexamethasone in experimental inflammatory bowel disease in guinea-pigs. *Journal of pharmacy and pharmacology, 43*(5), 353-355.

[108] Scheline, R. R. (1968). Drug metabolism by intestinal microorganisms. *Journal of pharmaceutical sciences*, *57*(12), 2021-2037.

[109] Simpkins, J. W., Smulkowski, M. A. C. I. E. J., Dixon, R. O. S. S., & Tuttle, R. O. N. A. L. D. (1988). Evidence for the delivery of narcotic antagonists to the colon as their glucuronide conjugates. *Journal of Pharmacology and Experimental Therapeutics*, *244*(1), 195-205.

[110] Haeberlin, B., Rubas, W., Nolen III, H. W., & Friend, D. R. (1993). In vitro evaluation of dexamethasone-β-D-glucuronide for colon-specific drug delivery. *Pharmaceutical research*, *10*(11), 1553-1562.

[111] Duchene, D., & Wouessidjewe, D. (1990). Pharmaceutical uses of cyclodextrins and derivatives. *Drug development and industrial pharmacy*, *16*(17), 2487-2499.

[112] Stella, V. J., & Rajewski, R. A. (1997). Cyclodextrins: their future in drug formulation and delivery. *Pharmaceutical research*, *14*(5), 556-567.

[113] Antenucci, R. N., & Palmer, J. K. (1984). Enzymic degradation of. alpha.-and. beta.-cyclodextrins by Bacteroides of the human colon. *Journal of agricultural and food chemistry*, *32*(6), 1316-1321.

[114] Minami, K., Hirayama, F., & Uekama, K. (1998). Colon-specific drug delivery based on a cyclodextrin prodrug: Release behavior of biphenylylacetic acid from its cyclodextrin conjugates in rat intestinal tracts after oral administration. *Journal of pharmaceutical sciences*, *87*(6), 715-720.

[115] Uekama, K., Minami, K., & Hirayama, F. (1997). 6A-O-[(4-Biphenylyl) acetyl]-α-,-β-, and-γ-cyclodextrins and 6 A-Deoxy-6 A-[[(4-biphenylyl) acetyl] amino]-α-,-β-, and-γ-cyclodextrins: Potential Prodrugs for Colon-Specific Delivery. *Journal of medicinal chemistry*, *40*(17), 2755-2761.

[116] Yano, H., Hirayama, F., Kamada, M., Arima, H., &Uekama, K. (2002). Colon-specific delivery of prednisolone-appended α-cyclodextrin conjugate: alleviation of systemic side effect after oral administration. *Journal of controlled Release*, *79*(1), 103-112.

[117] Yano, H., Hirayama, F., Arima, H., & Uekama, K. (2001). Preparation of prednisolone-appended α-, β-and γ-cyclodextrins: Substitution at secondary hydroxyl groups and in vitro hydrolysis behavior. *Journal of pharmaceutical sciences*, *90*(4), 493-503.

[118] Frank, D. W., Gray, J. E., & Weaver, R. N. (1976). Cyclodextrin nephrosis in the rat. *The American journal of pathology*, *83*(2), 367.

[119] Leroy-Lechat, F., Wouessidjewe, D., Andreux, J. P., Puisieux, F., & Duchêne, D. (1994). Evaluation of the cytotoxicity of cyclodextrins and hydroxypropylated derivatives. *International journal of pharmaceutics*, *101*(1), 97-103.

[120] Harboe, E., Larsen, C., Johansen, M., & Olesen, H. P. (1989). Macromolecular prodrugs. XIV. Absorption characteristics of naproxen after oral administration of a dextran T-70-naproxen ester prodrug in pigs. *International journal of pharmaceutics*, *53*(2), 157-165.

[121] McLeod, A. D., Friend, D. R., & Tozer, T. N. (1993). Synthesis and chemical stability of glucocorticoid-dextran esters: potential prodrugs for colon-specific delivery. *International journal of pharmaceutics*, *92*(1), 105-114.

[122] McLeod, A. D., Friend, D. R., & Tozer, T. N. (1994). Glucocorticoid–dextran conjugates as potential prodrugs for colon-specific delivery: Hydrolysis in rat gastrointestinal tract contents. *Journal of pharmaceutical sciences*, *83*(9), 1284-1288.

Targeted Prodrugs

[123] McLEOD, A. D., Fedorak, R. N., Friend, D. R., Tozer, T. N., & Cui, N. (1994). A glucocorticoid prodrug facilitates normal mucosal function in rat colitis without adrenal suppression. *Gastroenterology-Baltimore Then Philadelphia-*, *106*, 405-405.

[124] http://www.cdc.gov/hiv/topics/basic/.

[125] De Clercq, E. (2002). Strategies in the design of antiviral drugs. *Nature Reviews Drug Discovery*, *1*(1), 13-25.

[126] Huang, C. C., Tang, M., Zhang, M. Y., Majeed, S., Montabana, E., Stanfield, R. L. & Kwong, P. D. (2005). Structure of a V3-containing HIV-1 gp120 core. *Science*, *310*(5750), 1025-1028.

[127] Palombo, M. S., Singh, Y., & Sinko, P. J. (2009). Prodrug and conjugate drug delivery strategies for improving HIV/AIDS therapy. *Journal of drug delivery science and technology*, *19*(1), 3.

[128] De Clercq, E. (2007). The design of drugs for HIV and HCV. *Nature Reviews Drug Discovery*, *6*(12), 1001-1018.

[129] Pommier, Y., Johnson, A. A., & Marchand, C. (2005). Integrase inhibitors to treat HIV/AIDS. *Nature Reviews Drug Discovery*, *4*(3), 236-248.

[130] Update, A. E. (2007). December 2007. *Joint United Nations Programme on HIV/AIDS and World Health Organization*.

[131] Piot, P. (2006). AIDS: from crisis management to sustained strategic response. *The Lancet*, *368*(9534), 526-530.

[132] Merson, M. H. (2006). The HIV–AIDS pandemic at 25—the global response. *New England Journal of Medicine*, *354*(23), 2414-2417.

[133] Piot, P., Bartos, M., Ghys, P. D., Walker, N., & Schwartländer, B. (2001). The global impact of HIV/AIDS. *Nature*, *410*(6831), 968-973.

[134] Flexner, C. (2007). HIV drug development: the next 25 years. *Nature Reviews Drug Discovery*, *6*(12), 959-966.

[135] Struble, K., Murray, J., Cheng, B., Gegeny, T., Miller, V., & Gulick, R. (2005). Antiretroviral therapies for treatment-experienced patients: current status and research challenges. *Aids*, *19*(8), 747-756.

[136] Janssen, P. A., Lewi, P. J., Arnold, E., Daeyaert, F., de Jonge, M., Heeres, J. & Stoffels, P. (2005). In search of a novel anti-HIV drug: multidisciplinary coordination in the discovery of 4-[[4-[[4-[(1 E)-2-cyanoethenyl]-2, 6-dimethylphenyl] amino]-2-pyrimidinyl] amino] benzonitrile (R278474, rilpivirine).*Journal of medicinal chemistry*, *48*(6), 1901-1909.

[137] Rautio, J., Kumpulainen, H., Heimbach, T., Oliyai, R., Oh, D., Järvinen, T., & Savolainen, J. (2008). Prodrugs: design and clinical applications. *Nature Reviews Drug Discovery*, *7*(3), 255-270.

[138] Thomson Healthcare Inc. - Mayo Clinic.com: Fosamprenavir (Oral Route)-(http://www.mayoclinic.com/health/drug-information/ DR601699 - Accessed [June 19, 2008].

[139] Chapman, T. M., Plosker, G. L., & Perry, C. M. (2004). Fosamprenavir. *Drugs*, *64*(18), 2101-2124.

[140] Wire, M. B., Shelton, M. J., & Studenberg, S. (2006). Fosamprenavir. *Clinical pharmacokinetics*, *45*(2), 137-168.

[141] Furfine, E. S., Baker, C. T., Hale, M. R., Reynolds, D. J., Salisbury, J. A., Searle, A. D. & Spaltenstein, A. (2004). Preclinical pharmacology and pharmacokinetics of

GW433908, a water-soluble prodrug of the human immunodeficiency virus protease inhibitor amprenavir. *Antimicrobial agents and chemotherapy*, *48*(3), 791-798.

[142] Wood, R., Arasteh, K., Stellbrink, H. J., Teofilo, E., Raffi, F., Pollard, R. B. & Naderer, O. J. (2004). Six-week randomized controlled trial to compare the tolerabilities, pharmacokinetics, and antiviral activities of GW433908 and amprenavir in human immunodeficiency virus type 1-infected patients.*Antimicrobial agents and chemotherapy*, *48*(1), 116-123.

[143] Sadler, B. M., Chittick, G. E., Polk, R. E., Slain, D., Kerkering, T. M., Studenberg, S. D., & Stein, D. S. (2001). Metabolic Disposition and Pharmacokinetics of [14C]-Amprenavir, a Human Immunodeficiency Virus Type 1 (HIV-1) Protease Inhibitor, Administered As a Single Oral Dose to Healthy Male Subjects. *The Journal of Clinical Pharmacology*, *41*(4), 386-396.

[144] Wire, M. B., Shelton, M. J., & Studenberg, S. (2006). Fosamprenavir. *Clinical pharmacokinetics*, *45*(2), 137-168.

[145] Gilead Sciences INC. - Viread (tenofovir disoproxil fumarate) tablets: US package insert.-(http://www.gilead.com/pdf/viread_ pi.pdf -Accessed [January 23, 2007].

[146] Fung, H. B., Stone, E. A., & Piacenti, F. J. (2002). Tenofovir disoproxil fumarate: a nucleotide reverse transcriptase inhibitor for the treatment of HIV infection. *Clinical therapeutics*, *24*(10), 1515-1548.

[147] Chapman, T. M., McGavin, J. K., & Noble, S. (2003). Tenofovir disoproxil fumarate. *Drugs*, *63*(15), 1597-1608.

[148] Antoniou, T., Park-Wyllie, L. Y., & Tseng, A. L. (2003). Tenofovir: a nucleotide analog for the management of human immunodeficiency virus infection. *Pharmacotherapy: The Journal of Human Pharmacology and Drug Therapy*, *23*(1), 29-43.

[149] De Clercq, E. (1991). Broad-spectrum anti-DNA virus and anti-retrovirus activity of phosphonylmethoxyalkylpurines and-pyrimidines. *Biochemical pharmacology*, *42*(5), 963-972.

[150] De Clercq, E. (2003). Clinical potential of the acyclic nucleoside phosphonates cidofovir, adefovir, and tenofovir in treatment of DNA virus and retrovirus infections. *Clinical microbiology reviews*, *16*(4), 569-596.

[151] De Clercq, E. (2003). Clinical potential of the acyclic nucleoside phosphonates cidofovir, adefovir, and tenofovir in treatment of DNA virus and retrovirus infections. *Clinical microbiology reviews*, *16*(4), 569-596.

[152] Kearney, B. P., Flaherty, J. F., & Shah, J. (2004). Tenofovir disoproxilfumarate. *Clinical pharmacokinetics*, *43*(9), 595-612.

[153] Robbins, B. L., Srinivas, R. V., Kim, C., Bischofberger, N., & Fridland, A. (1998). Anti-human immunodeficiency virus activity and cellular metabolism of a potential prodrug of the acyclic nucleoside phosphonate 9-R-(2-phosphonomethoxypropyl) adenine (PMPA), bis (isopropyloxymethylcarbonyl) PMPA. *Antimicrobial agents and chemotherapy*, *42*(3), 612-617.

[154] Singh, Y., Palombo, M., & Sinko, P. J. (2008). Recent trends in targeted anticancer prodrug and conjugate design. *Current medicinal chemistry*, *15*(18), 1802.

[155] Kratz, F., Müller, I. A., Ryppa, C., & Warnecke, A. (2008). Prodrug strategies in anticancer chemotherapy. *Chem Med Chem*, *3*(1), 20-53.

[156] De Clercq, E. (2002). Strategies in the design of antiviral drugs. *Nature Reviews Drug Discovery*, *1*(1), 13-25.

[157] Park, S., & Sinko, P. J. (2005). P-glycoprotein and mutlidrug resistance-associated proteins limit the brain uptake of saquinavir in mice. *Journal of Pharmacology and Experimental Therapeutics*, *312*(3), 1249-1256.

[158] Sinko, P. J., Kunta, J. R., Usansky, H. H., & Perry, B. A. (2004). Differentiation of gut and hepatic first pass metabolism and secretion of saquinavir in ported rabbits. *Journal of Pharmacology and Experimental Therapeutics*, *310*(1), 359-366.

[159] Zhang, X., Wan, L., Pooyan, S., Su, Y., Gardner, C. R., Leibowitz, M. J. & Sinko, P. J. (2004). Quantitative assessment of the cell penetrating properties of RI-Tat-9: evidence for a cell type-specific barrier at the plasma membrane of epithelial cells. *Molecular Pharmaceutics*, *1*(2), 145-155.

[160] Ahsan, F., Rivas, I. P., Khan, M. A., & Torres Suárez, A. I. (2002). Targeting to macrophages: role of physicochemical properties of particulate carriers—liposomes and microspheres—on the phagocytosis by macrophages. *Journal of controlled release*, *79*(1), 29-40.

[161] Lewis, C. E., & McGee, J. O. (1992). *'D. Natural killer cells in tumourbiology* (pp. 176-203). Lewis CE, McGee JO'D, eds. The Natural Immune System: The Natural Killer Cell. Oxford: Oxford University Press.

[162] Fridkin, M., Tsubery, H., Tzehoval, E., Vonsover, A., Biondi, L., Filira, F., & Rocchi, R. (2005). Tuftsin-AZT conjugate: potential macrophage targeting for AIDS therapy. *Journal of Peptide Science*, *11*(1), 37-44.

[163] Pooyan, S., Qiu, B., Chan, M. M., Fong, D., Sinko, P. J., Leibowitz, M. J., & Stein, S. (2002). Conjugates bearing multiple formyl-methionyl peptides display enhanced binding to but not activation of phagocytic cells. *Bioconjugate chemistry*, *13*(2), 216-223.

[164] Nakai, T., Kanamori, T., Sando, S., & Aoyama, Y. (2003). Remarkably size-regulated cell invasion by artificial viruses. Saccharide-dependent self-aggregation of glycoviruses and its consequences in glycoviral gene delivery. *Journal of the American Chemical Society*, *125*(28), 8465-8475.

[165] Osaki, F., Kanamori, T., Sando, S., Sera, T., & Aoyama, Y. (2004). A quantum dot conjugated sugar ball and its cellular uptake. On the size effects of endocytosis in the subviral region. *Journal of the American Chemical Society*, *126*(21), 6520-6521.

[166] Desai, M. P., Labhasetwar, V., Walter, E., Levy, R. J., & Amidon, G. L. (1997). The mechanism of uptake of biodegradable microparticles in Caco-2 cells is size dependent. *Pharmaceutical research*, *14*(11), 1568-1573.

[167] Prabha, S., Zhou, W. Z., Panyam, J., & Labhasetwar, V. (2002). Size-dependency of nanoparticle-mediated gene transfection: studies with fractionated nanoparticles. *International Journal of Pharmaceutics*, *244*(1), 105-115.

[168] Stein, A., & Wild, J. (2002). *Kidney failure explained: everything you always wanted to know about dialysis and kidney transplants but were afraid to ask*. Class Pub.

[169] Benner, B. M. (2004). Benner & Rector's the Kidney. ; Vol. 1.

[170] M Huttunen, K., & Rautio, J. (2011). Prodrugs-an efficient way to breach delivery and targeting barriers. *Current Topics in Medicinal Chemistry*, *11*(18), 2265-2287.

[171] Wilk, S. H. E. R. W. I. N., Mizoguchi, H. A. R. U. K. O., & Orlowski, M. A. R. I. A. N. (1978). gamma-Glutamyldopa: a kidney-specific dopamine precursor. *Journal of Pharmacology and Experimental Therapeutics*, *206*(1), 227-232.

[172] Barthelmebs, M., Caillette, A., Ehrhardt, J. D., Velly, J., & Imbs, J. L. (1990). Metabolism and vascular effects of gamma-L-glutamyl-L-dopa on the isolated rat kidney. *Kidney international*, *37*(6), 1414-1422.

[173] Drieman, J. C., Kan, F. J. P. M., Thijssen, H. H. W., Essen, H., Smits, J. F. M., & Boudier, H. A. J. (1994). Regional haemodynamic effects of dopamine and its prodrugs l-dopa and gludopa in the rat and in the glycerol-treated rat as a model for acute renal failure. *British journal of pharmacology*, *111*(4), 1117-1122.

[174] Orlowski, M. A. R. I. A. N., Mizoguchi, H. A. R. U. K. O., &Wilk, S. H. E. R. W. I. N. (1980). N-acyl-gamma-glutamyl derivatives of sulfamethoxazole as models of kidney-selective prodrugs. *Journal of Pharmacology and Experimental Therapeutics*, *212*(1), 167-172.

[175] Drieman, J. C., Thijssen, H. H., & Struyker-Boudier, H. A. (1990). Renal selective N-acetyl-gamma-glutamyl prodrugs. II. Carrier-mediated transport and intracellular conversion as determinants in the renal selectivity of N-acetyl-gamma-glutamyl sulfamethoxazole. *Journal of Pharmacology and Experimental Therapeutics*, *252*(3), 1255-1260.

[176] Drieman, J. C., Thijssen, H. H. W., Zeegers, H. H. M., Smits, J. F. M., & Boudier, H. A. J. (1990). Renal selective N-acetyl-γ-glutamyl prodrugs: a study on the mechanism of activation of the renal vasodilator prodrug CGP 22979.*British journal of pharmacology*, *99*(1), 15-20.

[177] Drieman, J. C., & Thijssen, H. H. (1991). Renal selective N-acetyl-L-gamma-glutamyl prodrugs. III. N-acetyl-L-gamma-glutamyl-4'-aminowarfarin is not targeted to the kidney but is selectively excreted into the bile. *Journal of Pharmacology and Experimental Therapeutics*, *259*(2), 766-771.

[178] Drieman, J. C., Thijssen, H. H. W., & Struyker-Boudier, H. A. J. (1993). Renal selective N-acetyl-l-γ-glutamyl prodrugs: studies on the selectivity of some model prodrugs. *British journal of pharmacology*, *108*(1), 204-208.

In: Prodrugs Design – A New Era
Editor: Rafik Karaman

ISBN: 978-1-63117-701-9
© 2014 Nova Science Publishers, Inc.

Chapter V

Virus Directed Enzyme Prodrug Therapy (VDEPT)

Nidaa Habbabeh[1] and Rafik Karaman[1,2,]*
[1]Pharmaceutical Sciences Department, Faculty of Pharmacy
Al-Quds University, Jerusalem, Palestine
[2]Department of Science, University of Basilicata, Potenza, Italy

Abstract

The selective activation of prodrug in tumor tissues by exogenous enzyme for cancer therapy can be accomplished by several prodrugs therapies; gene-directed enzyme, virus-directed enzyme and antibody-directed enzyme. The main focus of enzyme/prodrug cancer therapy is to deliver drug-activating enzyme gene or functional protein to tumor tissues which is followed by a systemic administration of a prodrug.

Most of this chapter is devoted on the use of the virus-directed enzyme prodrug therapy (VDEPT), a pharmacologically oriented gene therapy strategy that uses viral vectors to deliver a gene that encodes an enzyme which is capable of converting a systemically administrated nontoxic prodrug into a cytotoxic agent within tumor cells. In order to modify specific cell type or tissue, viral vector is the most effective means of gene transfer that is currently used. It can be manipulated to express therapeutic genes and deliver genes to cells for providing either transient or permanent transgene expression. Several virus types are currently being investigated; including adenoviruses (Ads), retroviruses (γ-retroviruses and lentiviruses), adeno-associated viruses, and herpes simplex. The efficiency of transgene expression, ease of production, safety, toxicity, and stability all affected the choice of virus for routine clinical. This chapter provides an introductory overview of the general characteristics of viral vectors commonly used in gene transfer and their advantages and disadvantages.

Keywords: Virus directed enzyme prodrug therapy (ADEPT), Cancer therapy, Enzymes, Viruses, Genes

---

* Corresponding author: Rafik Karaman, Email: dr_karaman@yahoo.com; Tel and Fax +972-2-2790413.

List of Abbreviations

VDEPT = virus directed enzyme prodrug therapy
5-FC = 5-Fluorocytosine
6-MPDR = 6-Methylpurine deoxyriboside
AAV = Adeno-associated virus
ADEPT = Antibody-directed enzyme prodrug therapy
CAR = Coxsackie virus and adenovirus receptor
CD = Cytosine deaminase
CE = Carboxylesterase
CEA = Carcinoembryonic antigen
CPA = Cyclophosphamide
CPG2 = Carboxypeptidase G2
GCV = Ganciclovir
GDEPT = Gene-directed enzyme prodrug therapy
GPAT = Genetic prodrug activation therapy
HCC = Hepatocellular carcinoma
HIV = Human immunodeficiency virus
HSP = Heat shock protein
HSV-1 = Herpes simplex virus type 1
HTE = Human tyrosinase enhancer
hTR = Human telomerase RNA
HVJ = Hemagglutinating virus of Japan (Sendai virus)
IL-2 = Interleukin-2
i.p. = Intraperitoneal
i.s. = Intrasplenic
i.t. = Intratumoural
i.v. = Intravenous
MLV = Murine leukemia virus
NTR = Nitroreductase
PNP = Purine nucleotide phosphorylase
PSA = Prostate-specific antigen

Introduction

Cancer is a disease which is characterized by uncontrolled growth of abnormal cells [1]. The cancerous cells can invade the surrounded tissues and spread to other parts of the body through the blood and lymph systems (metastases) [2]. Mutation in cell's DNA, converts normal cells into cancer cells. This can be acquired, usually, by exposure to viruses or carcinogens (e.g., tobacco products, asbestos) or inherited such as in breast cancer where women who inherit a single defective copy of either the tumor suppress of genes BRCA1 or BRCA2 have a significantly increased risk of developing breast cancer. However, carcinogenesis is a complex multi-stage process. In order for a cancer to be developed more than one genetic change as well as many other epigenetic factor (hormonal, co-carcinogen and tumor promoter effects and etc.) must be involved. On the other hand, cancer cannot be produced by the above mentioned factors. However, they increased the likelihood of producing genetic mutation which will eventually result in cancer. Cancers are classified according to the type of cells that the tumor resembles and is therefore presumed to be the origin of the tumor. These types include solid tumors such as breast cancer, ovarian cancer, and tumors in the blood, such as polycythemia, leukemia and Hodkings disease. Tumors are generally classified as benign and malignant tumors. Benign tumors have well defined edge; usually it is covered by sheath which can be removed by surgery. In those cases chemotherapy is not necessary. However, if the benign tumor is untreated it might lead to malignant cancer. In malignant tumors the edge is not well defined; it has non-specific shape but it can be proliferated such that to look like a web of crab, hence it is called cancer. In this type of tumors surgery is difficult, therefore, chemotherapy is required and a secondary cancer can be developed by metastasis [3].

The main treatment for cancer is chemotherapy, which involves systemic anti-proliferative agents that kill dividing cells. These cytotoxic agents include antimetabolites, alkylating agents, DNA-complexing agents, mitosis inhibitors and hormones. They make disturbance with some aspects of DNA replication, repair, translation or cell division; by this way they exert their activity and treat the cancer. They interfere mainly with any highly proliferative cells like immune cells and hair cells, and therefore, are not truly selective for cancer cells. Lethal damage can be produced by prolonged use of chemotherapy to proliferating non-cancerous cells and this is particularly true in the treatment of solid tumors [4]. The importance of chemotherapy is as primary treatment for cancer patients. However, its success is limited by several drawbacks which include (i) insufficient drug concentrations in tumors, (ii) systemic toxicity, (iii) lack of selectivity to tumor cells such as in the case of bone marrow, and (iv) gut epithelia. This is particularly true in the treatment of solid tumors; re-growth and spread of more malignant and multi drug resistance forms of cancer have been observed after the use of cytotoxins in patients with appreciable tumor burdens that led to remissions of limited duration and the tumor cells became drug-resistant. This problem can be solved by a number of strategies such as, alternative formulations (e.g., liposomes), resistance modulation (e.g., PSC833), antidotes/toxicity modifiers (e.g., ICRF-18), and gene therapy [5, 6].

The Prodrug Approach

Less reactive and cytotoxic form of anticancer drugs can be achieved by using the prodrug approach therapy which provides an alternative approach for cancer treatment [7]. The term of prodrug was at first introduced by Albert [8] and Harper [9]. It was used to characterize pharmacologically inert derivative that can be converted *in vivo*, enzymatically or non-enzymatically, to exert a therapeutic effect of its active form [10- 15]. The prodrug approach is used to overcome many barriers such as: (i) pharmaceutical, such as poor solubility, insufficient chemical stability, unacceptable taste or odor, irritation and pain, (ii) pharmacokinetic, such as insufficient oral absorption, inadequate blood-brain barrier permeability, marked presystemic metabolism and toxicity, and (iii) pharmacodynamic, such as low therapeutic index and lack of selectivity at the site of action [7, 16, 17].

Thus, temporarily alteration of the physicochemical properties of drugs is the major objective of prodrug design for achieving the following characteristics:

1. To accomplish modification of drug pharmacokinetics.
2. To prolong drug's action.
3. To reduce toxicity and side effects.
4. To increased selectivity.
5. To resolve formulation challenges.

Enzyme prodrug therapy is a promising area for improving tumor selectivity. There are two steps which are involved in enzyme-activating prodrug therapy. In the first step, a drug-activating enzyme is targeted and expressed in tumors. In the second step, a nontoxic prodrug, a substrate of the exogenous enzyme that is now expressed in tumors, is administered systemically. As a result, a high local concentration of an active anticancer drug in tumors can be achieved by prodrug interconversion to its active form .

In order to make this approach clinically successful, certain requirements should be implemented in both enzymes and prodrugs:

For enzyme:

1. 1 The enzyme should be either a nonhuman origin or human protein that is absent or expressed only at low concentrations in normal tissue.
2. The protein must achieve sufficient expression in the tumors and must have high catalytic activity.

For prodrug:

1. The prodrug should be a good substrate for the expressed enzyme in tumors but not to be activated by endogenous enzyme in non-tumor tissues.
2. The prodrug must be able to cross tumor cell membranes for intracellular activation.
3. The cytotoxicity difference between the prodrug and its corresponding active drug should be as high as possible.
4. It is preferred that the activated drug be highly diffusible or be actively taken up by adjacent non expressing cancer cells for a "bystander" killing effect (the ability to kill any neighboring non expressing cells).
5. The half-life of the active drug should be long enough to induce a bystander effect but short enough to avoid drug leaking out into the systemic circulation.

Currently, there are two major ways to be used in the delivery for an enzyme/prodrug strategy:

(a) Delivery of genes that encode prodrug-activating enzymes into tumor tissues (GDEPT, VDEPT and etc.) (Figure 1) 18].
(b) Delivery of active enzymes onto tumor tissues (ADEPT).

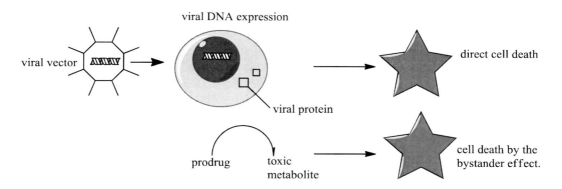

Figure 1. A schematic diagram showing how viral vector is used to direct enzyme prodrug therapy.

In order to enhance the selectivity of cancer chemotherapy, substantial efforts have been made. One approach that has been developed is suicide gene therapy, which is also known as gene-directed enzyme prodrug therapy (GDEPT) [19]. GDEPT is a two-step treatment. In this approach, a foreign enzyme is encoded to a gene which administered for selective expression in the tumor cells. The gene delivery vector can be administered locally at the tumor site or systemically to target metastasized cancer cells as well as solid tumors. The aim of this approach is to enable expression of the foreign enzyme only in the malignant cells prior to an administration of the prodrug.

For GDEPT a number of viral and non-viral gene delivery systems have been developed. Non-viral GDEPT vectors include naked DNA, liposomes, peptides and polymers [20]. Other strategies have been used for an expression of a prodrug converting enzyme by encapsulated cells that have been genetically modified [21, 22]. Another design involves hem agglutinating virus of Japan (HVJ, Sendai virus)-liposomes and polycation enhanced adenoviruses has been developed to obtain a combination of non-viral delivery system with viral vectors [23]. There are many advantages of using non-viral vectors, the most important one is the safety achieved upon their administration to humans. However, viruses are much more efficient at delivering genes into human cells. Consequently, the majority of current gene therapy clinical trials use viral gene therapy vectors and non-viral gene transfer has not been studied to the same extent in humans as much as the viral gene therapy.

When viral vector used in GDEPT systems the term to be referred to is VDEPT (virus direct enzyme prodrug therapy [24]. In VDEPT a virus targets the prodrug-activating enzyme to tumor cells selectively and transduces them efficiently.

In any gene therapy approach, it is important that viruses will be safe for administration to humans, and that the viral dose required for achieving a therapeutic effect has to be well below the dose that produces adverse side effects. Initial viral vectors for cancer gene therapy were engineered to be replication-defective [25], but new methods have been developed using replication selective oncolytic viruses (viro-therapy that replicate in and destroy cancer cells) [26, 27].

When these viruses are used many advantages are achieved: (1) the virus vectors can infect a tumor cell that generates progeny capable of spreading to other cells, (2) replicating viruses achieve higher efficiencies of gene delivery compared with replication-defective viruses [28] and (3) they are often oncolytic and have intrinsic antitumor activity.

The transcriptional regulatory domain of a tumor-associated marker gene and the protein coding domain of a non-mammalian enzyme chimeric gene are created in an artificial chimeric gene. The obtained artificial gene is delivered to the tumor cell for selective expression. When selectively is expressed, the nontoxic prodrug is converted metabolically to a toxic metabolite, by non-mammalian enzyme, selectively in the neoplastic cell. Much higher concentrations of the active cytotoxic drug within the microenvironment of the tumor can be achieved by this approach compared to systemic administration of the active moiety itself, potentially with increased tumor cell killing and reduced host toxicity [29]. Candidate enzyme/prodrug systems for cancer therapy are not, however, entirely cell-autonomous. However, bystander effect' should be demonstrated to involve spread of the cytotoxic species from cells which express the enzyme to kill adjacent, non-transduced cells [30]. This obviates the requirement for gene transfer to all tumor cells, which is an unrealistic goal with current vector technology.

There are several considerations for any viral vector:

1. The ability to attach to and enter the target cell,
2. successful transfer to the nucleus,
3. The ability to be expressed in the nucleus for a sustained period of time,
4. A general lack of toxicity.

Converting a Virus Into a Vector

In the case of gene therapy vectors, a modified genome carrying a therapeutic gene cassette is encapsulated in the viral particles in the place of the viral genome (Figure 2). The abortive (non-replicative or dead-end) infection that introduces functional genetic information expressed from the recombinant vectors into the target cell is called transduction (Figure 2).

Infection and replication phases are the two temporally distinct phases of the viral life. The early phase of gene expression, which is characterized by the appearance of viral regulatory products produced from the infection phase, allows the introduction of the viral genome into the cell. The late phase occurred, when structural genes are expressed and an assembly of new viral particles is accomplished.

The viral genome consists of genes and *cis*-acting gene regulatory sequences. Although some overlap exists, most *cis* acting sequences map is outside the viral coding sequences. The design of recombinant viral vectors with viral genome exploited this spatial segregation of genes and *cis*-acting sequences.

To generate a vector, the separation of coding genes and *cis*-acting sequences into distinct nucleic acid molecules should be made in order to prevent their reconstitution by recombination into productive viral particles. Heterologous plasmids can be used to express coding sequences.

The viral *cis*-acting sequences linked to the therapeutic gene can then be introduced into the same cell, leading to the production of replication-defective particles able to specifically transduce the new genetic information into target cells. An important factor that determines the efficiency and safety of a vector system is maintaining the separation of viral genes and *cis*-acting sequences during production. .

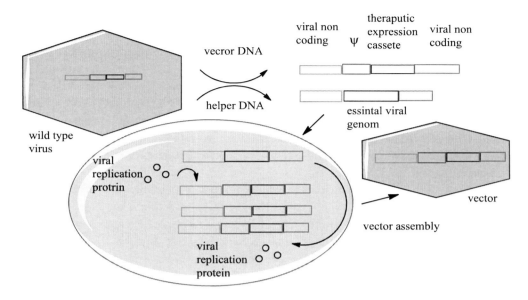

Figure 2. Genetic strategy for engineering a virus into a victor.

The degree of organizational complexity of the viral genome makes limitation to the genetic engineering which described above. The intact viral genome often ensures an appropriate balance of viral protein production by complex regulatory changes in gene expression. Moreover, in an engineered vector-packaging system, *cis*-interactions between the genome and its translation products were found to be missing. Inefficient packaging of vector genomes and the release of excess defective vector particles that not only are incapable of gene transfer but often interfere with the transduction of biologically active vector particles are resulted from these intrinsic limitations of vector design as compared to wild-type viruses.

The attempts to reconstitute vector particles from synthetic components are limited due to complex integration of the viral lifecycle with the cellular machinery. The use of *in vitro* assembly system for duplicating these processes has been proven to be a daunting challenge that would increase the biosafety of viral vectors if succeed.

The concentration of viral particles and/or the number of virions that are capable of transduction is used to measure the relative concentration of vectors which is expressed as a titer. There is small percentage of transducing particles from the total particles, and can vary between different preparations. Quantification is generally subjected to variation resulting from different methods used in different laboratories.

So standardized methods for determining the specific activity of vectors is strongly needed. Particle titer and an infectious or transducing titer are both important, because efficacy, toxicity and immunogenicity are affected by the presence of impurities and variations in infectious activity.

Properties of Vectors For Gene Therapy

For gene therapy to be successful, an appropriate amount of a therapeutic gene has to be delivered into the target tissue without substantial toxicity. The suitable application for specific gene therapy for each viral vector system is characterized by an inherent set of properties.

For some disorders, long term expression from a relatively small proportion of cells would be sufficient (for example, genetic disorders), whereas, high but transient gene expression for other pathologies would be required. For example, gene therapies designed to interfere with a viral infectious process or to inhibit the growth of cancer cells by reconstitution of inactivated tumor suppressor genes may require gene transfer into a large fraction of the abnormal cells. The bystander effect is utilized to enhance gene transfer strategies that are based on the delivery of tumor specific toxins or conversion of prodrugs into toxins.

This allows transportation of either the gene product or the converted prodrug between cells, such that even when targeting only a fraction of cells within a tumor the therapeutic efficacy may be achieved [31]. The induction of immune responses to tumor antigens and the interruption of the tumor vascular supply are used as other gene transfer strategies for cancer which may require intermediate levels of gene transfer in a cell-type specific subset of the cells within, or from, a tumor. Furthermore, oncolytic viruses, not containing transgenes but are genetically engineered to allow tumor-specific viral replication which induce cell lysis, and spread to neighboring malignant cells, are used in these approaches [32].

Regulated gene expression is required in some forms of gene therapy. In the state of diabetes, rapid changes in glucose concentrations and metabolic perturbations are important to regulate exogenous expression of insulin. Posttranslational processing that is responsive to these metabolic cues will be required in this situation. In other cases such as anemia, turning the erythropoietin gene on or off may make regulation to hematocrit by an administration of oral drugs (for example, tetracycline derivations) that regulate a specific trans activator that activate or repress a specific promoter [33].

Most pathological and immunological consequences of viral infection are influenced by the expression of viral genes, but gene transduction by recombinant vectors is often well tolerated. There are several problems that may be observed with gene transfer vectors:

1. Acute toxicity which results from the infusion of foreign materials.
2. Cellular immune responses directed against the transduced cells.
3. Humoral immune responses against the therapeutic gene product.
4. Insertional mutagenesis by certain integrating vectors.

The integration of currently used vector happens in a random manner. Integration which is a mutagenic event having well-established potential for disruption and transcriptional activation of cellular genes, including oncogenes. Nonetheless, most transduced cells are well tolerated for integration, and instrumental to ensure stability of the newly introduced genetic information in the recipient. It should be noted, that until now the vector which is used in human trials was integrated into a relatively small proportion of cells within a target tissue. The risks of viral integration might need to be reconsidered due to the generation of more efficient vectors having the ability for targeting a wider spectrum of cells, including stem cells capable of self-renewal and massive clonal outgrowth. Inadvertent transmission of vector sequences into germ cells is an additional undesirable potential effect. Though this risk is negligible especially with an integrating vector, and any such germ line event raises important safety and ethical issues.

These potential risks could be mitigated by some desirable properties to the vector which include the ability to infect selectively a specific target cell or tissue.

Current methods to circumvent some of the problems of promiscuous transduction include:

1. The tissue-specific promoters that have been used to drive expression of the transduced gene.
2. The surface recognition elements of recombinant viral particles which were modified to change their cell-recognition properties.

Type of Vector Used

Adenovirus

Dividing and non-dividing cells could be infected by human adenoviruses. In infected cells, the adenoviral genome remains episomal and does not usually integrate into the host DNA therefore the risk of Insertional mutagenesis is minimized. A gene expression mediated by adenovirus is relatively short-term, but it can last for up to several weeks. For cancer suicide gene therapy approaches, the aim is to destroy the target cells shortly after infection, in contrast to gene replacement therapies where long-term transgene expression is required. Moreover, the beneficial of GDEPT is shutting down the adenoviral gene expression by decreasing long-term pathogenicity. In GDEPT protocols, both replication-defective and replicating adenoviruses have been used. The first generation vectors that are made by substituting an expression cassette for the viral E1 and/or E3 region have contributed to the majority of non-replicating GDEPT adenoviruses. Subsequently, the development of second generation adenoviruses is important for reducing the toxicity and immune response to recombinant adenoviruses, which are mainly due to the *de novo* synthesis of viral proteins in infected cells [34].

In second-generation adenoviruses, in order to reduce toxicity and to minimize the risk of replication-selective viruses occurring during the viral production process, due to homologous recombination between the vector and the producer cell line, additional genes for viral replication have been inactivated. For example, the depletion of E1/E4-TK-expressing vectors have been constructed and showed a substantially decreased rate of recombination through production.

For several E1/E4 adenoviruses, good safety profiles and decreased immunogenicity have been reported, however, in a non-GDEPT clinical trial only one vector has led to a fatality event. It appeared that the activation of innate immunity in this trial have been triggered by the virus, resulting in systemic inflammation, multi-organ failure and acute respiratory distress syndrome, despite the fact that in animal models the virus performance was good; highlighting the limitations of preclinical studies in predicting human responses to gene therapy [35].

Thymidine Kinase and Cytosine Deaminase

Replication-defective adenoviruses for GDEPT have been assessed in numerous clinical trials. The prodrug-converting enzyme, TK in a combination with the prodrug ganciclovir (GCV) has been used in most of these studies. With TK mediated GDEPT there are various types of cancer that have been treated clinically, including malignant mesothelioma, malignant glioma, retinoblastoma, melanoma, metastatic colorectal liver carcinoma and ovarian cancer, where i.p. injection was used to deliver the vector Ad-OC-TK, a virus that employs the tissue-selective osteocalcin promoter to regulate expression of TK, and to target the enzyme to prostate tumors used in another clinical study. Human prostate tumor cells as well as the surrounding stromal cells express osteocalcin and therefore Ad-OC-TK is designed to target both cells types. The virus was injected directly into prostate cancer lymph nodes and bone metastases of patients, followed by an oral administration of the prodrug. The treatment was tolerated with no serious side effects. Moreover, TK was delivered to the tumors and in treated specimens, an evidence of apoptosis was observed. However, the use of Ad-OC-TK is limited to intralesional application since systemic administration is expected to lead to toxicity because osteocalcin is not only expressed in prostate tumors; Ad-OC-TK can also drive TK expression into normal osteoblasts [36].

Transcriptional targeting tumor-selective promoters have also been used. For instance, for liver cancer to restrict TK-expression (α-fetoprotein promoter) and melanoma (tyrosinase promoter) preclinical applications have been investigated.

Early attention was received for the use of recombinant adenoviruses as a vehicle to transfer genes into the respiratory epithelium for treating diseases such as cystic fibrosis. However, it was quickly realized that the most efficient gene transfer system in a variety of tissues was this class of vectors [37].

There are over 50 different human adenoviral sero-types, but the current vectors are primarily derived from the most common serotypes to which most adults have been exposed; those known as 2 and 5. However, many efforts have been made to avoid potential problems related to pre-existing immunity that may reduce the efficacy of vector administration. Therefore, other serotypes or even non-human adenoviruses were later exploited [38].

Both viral DNA strands encoding over 50 polypeptides containing approximately 36-kilobase viral dsDNA genome with overlapping transcriptional units. After cell entry, the genome enters into the nucleus; this happens by viral particle which contains proteins that allow for efficient endosomal lysis and escape. The process of viral gene expression leads to genome replication starts at region 1 (E1) genes which are quickly transcribed and serve in part as a master transcriptional regulator. For viral genome replication, the E1 genes in combination with the E2 and E4 genes are required. Late in the life cycle, for encapsulation of the newly replicated genomes, the viral structural proteins genes are needed to be transcribed. Viral-induced cell lysis can release as many as 10,000 virions which can be produced from one cell. Purified concentrations of 1×10^{13} vector particles/ml can be routinely achieved. For the viral life cycle the E3 genes is dispensable, and the wild-type infection plays a role in immune surveillance in infected hosts. Protection against some of the immune-mediated responses directed against the vector or vector-transduced cells in animal studies by these genes have been suggested, but due to differences in animal species and strains used for the studies this remains controversial. However, additional room for larger foreign DNA inserts in the range of 8 kb is allowed by the removal of this region [39].

In the first generation vectors, in order to make room for the therapeutic expression cassette, the E1 region is removed in order to prohibit transactivation of viral genes required for viral replication. For the vector to be made, the E1-deleted viral genome containing the transgene is added to a cell line that contains a stable E1a expression cassette allowing the added DNA to replicate and be packaged into E1 deleted vectors that are not capable of replication.

Low-level transcription of the remaining viral genes after the removal of E1 gene production is occurred resulting in early innate cytokine responses, followed by antigen-dependent immune responses that include cell-mediated destruction of transduced cells, reducing the period of gene expression. Second and third generation vectors with deletions of E1 and E2 and/or E4 genes were later studied [40]. Although these vectors gave reduced toxicity profiles in animals, toxicity from an E1/E4 deleted adenovirus vector infused into the hepatic artery of a young man with partial OTC deficiency was the first reported fatal event from gene therapy.

The removal of all the viral genes from the vector is a daunting task due to the complexity of adenovirus; this occurs because unlike retroviruses, it is not possible to make construction of a packaging cell line. Instead, a system of helper-dependent vector is developed in which all the viral genes required for replication are part of one virus (the helper) but these viral genes have in their packaging domain a conditional defect making them less likely to be packaged into a virions. The second vector contains only the viral inverted terminal repeats (ITRs), therapeutic gene sequences (up to 28–32kb) and the normal packaging recognition signal which allows this genome to be selectively packaged and released from cells. Purification to the helper virus and vector can be made by physical means [41].

After intravenous administration, the liver is the final station to the most of the adenovirus vector, but direct injection can transduce most tissues. Preclinical animal studies have used these vectors to transduce liver, skeletal muscle, heart, brain, lung, pancreas and tumors [42].

Retroviruses

Retroviruses are lipid-enveloped particles consisting of a homodimer of linear, positive-sense, single-stranded RNA genomes of 7 to 11 kilobases. The RNA genome is retro-transcribed into linear double stranded DNA which integrates into the cell chromatin; this occurs after entry of the virus into target cells. This family of viruses has several varieties that being exploited for gene therapy use: the mammalian and avian C-type retroviruses (hereafter also referred to as oncoretroviruses), lentiviruses, such as HIV and other immunodeficiency viruses, and spumaviruses. Chronic infection is tended to be establish by these viruses but it is usually well tolerated by the host, however, latent diseases may also be happened ranging from malignancy to immunodeficiency.

All retroviral genome at their ends have two long terminal repeat (LTR) sequences. During viral gene expression, LTR and neighboring sequences act in *cis* during packaging retro-transcription and integration of the genome. The structural proteins, nucleic-acid polymerases/integrases and surface glycoprotein are encoded by LTR sequences frame, the tandem *gag, pol* and *env* genes, respectively. A much more complex genome was found in lentiviruses; in addition to the *gag, pol,* and *env* genes, two regulatory genes *tat* and *rev*are encoded in these viruses. These regulatory genes are essential for expression of the genome and variable sets of accessory genes. Spumaviruses also contain *bel-1,* an essential gene regulating expression of the genome, and other genes of unknown functions.

An effective and simple retrovector design is achieved due to the location of most *cis*-acting sequences in the terminal regions; this makes these retrovector the most widely used vector system in gene therapy clinical trials. The viral glycoprotein envelope dictates the host range of retroviral particles through its interaction with receptors on target cells. The viral-envelope glycoproteins post-translational modification is a signature of the type and species of producer cell, and affects the stability of the particle when delivered into a specific species. The mechanism of particle assembly allows for substitution of one viral Env by another one from a different virus in a process referred to as pseudo typing. By Suchan approach, the host-range of retroviral vectors can be expanded by incorporating sequences from unrelated viruses. For example, vectors pseudo typed with G glycoprotein of the vesicular stomatitis virus (VSV-G), can infect most cells, and can be concentrated to titers up to 1×10^{10} t.u. /ml [43]

The ability to integrate efficiently into the chromatin of target cells is a useful property of retroviral vectors. Although stable expression of the transduced gene cannot be achieved by integration, however it is an effective way to maintain the genetic information in a self-renewing tissue and in the clonal outgrowth of a stem cell.

For the pre-integration complex to gain access to the chromatin, the disruption of the nuclear membrane is required, and the target cell mitosis after entry is strictly affected by the productive transduction of retroviral vectors. Because at any given time only a fraction of cells pass through mitosis, so the applications of retroviral vectors in gene therapy is largely limited to selected targets *ex vivo* such as, lymphocytes and hematopoietic progenitor cells [44].

The application of retrovectors *in vivo by* systemic delivery is limited because retrovectors are unstable in human serum and are rapidly inactivated by human complement.

This problem can be avoided by producing the vectors in a packaging cell based on a human cell line using the envelope gene from a cat virus RD114. Thus selection of both the cell line and the *env* gene might achieve resistance to human complement.

Lentiviruses

Lentiviruses are currently under preclinical development, they are promising vectors to be used. Unlike retroviruses, the nuclear import machinery of the target cell is crucially important for enabling lentiviruses active transport of the pre-integration complex through the nucleopore. The genetic information that found to be only a fraction of the parental genome is required to package a functional lentiviral core in the vector [45]. For viral pathogenesis, the non-required genes are critical to increase vector biosafety; new generations of "minimal" packaging constructs have been adopted. In order to alleviate such concerns an important approach relies on the use of self-inactivating transfer vectors was followed. Therefore, the risk of vector mobilization and recombination substantially diminishes by these vectors which contain a deletion in the downstream LTR which its transduction into target cells results in the transcriptional inactivation of the upstream LTR.

The non-human lentiviruses (for example, simian, equine, feline, caprine and bovine) have been used to derive hybrid lentiviral vectors, using similar approaches to those used for HIV-derived vectors, on the rationale that they would be more acceptable for clinical application because the parental viruses are not infectious to humans.

The vector of VSV-pseudo typed lentiviral can be delivered directly *in vivo*. The neurons and glial cells of the central nervous system (CNS) can be efficiently transduced in the rodents and non-human primates.

For this type of vectors, stable and long-term transgene expression was observed without detectable pathological consequences. In animal models of retinal photoreceptor degeneration, the long-term therapeutic efficacy of lentivirus-mediated gene transfer into the CNS has been reported. Several non-dividing, differentiated epithelial tissues of rodents, humans and other species, isolated or dissociated *ex vivo* are transduced efficiently by lentiviral vectors [40]. The lentiviral vector-mediated gene delivery *in vivo* actual potential and limitations still to be defined.

The transduction of the elusive long-term repopulating hematopoietic stem cells (HSC) is possibly a unique application of lentiviral vectors. Efficient marking of human and primate HSC originating long-term, and multi lineage reconstitution in xenogeneic or autologous hosts, respectively, is resulted from short *ex vivo* incubation with lentiviral vector, without a need for cytokine stimulation.

Great constraints on the viral genome and on its exploitation for gene transfer purposes are obtained by the obligatory RNA step in the retroviral lifecycle. The human foamy viruses (HFV) have been used to generate replication-competent and replication-defective vectors. Further studies are required to appreciate their value in clinical applications [42].

Adeno-Associated Virus

Adeno-associated viruses (AAVs) are human parvoviruses that normally require a helper virus, such as adenovirus to mediate their productive infection. They were initially discovered as a contaminant in adenoviruses preparation. There are six known human viral serotypes, each of which may have different tropic properties. Most studies to date have focused on AAV-2. This kind of virus is an ideal candidate for gene therapy because there is no known disease associated with AAV infection [45].

There are two genes in the viral genome, each producing multiple polypeptides: *rep*, required for viral genome replication; and *cap*, encoding structural proteins. The major limitation of this vector system is that its packaging capacity is about 5.0 kb. For the wild-type virus to integrate into a specific region of human chromosome it needs the presence of *rep* gene. Due to the absence of this *rep* gene the integration property is lost in vectors.

Production of AAV vectors can be obtained by an addition of the following: separate plasmids containing the ITRs flanking the therapeutic gene cassette, the *rep/cap* genes, and a helper adenovirus or a third plasmid with the essential adenoviral helper genes. This approach does not require the input of any viruses.

Episomal transgene expression and random chromosomal integration are the two ways that AAV vectors use to transduce cells. A slow rise in gene expression was resulted after gene transfer in animals; the level of expression reached a steady-state level after a period of weeks. This is due, perhaps in part to a requirement for either vector ssDNA annealing, or second strand-synthesis followed by vector genome linking to form concatemers for generation of dsDNA genomes. It is difficult to elucidate the mechanistic process of transduction because of the numerous and complex genome vector forms found *in vivo* in the different tissues. Nevertheless, different groups overcome the limited coding capacity by splitting a gene or expression cassette into two vectors and simultaneously administering them to muscle or liver [42].

Since the viral coding sequences are lacked in AAV vector genome, the toxicity or any inflammatory response (except for the generation of neutralizing antibodies that may limit re-administration) is not associated with the vector itself. By *in vivo* administration, the vector particle can be delivered to many different organs (for example, the CNS, liver, lung and muscle) and efficient transduction to non-dividing cells can be achieved by AAV vectors. Moreover, there have been reports indicating preclinical efficacy in different animal models of genetic and acquired diseases.

AAV vector has been used in clinical trials for the treatment of cystic fibrosis, hemophilia and muscular dystrophy [45]. It is likely that treating some diseases will be applied by this vector and so more clinical trials with this vector are expected soon.

Herpes Simplex Virus

Herpes viruses according to their ability to persist after primary infection in humans, in a state of latency where disease is absent in human hosts with normal immune status, are promising for the use as vehicles for *in vivo* transfer genes to cells.

For purposes of gene transfer, herpes simplex virus type 1 (HSV-1) is currently the most extensively engineered herpes virus. There are many features in this type of virus which provide for multiple sites of foreign gene insertion, making HSV a large capacity vector capable of harboring at least 30 kb of non-HSV sequences representing large single genes or multiple transgenes that may be coordinately or simultaneously expressed. These features include the HSV, a large genome composed of 152 kb of linear dsDNA containing at least 84 almost entirely contiguous (unspliced) genes, approximately half of which are nonessential for virus replication in cell culture. The expression of the remaining lytic viral functions is not achieved in highly defective mutants deleted for the five immediate early (IE) genes which are essentially silent except for transgene expression.

Without the production of detectable replication competent virus these vectors can be grown to high titer in complementing cell lines. The IE gene deletion vectors are capable of persisting in a state similar to latency in neurons and other cell types within non-neuronal tissue, therefore these vectors are non-cytotoxic. A most attractive feature, which results in an efficient gene transduction, is the efficient infectivity of HSV. Repeated vector administration even in immune hosts can be applied due to efficient infectivity and transduction. Limitations of these vectors include:

1. The experience with recombinant herpes viruses in patients is limited.
2. Difficulties related to long-term transgene expression in certain tissues including brain.
3. Difficulties related to vector targeting, since the mechanism of HSV attachment and entry is complex, involving multiple viral envelope glycoproteins.

HSV amplicon vectors represent an alternative to replication defective and recombinant genomic vectors. Amplicon plasmids are based on defective interfering virus genomes that arise on high passage of virus stocks. The lengths of the amplicon plasmids are in general approximately 15 kb and minimally possess a viral origin of replication and packaging sequences. For particle production and packaging of genome length concatemerized vector DNA, the standard amplicon system requires the functions of helper HSV. The use of helper virus genome plasmids deleted for packaging signals has been used to improve the production of amplicon vector; the propagation of helper genomes is occurred in bacteria and bacterial artificial chromosomes. The advantage of these preparations is being nearly helper-free; however, until the helper DNA is completely devoid of sequences shared with the amplicon vector (for example, origin of replication), the possibility of contamination of vector stocks with unwanted recombinants is increased.

Transfection Production systems are also difficult to scale–up, and have not yet produced high titer vector. Thus far, production of replication–competent virus-free genomic vectors using complementing cells resulted in a 2–3 log higher vector particle yield, using a less complicated production system

The treatment of animal models with HSV vectors has been successfully applied for many diseases such as cancer, PNS disease, certain brain diseases, spinal nerve injury and pain. Perhaps using these vectors as gene transfer sensory neurons is the most promising current use of these vectors. Because similar hosts have been found for wild-type virus, HSV is already highly evolved for this purpose. Sensory neurons can take up highly defective vectors following direct inter-dermal injection by sensory neurons where they persist, apparently for life, in nerve cell bodies. For long-term expression of therapeutic genes the latency promoter can be applied in a separate virus locus [46].

The safety and effectiveness of HSV vectors in the clinical setting is going be tested in the coming years. Further improvements of the vector design should be forthcoming and should include:

1. The development of HSV packaging line for an efficient production of amplicons,
2. Methods to improve transgene control in the HSV vector.

Sindbis Virus

Sindbis virus is a blood-born RNA virus. The transmission of the virus occurs through mosquito bites and selectively infects the tumor cells. The 67-kDa high-affinity laminin receptor (LAMR) is probably mediates the tumor-selectivity of Sindbis virus; the up regulation of this receptor occurs in numerous human cancers. Cytotoxic genes are not carried by sindbis vectors and they are replication defective viruses, however, apoptosis in infected cells *are* induced by them. Sindbis vectors retain the blood-born attribute, and a systemic delivery to the virus can be applied.

Efficient gene delivery vectors are produced by this virus, and Sindbis vector which expresses TK (Sindbis/tk) has been developed for the GDEPT approach. Furthermore, the apoptotic nature of the virus influences the virus therapeutic effect. However, the anti-tumor efficacy is enhanced significantly by co-administration of GCV, providing a proof that Sindbis virus is a suitable vector for GDEPT [47].

Vaccinia Virus

The vaccinia virus (VV) is used over the world as a vaccine against smallpox; for this reason it has been tested in humans as a vaccine in clinical trials for cancer immunotherapy. A good safety record was reported for this virus since it does not cause any known human disease.

The integration process by VV has never been observed; it spends its entire lifecycle in the cytoplasm of infected cells, so the risk of Insertional mutations is minimized. VV is a cytolytic virus with a short life-cycle, and it spreads rapidly through infected tissues. The virus can infect laboratory animals and almost all types of cells however, after *in vivo* systemic administration of VV, it inherently targets tumors. It is believed that the virus size is responsible for this natural tumor tropism. From all oncolytic viruses the VV is the largest one (>200 nm) and it has been hypothesized that the extravasation of the viral particles is only due to leaky vasculature (such as in tumors and ovaries).

In order to enhance the VV tumor-selectivity at the genetic level many approaches have been described. The employment of transcriptional targeting strategies is not possible due to the fact that the replication of the viral occurs in the cytoplasm and independently of the host DNA synthesis machinery. However, gene deletion method can be used to make VV targeted to tumor cells, i.e., the modification of genes that is necessary for viral replication in normal, quiescent cells.

VV has a linear, double-stranded DNA genome, which is accessible to manipulations and mutant strains that replicate only in dividing cells. Double deleted vaccinia virus that lack the genes for the viral thymidine kinase (TK) and vaccinia growth factor (VGF) are generated. The host thymidine kinase or host cell nucleotides, which are more available in proliferating cells compared to resting tissues, are responsible for the resulting virus vvDD replication, thus, inhibiting the viral replication in non-dividing cells. When vvDD was delivered intravenously at doses up to109 pfu the tumor-selectivity in mice was shown to be enhanced and a good safety profile in rhesus macaques was achieved [42].

Replicating RNA Viruses

Many RNA viruses are naturally oncolytic, for tumor-selective replication, they often rely on defective signaling pathways in malignant cells. The examination of some RNA viruses has already been started in clinical studies. The phase I clinical trials have been safely completed for two different strains of Newcastle disease virus, PV701 and MTH-68/H, and in patients with cervical and colorectal cancer. The PV701 strain is currently in phase II studies. The administration of Newcastle disease virus can be repeated by intravenous infusion and tumor responses to virus treatment have been reported. Reovirus is another oncolytic RNA virus, a couple of phase I and phase II studies have been completed and two additional phase I trials have been initiated. The results of these studies indicate that one intratumoural injection of reovirus was well tolerated. The safety of systemic reovirus administration is currently under investigation [48].

The fact that the genomes of RNA viruses can only be manipulated in their DNA forms, maks RNA virus engineering for transgene delivery or tumor targeting is hampered. This is contrarily to DNA viruses.

However, in order to rescue several positive and negative-strand RNA viruses "reverse genetics" many systems have been developed. For instance, measles virus has been shown to express foreign proteins effectively, and retargeted measles virus displaying single-chain antibodies for tumor selective targeting has been generated. Furthermore, in order to deliver foreign genes and to target tumor cells it has been demonstrated that Newcastle disease virus can be engineered. Whilst for other RNA viruses (including influenza, polio and mumps), virus engineering is available, but the challenge of genetic engineering of segmented, double-stranded RNA viruses, such as reovirus, remain to be accomplished [42].

Current evidence suggests that fighting cancer is more successful when these oncolytic viruses are used with therapeutic genes that employ an additional cytotoxic mechanism, such as GDEPT. Attacking the tumors using this approach has a multi-faceted mode [42]:

(1) There are successive rounds of virus-mediated cancer cell killing.

(2) Relatively long-lived expressions of the prodrug-converting enzymes are delivered by replicating viruses which are then able to activate a large number of prodrug molecules, providing an amplification effect. The viruses are expected to improve enzyme delivery and expression by spreading throughout the tumors, independently of vascularization or necrosis, compared with replication-defective vectors.

(3) The bystander effect is important because it leads to killing of uninfected cancer and importantly, will also target the stromal cells that support the tumor, such as the vasculature.

(4) In order to enhance the efficacy of monotherapy, the use of virus/prodrug combinations tailored has the potential to act synergistically.

(5) Different mechanisms are used by oncolytic viruses and GDEPT to kill cells by making them less resistant to the treatment.

Hybrid Vectors

In order to get better vectors, attempts to combine the best features of different viruses in hybrid vectors have been applied. The site-specific integration machinery of wild-type AAV with the efficient internalization and nuclear targeting properties of adenovirus is one of the most interesting hybrid couples that are applied. In the presence of adenovirus or herpes virus infection, AAV undergoes a productive replication cycle; this is because AAV is a helper-dependent parvovirus; so in the absence of the helper functions the virus genome integrates into a specific site on the chromosome, 19.13.3-qtr, AAVS1. Integration of the AAV genome into AAVS1 requires expression of the AAV Rep protein. As conventional rAAV vectors are deleted for all viral genes, including *rep*, they are not able to specifically integrate into AAVS1, but this potentially a useful feature of the parental wild-type virus which has been harnessed in hybrid vectors.

Although hybrid vectors that contain AAV Rep could be useful for *ex vivo* transduction, their use for *in vivo* gene transfer might be limited. A transposon approach has been used to achieve integration from an adenovirus vector; a gene-deleted adenovirus vector that carried an hFIX transposon flanked by *Flp* motifs was constructed. The generation of transposon circles and the random integration of the *hFIX* gene in mouse liver have been achieved by systemic delivery of this vector with a second gene-deleted vector that expressed the *Flp* and *Sleeping Beauty* recombinases. Therapeutic levels of hFIX were maintained for more than 6 months in the presence of extensive liver proliferation [49].

Prodrugs Activated by Virus-Directed Enzyme Prodrug Therapy Approaches

The availability of the genes encoding for the respective enzymes have led to the development of GDEPT and VDEPT approaches. The most important examples of VDEPT approaches are discussed in the following sections.

Nitroreductase

Enzymology of Nitroreductase

The reduction of nitro group to hydroxylamino group is catalyzed by nitroreductase. In addition, the reduction of nitro compounds and quinones such as menadion is also mediated by this enzyme. The isolation of this enzyme from E. coli is applied by using NADH or NADPH as a cofactor, and the inhibition is mediated by the DT-diaphorase inhibitor, dicoumarol.

Nitroreductase has a molecular weight of 24 kDa.. The Km of nitroreductase for menadione is 80 μM, and the Km for CB 1954 is 862 μM.

Activation of CB 1954 by Nitroreductase

The activation of 5-(Aziridin-1-yl)-2,4-dinitrobenzamide (CB 1954) (Figure 3) to the cytotoxic metabolite 5-(aziridin-1-yl)-4-hydroxylamino-2-nitrobenzamide is occurred by both *Escherichia coli* nitroreductase and rat DT diaphorase.

The 4-nitro group of CB 1954 is reduced by the rat DT-diaphorase, whereas the reduction of either of the 2-nitro groups is accomplished by *E. coli* nitroreductase. Both rat and human DT-diaphorase have been shown to reduce CB 1954 with four electrons, preferentially to the highly cytotoxic 4-hydroxylamine. However, bioactivation of CB 1954 in human tumor cells is too slow. The development of a novel antitumor prodrug therapy was established. It was shown that the DT-diaphorase enzyme NQO2 have the ability to bioactivate CB 1954. This enzyme is present in inactive form in human tumor cells. The activation of the enzyme NQO2 is happened upon cell exposure to reduced nicotinamide riboside or other reduced pyridinium compounds, which leads to 100- to 3000-fold increase in the cytotoxicity of CB 1954. The expression of NAD (P) H dehydrogenase (quinone) (DT-diaphorase; NQO1) is responsible for the NQO2 activity.

CB1954

Figure 3. Chemical structure of CB1945.

However, the activation of CB 1954 by E. coli nitroreductase with k_{cat} value of 360 min^{-1} is much more efficient than its activation by rat DT-diaphorase, with k_{cat} value of 4 min^{-1}. The activity of human DT-diaphorase is less than the activity of rat DT-diaphorase, and CB 1954 appears to inhibit the enzyme rather than to activate it (as a substrate). In combination with purified E. coli nitroreductase, CB 1954 was cytotoxic to V79 cells that were insensitive toward CB 1954. It should be indicated that cloning of E. coli nitroreductase led to the use of the enzyme in GDEPT. CB 1954 sensitivity with a bystander effect is enhanced by infection of mammalian cells with a recombinant retrovirus containing the nitroreductase cDNA.

Purine-Nucleoside Phosphorylase

Enzymology of Purine-Nucleoside Phosphorylase

The conversion of purine nucleoside to purine and α-d-ribose-1-phosphate in the presence of phosphorus is catalyzed by purine-nucleoside phosphorylase. The substrates for this enzyme are adenosine, guanosine, inosine, and their analogs. The reaction for the natural substrates is reversible. The phosphorylase enzyme is present in bacteria, such as E. coli, and mammals. The location of this enzyme in mammals is mainly in the liver, brain, thyroid, kidney, and spleen. The highest concentrations of the enzyme are found in the kidney, peripheral lymphocytes, and granulocytes.

Activation of Prodrugs by Purine-Nucleoside Phosphorylase

The Purine-Nucleoside Phosphorylase enzyme can be used in ADEPT, GDEPT, and VDEPT approaches that use prodrugs that cannot be activated by human purine-nucleoside phosphorylases. Purine-nucleoside phosphorylase from E. coli catalyzes the activation of the antitumor agent, 9-β-D-arabinofuranosyl-2-fluoroadenine (fludarabine, Figure 4) to 2-fluoroadenine with a K_m of 1.35 mM and a V_{max} of 7.7 nmol/min/mg of protein.

Figure 4. Chemical structure of fludarabine.

Although the mechanism of the antitumor activity for 2-fluoroadenine is unknown, it is believed that 2-fluoroadenine is phosphorylated to the toxic 2-fluoroadenine-triphosphate. Mammalian purine-nucleoside phosphorylases do not activate fludarabine similar to that seen with other adenine and adenine nucleosides. Therefore, the treatment of hepatocellular carcinoma was applied using fludarabine and purine-nucleoside phosphorylase. The gene-encoding E. coli purine-nucleoside phosphorylase is delivered by adenoviral followed by administration of fludarabine which prevented subcutaneous and intrahepatic tumor formation in nude mice and was also effective for the treatment of established tumors.

Thymidine Kinase

Enzymology of Thymidine Kinase

The phosphorylation of thymidine is accomplished by thymidine kinase using ATP. Thymidine-5-phosphate and ADP are the products of this process. Phosphor- group has also been observed with uridine and cytidine analogs. This enzyme is also involved in the salvage pathway of nucleotide biosynthesis. The Km values of natural ligands are generally in the low micromolar range. The cytosolic enzyme is found in bacteria such as E. coli, viruses such as herpes simplex, and mammals. Thymidine kinase is present in all tissues containing proliferating cells, and high activity levels are present in thymus and spleen.

The activity level of thymidine kinase is high in some leukemias, lymphomas, and other tumors, and increased serum levels have been observed in malignancies. The correlation between a high thymidine kinase activity and a rapid tumor proliferation is still unknown.

Activation of Ganciclovir by Thymidine Kinase

The activation of ganciclovir which is an ant herpetic prodrug is mediated by thymidine kinase (Figure 5). Then the cellular kinases subsequently convert the resulting ganciclovir monophosphate into the toxic ganciclovirtriphosphate nucleotide. Herpes simplex virus type 1 thymidine kinase (HSV-TK) activates ganciclovir which was found to be 3 orders of magnitude more efficient than any human kinase. Recently several gene therapy approaches have been developed with HSV-TK and ganciclovir.

Figure 5. Ganciclovir activation.

Alkaline Phosphatase

Enzymology and Localization of Alkaline Phosphatase

The hydrolysis of phosphate esters to the corresponding alcohols and phosphate is catalyzed by alkaline phosphatases. Zinc and magnesium have been found in the active centers of these metalloenzyme. Nearly all living organisms have the type of enzymes. These enzymes are found in liver, bone, kidney, and many other tissues in several species, including humans. The highest activity for these enzymes was fond in liver. In malignancies and renal diseases the differences in isoenzyme patterns of liver and bone have been found. Many placental, intestinal alkaline phosphatase and tissue-nonspecific isoenzymes have been cloned and sequenced.

Activation of Prodrugs by Alkaline Phosphatase

The wide distribution of alkaline phosphatases make these enzymes not usable to locally activate prodrugs except when targeting the enzyme by ADEPT, GDEPT, or VDEPT approaches. Therefore, alkaline phosphatase prodrugs have been developed primarily to increase the bioavailability of antitumor drugs.

β-Glucuronidase

Enzymology and Localization of β-Glucuronidase

The hydrolysis of D-glucuronides to the corresponding alcohol and D-glucuronate is catalyzed by a group of isoenzymes of the β-glucuronidase enzymes. β-glucuronidase enzymes are virtually present in all tissues and can be found in microsomes (endoplasmic reticulum) and lysosomes. The highest concentrations of β-glucuronidase activity can be found in the liver and spleen although. In humans considerable β-glucuronidase activity is also present in intestinal microflora. The enzyme has been extensively used in prodrug approaches because the levels of β-glucuronidase are elevated in necrotic areas of tumors.

Activation of Prodrugs by β-Glucuronidase

β-glucuronidase enzymes cannot be used to locally activate prodrugs without ADEPT GDEPT or VDEPT approaches. The bioavailability of antitumor agents has been improved by the development of β-glucuronidase prodrugs. Most prodrugs consist of the general structure drug-spacer- glucuronic acid. When β-glucuronidase catalyzes a prodrug hydrolysis reaction the fragmentation of the self-immolative spacer occurs and the drug is released.

Cytochrome P450

Enzymology of Cytochrome P450

The mono-oxygenation of substrates is catalyzed by the superfamily of P450 enzymes; in this process one atom of molecular oxygen is incorporated into a substrate and the other is reduced to water, and NADPH is used as a cofactor. Several types of oxidation reactions are catalyzed by these enzymes which have abroad substrate specificity. These reactions include hydroxylations, epoxidations, heteroatom oxidations, heteroatom dealkylations, oxidative group transfer, cleavage of esters, and dehydrogenations.

The biosynthesis or catabolism of steroid hormones, bile acids, fat-soluble vitamins, fatty acids, and eicosanoids are mediated by mammalian P450s, which are heme-containing microsomal proteins. Based on the P450 enzymes homology of their amino acid sequence they are divided into families. For the metabolism of drugs and other xenobiotics the most important human isoenzymes are CYP1A1/2, 2C9/19, 2D6, 2E1, and 3A4.

Localization of Cytochrome P450

The most important drug-metabolizing enzymes of mammals are P450 enzymes. Despite the highest concentration of the enzyme in the liver, they are present in virtually all mammalian tissues. In liver, the enzyme system is located on the endoplasmic reticulum (microsomes).

The enzymes system of P450 is not just found in the liver, it can be present in many other tissues such as the adrenal gland, the kidney, intestine, brain, lung, testis, skin, and spleen but the concentration of the enzyme in these tissue are lower than those in liver. The tissue distribution between humans and rodents is very much comparable. The P450 has been observed in a variety of tumors, but with lower relative levels compared with normal tissue. These types of tumor include the central nervous system, breast, colon, lung, ovarian, prostate, and kidney. The expression of CYP1A1, 2A6, 2B6, 2C8/9, 3A4 and 4A has been detected in primary and secondary liver tumors by using immuno histochemical staining, however, those levels are much lower than that present in normal liver tissue. Other tumor cells, such as colon adenocarcinoma and stomach, breast, bladder, prostate, and lung cancers express CYP3A enzymes. Expression of P450s in colon and lung tumors is lower than in normal tissues. In contrast, several reports have shown higher levels of CYP1A and CYP3A in tumors than in their corresponding normal tissues.

Cytosine Deaminase

Enzymology of Cytosine Deaminase

The amidine hydrolysis of cytosine to uracil and ammonia is catalyzed by cytosine deaminase. Other substrates for these enzymes are cytosine analogs, such as 5-methylcytosine and halogenated cytosines. The enzyme is not present in mammalian cells but it can be found in several bacteria and fungi. Therefore, ADEPT, GDEPT and VDEPT prodrug approaches have been developed.

Activation of 5-Fluorocytosine by Cytosine Deaminase

Cytosine deaminase activates the prodrug 5-fluorocytosine (5-FC) to 5-FU (Figure 6). The latter affects and kills cancer cells by incorporation into DNA and RNA and by inhibition of thymidylate synthetase. Several ADEPT, GDEPT and VDEPT approaches have been developed, since cytosine deaminase is not expressed in human cells.

Figure 6. Activation of 5-flurocytosine prodrug.

Methionine γ-Lyase

Enzymology of Methionine γ-Lyase

The stereo selective α, γ-elimination of L-methionine to methanethiol, ammonia, and α-ketobutyrate is catalyzed by methionine γ-lyase (2-oxobutanoate). The production of several other amino acids such as L-ethionine, L-homocysteine, and selenomethionine are also mediated by the pyridoxal 5-phosphate-dependent enzyme. In addition, the γ-replacement reaction of these substrates and thiols, such as 2-mercaptoethanol, is catalyzed by methionine γ-lyase. The gene therapy approaches, GDEPT and VDEPT utilize methionine γ-lyase enzyme for the delivery of anti-tumor agents.

Activation of Prodrugs by Methionine γ-Lyase

The activation of selenomethionine to γ-ketobutyrate, ammonia, and toxic methylselenol is activated by methionine γ-lyase (Figure 7).

Figure 7. Activation of selenomethionine by methionine γ lyase.

Selenomethionine is a better substrate than natural methionine. Recently a GDEPT and VDEPT approaches have utilized this enzyme because selenomethionine cannot be converted into methylselenol by mammalian cells. The recombinant adenovirus which-encodes methionine γ-lyase gene from *Pseudomonas putida* is used to transduce cancer cells, such as human lung, ovarian, pancreatic, head and neck. The cytotoxicity increased to a 1000-fold compared with non-transduced cells due to the addition of selenomethionine. In ovarian carcinoma cells methylselenol produces superoxide anion radical which damages the mitochondria and releases cytochrome *c*, resulting in activation of the caspase cascade and apoptosis. In vivo experiments revealed that selenomethionine in combination with recombinant adenovirus-encoding methionine γ-lyase gene was effective against rat hepatoma tumor cells implanted in mice [50].

Hazards and Hurdles

The Immune Response

The main limitation of gene therapy is the activation of many of the immunological defense systems that are used to tackle wild-type infections against the vectors and/or new transgene products that might be recognized as foreign.

The most immunogenic of all viral vector groups are adenovirus vectors, and overcoming this immunogenicity is the largest problem that gene therapists who using adenovirus vectors has faced. Multiple components of the immune response has been induced by adenovirus vectors including: cytotoxic T-lymphocyte (CTL) responses that can be applied against viral gene products or 'foreign' transgene products that are expressed by transduced cells, the induction of humoral virus-neutralizing antibody responses, and the potent cytokine-mediated inflammatory responses.

In order to reduce T-cell responses against viral gene products that are expressed by transduced cells many attempt have been made, such as by engineering helper-dependent (HD) vectors that are stripped of all viral genes. An improvement has been achieved by this advance, in the prospects of adenovirus vectors, long-term gene transfer and HD adenoviruses (HD-Ads) have facilitated life-long phenotypic correction in mouse models with negligible toxicity.

The reduction of the vector-mediated cytokine responses after a systemic administration of HD have been applied by the elimination of all viral genes from the adenoviral vector genome, but studies in the rat brain showed that caution must be taken because these highly disabled vectors still retain a potential to induce a capsid-mediated inflammatory response. It is highly danger to make inappropriate activation of inflammatory responses, these danger includes; a massive systemic inflammatory response that was induced by an adenovirus vector led to fever, disseminated intravascular coagulation, multi organ failure and eventual death of a patient during a trial for ornithine transcarbamylase (OTC) deficiency.

As with all drug-induced toxicities, the dose of the vector that is administrated affects the degree to which viral vectors induce harmful immune- and inflammatory responses and other toxic side effects. Studies which were applied on the immuno privileged rodent brain (in which the responses of innate immunity can be studied in isolation from adaptive cellular immune responses) have shown a linear increase of the inflammatory responses to the adenovirus capsid with an escalation in vector dose, but in other organs the situation could be more complicated, especially if the vector particles become disseminated into the circulation. The relationship between adenovirus vector dose and direct cellular toxicity has been specified in dose-escalation studies.

The degree of variability between immune responses in different individuals affects the ability to accurately predict vector-related side effects at a particular dose in human studies. It is clear that different patients have markedly different inflammatory and immune responses to the same dose of adenovirus vector. This was observed in the disastrous OTC trial of 1999.

It is difficult to predict which patients will have severe inflammatory reactions, but due to what occurred in the OTC trial, a National Institutes of Health (NIH) report recommended that "all research participants enrolled in gene-transfer clinical trials should be monitored for several types of acute toxicities before and after vector administration" and that monitoring "should routinely include a research participant's immune status, cytokine profile, and predisposing or underlying conditions that might elevate an individual's sensitivity to a particular vector" [51].

The vector system other than adenovirus vectors is less inflammatory and immunogenic. The induction of inflammatory or immune responses against viral proteins was not observed by using lentivirus and AAV vectors.

All classes of viral vectors have faced another obstacle which was raised from pe-existing humoral immunity to the parental wild type viruses. Efficient transduction with the viral vector can be precluded by circulating virus-neutralizing antibodies.

Switching the capsid serotypes was used to address the humoral immune responses against adenovirus and AAV vectors, but antibody responses towards secreted therapeutic proteins remain a theoretical problem for the long-term therapy of certain disorders.

Specificity of Transgene Delivery

Natural infections with wild-type viruses are restricted to those tissues that are accessible through the route of transmission however, recombinant vectors are not subject to the same physical limitations. For example, adenoviruses and AAVs do not naturally infect the CNS system; but, both vectors can efficiently infect neurons if they are injected into the brain. From certain perspectives, the promiscuity of viral vectors is more of a liability than a benefit, as the systemic delivery of vector generally leads to unwanted vector uptake by many different cell types in multiple organs.

The leakage and dissemination to other tissues can be resulted even from a local delivery of vector. Transgene expression can be restricted to specific cell types and even switched on and off using tissue-specific and/or regulation promoters, but harmful consequences can be resulted from dissemination of the vector particle itself which include among other the induction of the massive systemic immune response which resulted from the lack of adenovirus vector specificity.

As discussed previously, the vector dose primary influences the severity and risk of eliciting harmful immune responses and other toxic side effects. The safety of gene therapy will be increased by administration of lower viral loads, and this can be achieved by increasing the efficiency for viral vectors to infect specific cell populations. Transductional targeting can be applied by modifying the vector capsid, to address the significant problem of nonspecific and/or inefficient uptake.

For cancer gene-therapy research, transductional targeting is a particular focus; this is because the tumor cells often down regulate the expression of the cellular receptors that are normally used by the virus for infection.

Pseudo typing is the simplest form of transductional retargeting, which requires little prior information of specific virus–receptor interactions. Retroviruses pseudo typing has been well established, but pseudo typing has been used to create a chimeric adenovirus vector comprising the adenovirus type-35 fiber protein incorporated in a type-5 capsid. The main limitation of pseudo typing for achieving transductional retargeting is that tropism is determined by the pre-existing specificities of the parental viruses.

Conjugation the capsids with molecular adaptors is a second approach used for targeting vector capsids to distinct cell populations (usually bi-specific antibodies) with particular receptor-binding properties in order to enhance the transduction of various cultured cell types by using adenovirus, retrovirus and AAV vectors. A third approach that has been used is engineering the capsid genes genetically in such a way that normal receptor binding is abolished and/or a small peptide ligand for alternative receptor binding is incorporated into the capsid structure.

Alternative internalization pathways are applied to re-route the adenovirus vectors, but the genetic retargeting of other vectors is more difficult. Different viral glycoproteins are used for internalization of herpes viruses into cells which is a complex process. Similarly, it is difficult to modify retrovirus binding without negatively affecting internalization, this is because that retrovirus receptor binding exposes fusogenic domains in the viral envelope .The genetically engineering of AAV capsid has been successfully made but, in general, AAV engineering has been more difficult, as the AAV capsid does not easily accommodate heterologous peptides and modified vector particles are often unstable at a step subsequent to internalization. This type of approach might be facilitated in the future by the recent determination of the crystal structure of the AAV2.

In order to design and select functional and stable targeted viruses, two novel approaches of genetic targeting have been used. DNA family shuffling has been used in the first approach, to genetically recombine envelope genes from six different strains of MLV, producing a library of 1×106MLV variants containing chimeric enveloped proteins.

It is possible to make target vectors to new cell types, this result has been shown from the data of many different studies, but it is difficult to prevent nonspecific uptake by other cell populations. Nevertheless, the reduction of the potential for toxic side effects could be achieved by increasing the efficiency of transduction of the appropriate cell type through a combination of transductional targeting and the use of optimal promoters by administration of lower doses of the virus [52].

Insertional Mutagenesis

An attempt to obtain stable gene transfer in proliferating cells such as haematopoietic cells was applied by using integrating viral vectors, which are mostly derived from retroviruses that have been used for more than 10 years in clinical trials. When the retroviral vector genomes integrated randomly into host chromatin the risk of disrupting a cellular sequence connected with malignancy was predicted to be in the region of 1 in 10 million insertions. During *ex vivo* gene transfer, even though more than 10 million cells are typically modified with retroviral vectors, the risk of inducing cancer was considered to be negligible, this is because oncogenes is usually requires multiple genetic lesions.

The fact that vector induced cancer had never been observed in any of the hundreds of patients that were treated with retroviral vectors in many different gene-therapy trials reinforced this viewpoint.

Our perception about the risks of using integrating retrovirus vectors for certain types of gene therapy has been challenged by the recent evidence from a number of separate studies. One study showed that leukemia had been induced in mice through the transplantation and expansion of a clone of retro virally transduced bone-marrow cells.

Clonal expansion (required in *ex vivo* hematopoietic gene therapy applications) seems to be a risk factor that contributes to cellular transformation and it is improbable that integrating vectors would induce cancer in non-dividing tissues in individuals with functional immune systems, in which cell proliferation was not a therapeutic end point.

Nevertheless, much interest will probably focus on making existing integrating vectors safer (for example, by engineering SUICIDE GENES into the vector backbone to provide a self-destruct mechanism in case of oncogenesis) and on developing new vector systems that are capable of mediating integration into specific predetermined sites. Recently, the site-specific integration machinery of bacteriophage ΦC31 has been exploited in non-viral delivery approaches to achieve the targeted integration of transgenes in mice and human cells. Incorporating of the ΦC31 integrase system into a viral vector is an obvious next step.

rAAV vector integration, initially hailed as the safest of gene-therapy vectors, has received a share of scrutiny.

The risks that are associated with rAAV integration will be much lower than those for retroviral vector applications, this is because the frequency of rAAV integration *in vivo* is low (<10% of persistent vector genomes are integrated in the liver) and most applications of rAAV vectors target non-proliferating cells. The analysis of rAAV integration sites has shown that the integrated rAAV genomes are frequently associated with chromosomal rearrangements and deletions of large segments of chromosomal DNA, this is unlike retrovirus integration. Integration of rAAV genomes into the host chromosomes is thought to happen through NON-HOMOLOGOUS END-JOINING (NHEJ) of rAAV free-ends with broken chromosomes.

Whether the rAAV free DNA ends induce chromosomal damage, or whether they are simply fused by NHEJ to pre-existing chromosomal breaks, it is a current topic of study. Two pieces of evidence from cell culture and mouse studies indicate that the induction of double-strand breaks by geno toxic agents will increase rAAV integration in cell culture and increasing and the dose of rAAV vector above a threshold level does not increase the number of integrated genomes in mice [52].

Perspectives and Future Directions

The work that have been done in the past few years on developing better vectors is beginning to be translated into some encouraging preliminary results in the clinic. The followings describe some advances in this area of research:

1. The development of new systems which allow efficient production of gene-deleted less immunogenic vectors.
2. The efficiency of the *ex vivo* transduction of hematopoietic cells have been Improved.
3. The specificity and efficiency of *in vivo* transgene expression have been improved through the optimization of tissue-specific and inducible promoters.
4. The development of alternative viral serotypes, which allow expansion of the repertoire of vector tropisms and the evasion of pre-existing immune responses.
5. For vector development, new virus species have been identified (for example, Epstein–Barr virus, foamy viruses, SV-40, α-viruses and negative-strand RNA viruses).

There are many hurdles that remain to be overcome. The safety of present integrating vector systems that are based on retrovirus vectors is an important concern that has been emerged.

Integrating vectors that are based on transposes or other integrases remain to be studied. The presence of large amount of genetic information that has become available from the sequencing of the mouse and human genomes will be important for addressing these issues.

As more work is needed to develop site-specific integrating vectors, the improvement of the ability of vectors to home in and infect specific target-cell populations is also needed more work.

Another substantial challenge that remains is how to predict the response of individual patients to inflammatory vectors. For evaluating vector performance and efficacy, preclinical studies in large-animal models are important, but it is difficult to make complete predictions on the basis of preclinical trials, this is because human immune responses are more variable than those observed in animal models. An important component of patient evaluation in future clinical trials is monitoring pre-existing immunity to parental wild-type viruses. For measuring vector potency and concentration many rigorous and uniformly recognized standards need to be introduced in order to allow meaningful data comparison across different clinical studies.

RNA interference (RNAi) is new technologies that allow new disease targets to become amenable to gene therapy through the fusion of viral vector-mediated gene transfer. RNAi technology has already been incorporated into adenovirus, lentivirus and retrovirus vectors and used to knockdown gene expression in cell culture and in experimental animals.

This powerful tool has been used to evaluate many viral vector systems, and was used to develop therapies for a range of diseases, including dominantly-inherited genetic disorders, infectious disease and cancer.

At the present time, for efficient gene transfer into most tissues, viral vectors have been used as the best available vehicles. In order to develop more efficient non-viral vectors that will ultimately rival virus-based systems, we have to continue unravel and understand the biological mechanisms that underlie virus entry into cells, transport of viral particles to the cell nucleus and the persistence of viral DNA, such that we will be able to apply this knowledge to make development in non-viral delivery system.

All the gene therapy vectors must achieve a specific set of functions, whatever they look like in the future, these functions include:

1. After delivery by a non-invasive route, they preferably must target specific populations of cells in a target tissue.
2. They must express therapeutic levels of transgene expression in a safe and regulated manner for the appropriate length of time.

In gene-therapy research, there is still a huge amount of work to be done. So far many obstacles have been encountered, and more will be probably in the way, but these obstacles are not insurmountable.

The outcome of a range of diseases will be surely improved by maintaining a strong focus on improving vectors gene therapy and by continuing to identify and address potential hurdles [52].

Summary and Conclusion

For the treatment of cancer, viral vectors have rapidly become important therapeutic agents. However, conventional gene therapy is less complex than GDEPT because it utilizes two components, the virus and the prodrug.

Thus, for successful therapy the dosing and the timing of vector and prodrug administration are very crucial. In order to mimic the clinical situation, preclinical time course experiments in animal models are useful tools, but, the resulting data cannot always be extrapolated to humans.

The difficultly to predict how long it takes to achieve sufficient levels of gene expression after virus administration, makes clinical study design for GDEPT much more complicated. The route of vector delivery is another issue for clinical GDEPT applications. It is more effective if the virus is administrated systemically, but due to inefficient targeting of the extratumoral, expression of the enzyme may occur which leads to systemic toxicity upon prodrug administration.

To overcome this hurdle, transcriptionally targeted, replicating viruses are designed. These vectors should neither express the prodrug-converting enzyme nor amplify in normal cells. They might even be cleared from healthy tissues, whilst spreading throughout the tumors, creating a differential of enzyme expression between tumors and normal tissues.

In the ideal clinical setting, for each individual patient the timing of virus and prodrug should be carefully tailored, for example by monitoring blood samples for the presence of the enzyme or by using imaging techniques. VDEPT undoubtedly has a potential as a cancer therapy. Preclinical and clinical data are promising and more VDEPT trials can be expected in the near future. We believe that these studies will feed our knowledge of the behavior of viral GDEPT vectors in patients and help to increase the safety and efficacy of virus-mediated GDEPT.

References

[1] Hanahan, D. and Weinberg R.A., (2000)The hallmarks of cancer. *Cell*. 100(1), 57-70.

[2] Chambers A.F., Groom A.C. and MacDonald I.C.,(2002) Dissemination and growth of cancer cells in metastatic sites. *Nat Rev Cancer*, 2(8), 563-72.

[3] Rang HP, Dale MM, Ritter JM, Flower RJ, Henderson G, Rang and Dales (2011). Pharmacology seventh edition, 675.

[4] Skeel, R.T. and Khleif S.N., (2011) Handbook of cancer chemotherapy: Wolters Kluwer Health.

[5] Gottesman, M.M., T. Fojo, and S.E. Bates,(2002) Multidrug resistance in cancer: role of ATP–dependent transporters. *Nature Reviews Cancer*, 2(1), 48-58.

[6] Frei, E, (1988) Preclinical studies and clinical correlation of the effect of alkylating dose. *Cancer research*, 48(22), 6417-6423.

[7] Rautio, J.(2008) Prodrugs: design and clinical applications. *Nat. Rev. Drug Discov*.,. 7(3), 255-270.

[8] Albert, A., (1958) Chemical aspects of selective toxicity. *Nature*. 182(4633), 421.

[9] Tegeli, V., (2010) Review on Concepts and Advances in Prodrug Technology. *International Journal of Drug Formulation & Research*, 1(3), 32-57.

[10] Connors, T.A., (1995)The choice of prodrugs for gene directed enzyme prodrug therapy of cancer. *Gene Ther.*, 2(10), 702-709.

[11] Friis, G.,(1996) , A text book of drug design and development. A textbook of drug design and development.

[12] Dahan A., Khamis M., Agbaria R., and Karaman R.(2012). Targeted prodrugs in oral delivery: the modern molecular biopharmaceutical approach. *Expert Opinion on Drug Delivery*, 9, 1001–1013.

[13] Karaman R., Fattash B. and Qtait A. (2013) The future of prodrugs – design by quantum mechanics methods. *Expert Opinion on Drug Delivery.*, 10, 713–729.

[14] Karaman R. (2013) Prodrugs design based on inter- and intramolecular processes. *Chem. Biol. Drug.Des.* 82, 643–668.

[15] Karaman ,R.(2013)The Prodrug Naming Dilemma. *Journal of Drug Designing*, 2: e115.doi:10.4172/2169-0138.1000e115.

[16] Testa, B., (2004) Prodrug research: futile or fertile? . *Biochem Pharmacol.*, 68(11), 2097-106.

[17] Ettmayer, P.,(2004) Lessons Learned from Marketed and Investigational Prodrugs. *J. Med. Chem.*, 47(10), 2393-2404.

[18] Huber, B.E., C.A. Richards, and E.A. Austin, (1994) Virus-directed enzyme/prodrug therapy (VDEPT). Selectively engineering drug sensitivity into tumors. *Ann. N Y Acad. Sci.*, 716, 104-14; discussion 140-3.

[19] Bridgewater, J.A., (1995) Expression of the bacterial nitroreductase enzyme in mammalian cells renders them selectively sensitive to killing by the prodrug CB1954. *Eur. J Cancer*, 31A(13- 14), 2362-70.

[20] Springer, C.J.,(2004) Introduction to vectors for suicide gene therapy, *in Suicide Gene Therapy,Springer.* p.29-45 [21] Salmons, B., M. Lohr, and W.H. Gunzburg, (2003) Treatment of inoperable pancreatic carcinoma using a cell-based local chemotherapy: results of a phase I/II clinical trial. *J. Gastroenterol.*, 38 (15), 78-84.

[21] Sakai, S.., (2005) Subsieve-size agarose capsules enclosing ifosfamide-activating cells: a strategy toward chemotherapeutic targeting to tumors. *Mol. Cancer Ther.*, 4(11),1786-90.

[22] Springer, C.J., (2004) Suicide Gene Therapy: Methods and Reviews. *Springer,* Vol. 90.

[23] Huber, B.E., C.A. Richards, and T.A. Krenitsky,(1991) Retroviral-mediated gene therapy for the treatment of hepatocellular carcinoma: an innovative approach for cancer therapy. *Proceedings of the National Academy of Sciences,*. 88(18), 8039-8043.

[24] Kirn, D., R.L. Martuza, and J. Zwiebel, (2001) Replication-selective virotherapy for cancer: Biological principles, risk management and future directions. *Nat. Med.*, 7(7), 781-787.

[25] Kirn, D.H. and F. McCormick,(1996) Replicating viruses as selective cancer therapeutics. *Molecular Medicine Today.*, 2(12), 519-527.

[26] Kirn, D., (2002) The emerging fields of suicide gene therapy and virotherapy. *Trends Mol. Med.*, 8(4), S68-73.

[27] Ichikawa, T. and E.A. Chiocca, (2001) Comparative analyses of transgene delivery and expression in tumors inoculated with a replication-conditional or -defective viral vector. *Cancer Res.*, 61(14), 5336-9.

[28] Huber, B.E.,,(1994) Metabolism of 5-fluorocytosine to 5-fluorouracil in human colorectal tumor cells transduced with the cytosine deaminase gene: significant antitumor effects when only a small percentage of tumor cells express cytosine deaminase. *Proceedings of the National Academy of Sciences,* 91(17), 8302-8306.

[29] Freeman, S.M., (1993) The "bystander effect": tumor regression when a fraction of the tumor mass is genetically modified. *Cancer research*, 53(21), 5274-5283.

[30] Aghi, M., F. Hochberg, and X.O. (2000) Breakefield, Prodrug activation enzymes in cancer gene therapy. *The Journal of Gene Medicine*, 2(3), 148-164.

[31] Hermiston, T., (2000) Gene delivery from replication-selective viruses: arming guided missiles in the war against cancer. *Journal of Clinical Investigation,* 105(9), 1169-1172.

[32] Clackson, T., (2000) Regulated gene expression systems. *Gene Ther.*, 7(2), 120-125.

[33] Danthinne, X. and M.J. (2000) Imperiale, Production of first generation adenovirus vectors: a review. *Gene Ther.*, 7(20), 1707-14.

[34] Raper, S.E., (2003) Fatal systemic inflammatory response syndrome in a ornithine transcarbamylase deficient patient following adenoviral gene transfer. *Mol. Genet. Metab.*, 80(1-2), 148-58.

[35] Schepelmann, S. and C.J. Springer, (2006) Viral Vectors for Gene-Directed Enzyme Prodrug Therapy. *Current Gene Therapy,* 6(6), 647-670.

[36] Kovesdi, I., (1997) Adenoviral vectors for gene transfer. *Current Opinion in Biotechnology,* 8(5), 583-589.

[37] Wickham, T.J., (2000) Targeting adenovirus. *Gene Ther.*, 7(2), 110-4.

[38] Barr, D.., (1995) Strain related variations in adenovirally mediated transgene expression from mouse hepatocytes in vivo: comparisons between immunocompetent and immunodeficient inbred strains. *Gene Ther.*, 2(2), 151-5.

[39] Christ, M., (2000) Modulation of the inflammatory properties and hepatotoxicity of recombinant adenovirus vectors by the viral E4 gene products. *Hum. Gene Ther.*, 11(3), 415-27.

[40] Balague, C., (2000) Sustained high-level expression of full-length human factor VIII and restoration of clotting activity in hemophilic mice using a minimal adenovirus vector. *Blood,* 95(3), 820-8.

[41] Kay, M.A., J.C. Glorioso, and L. Naldini, (2001) Viral vectors for gene therapy: the art of turning infectious agents into vehicles of therapeutics. *Nat. Med.*, 7(1), 33-40.

[42] Burns, J.C.,(1993) Vesicular stomatitis virus G glycoprotein pseudotyped retroviral vectors: concentration to very high titer and efficient gene transfer into mammalian and nonmammalian cells. *Proc. Natl. Acad. Sci. USA,* 90(17), 8033-7.

[43] Vigna, E. and L. Naldini, (2000) Lentiviral vectors: excellent tools for experimental gene transfer and promising candidates for gene therapy. *The Journal of Gene Medicine,* 2(5), 308-316.

[44] Muzyczka, N., (1992) Use of adeno-associated virus as a general transduction vector for mammalian cells, in Viral Expression Vectors, *Springer*, 97-129.

[45] Wagner, J.A.,(1999) Safety and biological efficacy of an adeno-associated virus vector-cystic fibrosis transmembrane regulator (AAV-CFTR) in the cystic fibrosis maxillary sinus. *Laryngoscope*, 109(2 Pt 1), 266-74.

[46] Tseng, J.C., (2006) Tumor-specific in vivo transfection with HSV-1 thymidine kinase gene using a Sindbis viral vector as a basis for prodrug ganciclovir activation and PET. *J. Nucl. Med.*, 47(7), 1136-43.

[47] Norman, K.L. and P.W. Lee, (2005) Not all viruses are bad guys: the case for reovirus in cancer therapy. *Drug Discov Today.,* 10(12), 847-55.

[48] Yant, S.R., (2002) Transposition from a gutless adeno-transposon vector stabilizes transgene expression in vivo. *Nat. Biotechnol.,* 20(10), 999-1005.

[49] Rooseboom, M., J.N. Commandeur, and N.P. Vermeulen,(2004) Enzyme-catalyzed activation of anticancer prodrugs. *Pharmacol. Rev.,* 56(1), 53-102.

[50] Andeson, W.F.,(2002) Assessment of adenoviral vector safety and toxicity: report of the National Institutes of Health Recombinant DNA Advisory Committee. *Hum. Gene Ther.,* 13(1), 3-13.

[51] Thomas, C.E., A. Ehrhardt, and M.A. Kay, (2003) Progress and problems with the use of viral vectors for gene therapy. *Nat. Rev. Genet.,* 4(5), 346-58.

In: Prodrugs Design – A New Era
Editor: Rafik Karaman

ISBN: 978-1-63117-701-9
© 2014 Nova Science Publishers, Inc.

Chapter VI

Gene Directed Enzyme Prodrug Therapy (GDEPT)

Jawna' Sirhan[1] and Rafik Karaman[*,1,2]

[1]Pharmaceutical Sciences Department, Faculty of Pharmacy,
Al-Quds University, Jerusalem, Palestine
[2]Department of Science, University of Basilicata, Potenza, Italy

Abstract

The majority of this chapter is devoted to gene-directed enzyme prodrug therapy (GDEPT) which is considered one of the important strategies for the treatment of cancer. It is based on the delivery of a suicide gene that is considered as being a cancer treatment without affecting normal tissues.

GDEPT is a promising strategy that aims to limit the systemic toxicity and improve the selectivity of chemotherapy use through the expression of a gene that encodes an enzyme which converts nontoxic prodrug into an activated cytotoxic agent.

In the treatment for cancer chemotherapy using GDEPT there are two steps:(i) a gene of a foreign enzyme is delivered to a tumor by a vector and (ii) a prodrug is then administered which is selectivity activated inside the tumor site. The implementation of a prodrug strategy has an improvement in the physicochemical and pharmacokinetic properties over the pharmacologically active compounds. The most widely used enzyme/prodrug combinations in GDEPT which have been investigated for applications in cancer therapy include herpes simplex virus thymidine kinase with ganciclovir, and cytosine deaminase, the bacterial enzyme carboxypeptidase G2 and E. coli nitroreductase, which activates the prodrug CB1954 and related mustard prodrug analogs: some of which may be superior to CB1954. Synergies between different GDEPTs and other modalities are needed to be explored to maximize therapeutic benefit with minimal toxicity.

Keywords: GDEPT, Bystander effect, Cancer, Chemotherapy, Enzymes, Prodrugs.

---

* Corresponding author: Rafik Karaman, e-mail: dr_karaman@yahoo.com; Tel and Fax +972-2-2790413.

List of Abbreviations

GDEPT	Gene-directed enzyme prodrug therapy
ADME	Absorption, distribution, metabolism, excretion
2FU	2-Fluoroadenine
PNP	Purine nucleoside phosphorylase
GCV	Ganciclovir
ACV	Acyclovir
Cx	Connexins
HSV1	Herpes simplex virus 1
HSV TK	Herpes simplex virusthymidine kinase
VP22	Virus protein
CD	Cytosine deaminase
CB1954	5-(Aziridin-1-yl)-2,4-dinitrobenzamide
CYP450	Cytochrome P450
DNA	Deoxyribonucleic acid
IL	Interleukin
FC	*5-Fluorocytosine*
FU	5-Fluorouracil
FDA	Food and drug administration
5-FdUMP	5-Fluoro-2′-deoxyuridine 5′-monophosphate
5-FdUTP	5-Fluorodeoxyuridinetriphosphate
5-FUTP	5-Fluorouridine triphosphate
5-FUMP	5-Fluorouridine monophosphate
RNA	Ribonucleic acid
UTP	Uridine triphosphate
NADH	Nicotinamide adenine dinucleotide
NADPH	Nicotinamide adenine dinucleotide phosphate
ADEPT	Antibody directed enzyme prodrug therapy
FMN	Flavin mononucleotide
IAA	Indole-3-acetic acid
HRP	Horseradish peroxidase
FIAA	5-Fluoroindole-3-acetic acid
CP	Cyclophosphamide prodrug
IP	Isophosphamide
CPA	Cyclophosphamide
IFO	Ifosfamide
CPG2	CarboxypeptidaseG2
CMDA	4-[(2-Chloroethyl)(2-mesyloxyethyl)amino]benzoyl-L-glutamic acid
MTX	PheMethotrexate phenylalanine

Introduction

A conventional chemotherapy suffers from many limitations. One of such limitations is the lack of selectivity for tumor cells which results in dose-limiting and toxic side-effects. One of the approaches to overcome these problems is the use of prodrugs; non-toxic forms of cytotoxic agents that are selectively converted to the toxic drug at the tumor site. Strategies used to guide the enzyme to tumor sites have been replaced to a large extent by gene-directed approaches [1].

The use of chemotherapy against advanced solid tumors is limited because of host toxicity and tumor resistance. As an approach to meet this challenge is the use of a combination chemotherapy by which the timing and sequence of drugs administration may be critical [2].

The inefficacy of cancer chemotherapy is largely due to limitations arising from dose-limiting, toxic side-effects and the generation of multidrug-resistant tumor cells as a result of insufficient drug concentrations at the tumor site. The gene-directed enzyme prodrug therapy has shown promising results for overcoming these sorts of problems. The driving force for this approach is the tumor-directed delivery of a gene encoding an enzyme that cleaves in a systematic manner the administered inactive prodrug to a toxic drug. Prodrugs usually possess little toxicity; therefore, large amounts of the prodrugs can be administered, which in turn might lead to high drug concentrations at the tumor sites. The most common GDEPT system that is available at present is the herpes simplex virus thymidine kinase/ganciclovir system; functions intracellularly and thereby limits the drug efficacy since the prodrug permeability is restricted. In an attempt to improve this method, prokaryotic carboxypeptidase G2 displayed on the cell surface has been developed to be utilized in the GDEPT. Nevertheless, by using a non-human enzyme this may provoke undesired immune responses, particularly if multiple applications are required [3, 4].

Various targeted therapies are being developed in order to minimize unwanted toxicity to non-cancerous cells, and to maximize the concentration of chemotherapeutic drugs at tumor sites. GDEPT is a suicide gene therapy based on anticancer strategy that relies on selective introduction and expression of foreign gene(s) into tumor cells which is followed by gene product mediated activation of inert prodrugs into cytotoxic agents, resulting in localized tumor cell death and providing therapeutic selectivity [5]. Prodrug activation usually generates: (1) toxic levels of drug concentrations only at the tumor cells, (2) minimum toxicity to normal cells and (3) improvement of therapeutic index during cancer therapy. The active drug can kill the tumor cells, but also it can create a zone of dead cells around the cancer cells which are modified to express transgenes through bystander effect. For a success of GDEPT in a clinical setting, it is essential to be able to in vivo monitor the transgene expression and function. Gene transfer optimization protocols; vector development and prodrug dosing schedules are some of the key criteria essential for translation of a GDEPT candidate to human applications. The assessment of location, magnitude and duration of transgene expression in vivo through various modern noninvasive imaging technologies may help in developing an efficient and safe gene therapy protocols [6].

However, new treatment options are required, and during the last few decades, a number of investigators have started to evaluate unconventional strategies for the treatment of a variety of cancers. These include novel immunological strategies and therapeutic vaccines, as well as gene-based approaches such as antisense nucleic acids, expression of tumor suppressor genes and gene-directed enzyme prodrug therapy. In GDEPT, when a specific, heterologous gene is introduced into tumor cells, the respective gene product is able to locally converts a systemically administered non-toxic prodrug into its active -toxic form, exerting the therapeutic effect in the tumor cells as well as in the surrounding cells due to bystander effect mediated by diffusion of the toxic metabolites [7].

The major goal of using antitumor therapies is to target specifically and selectively toxic agents to tumors, whereas sparing normal tissue from damage. This may be achieved by gene therapy that can combine highly specific gene delivery with highly specific gene expression.

Gene therapy of cancer is a novel approach that has the possibility to selectively eradicate tumor cells, while leaves normal tissue from any damage effects.

Three issues needed to be considered for gene therapy: (1) the delivery mode of a gene to the tumor, (2) the regulation of gene expression and (3) the therapeutic efficacy [8].

In particular, gene directed enzyme prodrug therapy (GDEPT) is a promising and new strategy that aims to limit the systemic toxicity and improve the selectivity of chemotherapy, through the expression of a gene that encodes an enzyme,which converts non-toxic prodrug into activated cytotoxic agents [8-11]. It is a two steps treatment for cancer chemotherapy: in the first step, a gene of a foreign enzyme is delivered to the tumor by a vector, followed by the expression of foreign enzyme where it is expressed by the use of specific promoters, in the second step, a prodrug is administered which is selectivity activated in the tumor [10, 12-17].

Several GDEPT combinations have been proposed, the most studied one is the Herpes Simplex virus thymidine kinase/gancyclovir system. This combination has shown safety and a reasonable efficacy. Tumor tissue can be selectively targeted by GDEPT using tissue or environmentally controlled gene expression. In particular, an attractive target is the hypoxic regions of tumors, since severe hypoxia is a tumor specific condition, and an adverse prognostic factor [13].

In the following sections, the most widely used enzyme/prodrug combinations in GDEPT are described [8].

The Prodrug Concept

According to Albert's definition, a prodrug is the inactive form of its parent drug [18-21]. However, Prodrugs are chemicals that are inert even at relatively high doses, but can be converted to toxic species at the intended target [8].

The prodrug strategy is usually implemented when an improvement in the physicochemical, biopharmaceutical and/or pharmacokinetic properties of pharmacologically active compounds is required. It is estimated that about 10% of worldwide marketed drugs can be classified as prodrugs[22].

Improving or eliminating the undesirable drug properties such as undesirable taste, low target selectivity, low solubility in water or lipid membranes, chemical instability, irritation or pain after local administration, presystemic metabolism and toxicity is the main aim of prodrug design,. In general, the goal of using prodrugs is to optimize the absorption, distribution, metabolism, excretion, and unwanted toxicity of the parent drugs [22].

Classically, prodrug relates to biologically inert derivatives of drug molecules that undergo an enzymatic and/or chemical conversion *in vivo* in order to release the pharmacologically active parent drug. The active drug is released from its inactive form before, during or after absorption of the prodrug. Some drugs are released only after reaching the targets of their actions. The aim of a prodrug is to increase the bioavailability and therapeutic effectiveness of its parent drug [22].

In cancer chemotherapy, the prodrug should be able to diffuse throughout the tumor site; a good substrate for the enzyme,located within the tumor site, to form a drug that is highly cytotoxic, and metabolically stable under physiological conditions and has suitable pharmacological and pharmacokinetic properties; in order to diffuse efficiently [8, 23]. For achieving a therapeutic response, the released anti-cancer drug should be at least a 100-fold more toxic than the prodrug itself. The toxic agent should also have a half-life that allows diffusion to the surrounding non-transfected cells, but ensures that any drug escaping into the circulation will be inactive. Moreover, the induced cytotoxicity should be proliferation-independent, in order to kill a wide range of tumor cell's populations [8].

The physicochemical properties including overall lipophilicity, charge, rate of metabolism and ability to form reversible/irreversible complexes with cellular macromolecules govern the pharmacokinetic characteristics of prodrugs and their effectors. There is also a need for high differentiation between the prodrug and its corresponding drug. [23]

Most importantly, the prodrug when given systemically it should be characterized with low cytotoxicity to normal tissues [23].

In order to convert the prodrug into its active drug in the GDEPT approach, the conversion should be catalyzed by specific enzymes that is either unique to the tissue or are at higher concentrations at the tumor sites, without any dependence on catalysis by other enzymes. The prodrug conversion pathway should be different from any endogenous enzyme for avoiding cytotoxic activation of the prodrug in normal tissues. The prodrug should not be catalyzed by endogenous enzymes, and should be delivered in sufficient amounts to affect the prodrug conversion [8, 23].

The prodrugs utilized in the suicide gene therapy need to satisfy a number of criteria; they must work efficiently and be selective substrates to the activating enzyme, and have the ability to be metabolized to potent cytotoxins that kill cells at all stages of the cell cycle. Both prodrugs and their activated drugs should have good distribution properties such that the resulting bystander effects can maximize the effectiveness of the therapy [24, 25].

In the selection of the appropriate enzyme/prodrug combination, priority should be given to the enzyme. The enzyme should be monomeric, for ease of handling and possible protein modification, with low molecular weight and with no need for glycosylation. Even at low concentrations of the substrate, the enzyme should have high catalytic activity under physiological conditions; fast and efficient prodrug activation. Expression of the enzyme itself should not lead to cytotoxic effects; the bystander effect required would not be achievable if the cells were to be killed by the action of the enzyme alone [8].

The location of gene expression (cytoplasmic/nuclear or mitochondrial) in the cell was found to be critical for the efficiency of the prodrug activation with NTR–CB1954–GDEPT.

GDEPT allows a concentration of the toxic drug in the tumor microenvironment; the retention of the prodrug and its toxic products in the cell for a long time is important for achieving high cell toxicity levels which further enhance the anti-cancer drug efficacy. The significant advantage of GDEPT is that once the active drug is formed it can enter nearby cells to elicit a local bystander effect which is strongly influenced by the size and metabolism of the active drug formed [23, 24]. If the drug is a small molecule, such as 2-fluoroadenine (2FU), a toxic drug formed from the activity of PNP on fludarabine phosphate, it is most likely to diffuse passively near cells providing a strong local bystander effect. On the other hand, drugs that are highly phosphorylated may require active transport or gap junctions to allow toxicity to occur in neighbouring cells, such as triphosphates of ganciclovir (GCV) or its analogue, acyclovir (ACV) when activated by HSV-tk. Such drugs may have a variable bystander effect based on the targeted cancer cell's type [23, 26].

In general, two classes of anticancer agents are used in the GDEPT approach: antimetabolites and alkylating agents. Alkylating agents have the advantage of crosslinking non-cycling and cycling cells, and by this way, larger population of tumor cells will be targeted. However, the antimetabolites have a complex pathway of activation and can induce resistance. Prodrugs of alkylating agents, that are less cell cycle-specific than antimetabolites and more effective against non-cycling tumor cells, appear to be more active prodrugs, requiring less prolonged dosing schedules for achieving desirable effectiveness [12, 23, 24].

The Bystander Effect

The main scientific attraction of GDEPT is the local bystander effect that is crucial for a successful GDEPT strategy [8, 23].

The bystander effect is the ability to kill any neighboring non-expressing cells, an extension of the killing effects of the active drug to non-transduced cells passively or via gap junctions, leading to their death. This results in an in situ amplification of cytotoxicity. It is preferred that the activated drug be highly diffusible or be actively taken up by adjacent non-expressing cancer cells, as cell-cell contact is not required for a bystander effect. The killing ability of the anti-cancer drug system is enhanced by the bystander effect (Figure 1) [8, 23, 27-29].

In addition, it is clear that a lack of cytotoxicity of the enzyme itself is a prerequisite for a substantial bystander effect, even when produced at a high rate [8].

Two major categories of bystander effect have been specified: local and immune mediated [8]. In the local bystander effect, the killing of neighbouring cells is because of a toxic metabolic product transfer via gap junctions, apoptotic vesicles, or through the diffusion of soluble toxic metabolites. The dependence only on gap junctions could be a limitation, because cell-to-cell contact is required, and the number of tumor tissues have shown to down-regulate intercellular gap junction communication. Due to the transfer of apoptotic factors, the local bystander effect can also be induced by a contact with dead or dying cells (kiss of death) [8, 30, 31].

Lipophilicity of the drug activated form is an important parameter in determining the bystander effect generated by a passive diffusion. Many of the early antimetabolite-based prodrugs provide very polar activated forms, thus, limiting their ability to diffuse across cell membranes, and their transfer relies on gap junctions between cells [24].

In the case of freely diffusing species a key role to obtain a considerable but localized bystander effect is determined by the drug half-life. In addition, the half-life of an active drug should be long enough to induce a bystander effect. On the other hand, it should be short enough to avoid the drug leaking out into the systemic circulation [8, 32].

The systemic immune response plays a crucial role in inducing bystander killing. The presence of an intense inflammatory infiltrate has a respected role in regressing tumors of immune-competent animals treated with GDEPT systems. Moreover, the bystander effect was significantly reduced in immune-deficient athymic mice after sublethal irradiation. The immune stimulation does not only enhance local tumor killing, but it also induces the regression of distant tumor deposits (distant bystander effect) [8].

Gap junctional communication, can be enhanced by regulating the production of connexins (Cx); membrane proteins considered to be the building blocks for gap junctions and the major factors responsible for the gap junction mediated bystander phenomenon [8].The Cx-encoding or chemically induced Cx-genes increase intercellular communication and transfer of toxic agents. In some human-tumor cells expression also corrects surface localization of Cx43; necessary components of the bystander effect.

HSV1 virion protein VP22 is an attractive tool to enhance the bystander effect. When synthesized in infected cells, VP22 can spread very efficiently via a Golgi-independent pathway to surround uninfected cells, where it accumulates in the nucleus. Therapeutic advantage of this biologically active bystander effect for GDEPT was demonstrated by coupling the VP22 gene to the HSV TK gene, which produced significant bystander killing in vitro and tumor regression in vivo, regardless of cellular gap junction activity [8].

The combination of tumor immunization with GDEPT systems is a strategy to improve the in vivo bystander effect and enhance the immunological response to the tumor. Co-transfection of cytokine and suicide gene based vectors followed by prodrug treatment has been proven to be successful with varying results.This method induced more potent tumor growth inhibition and longer survival than the separate treatments [8, 23].

Distant bystander effect on the other hand, is known as killing tumor cells that can be obtained using the GDEPT approach. In addition, it induces systemic antitumor responses including host immune responses that can decrease metastatic growth of cancer cells at distant sites [23].

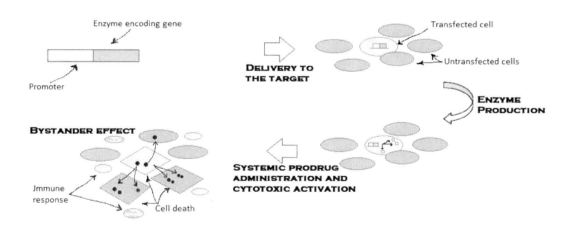

Figure 1. Schematic diagram for gene directed enzyme prodrug therapy (GDEPT).

Prodrug Activation-Based Cancer Gene Therapy

The principle of prodrug activation gene therapy is that transduction of a tumor cell population with a foreign gene provides a unique prodrug activation capacity along with a chemo-sensitivity which is absent from host cells that do not express the gene [33].

Several prodrug-activating enzyme systems have been investigated for applications in cancer therapy include herpes simplex virus thymidine kinase (HSV-TK) in combination with ganciclovir, and cytosine deaminase (CD), a bacterial gene that can sensitize tumor cells to 5-fluorocytosine by transforming it to a known cancer chemotherapeutic drug, 5-fluorouracil, the bacterial enzyme, carboxypeptidase G2, not having a mammalian homolog, and can be used to activate certain synthetic mustard prodrugs by cleaving the glutamic acid moiety to release an active cytotoxic mustard metabolite and E. coli nitroreductase. The latter activates the prodrug CB1954 and related mustard prodrug analogs; some of which may be superior to CB1954 [8, 33].

Few limitations may demolish the efficacy of prodrug/gene combinations and may limit their application to cancer chemotherapy. These limitations include (i) the non-mammalian nature of these genes, in which the gene products can elicit immune responses that intervene with prodrug activation, (ii) the dependence on certain drugs such as antiviral and antifungal agents that were developed without testing their activity for cancer chemotherapeutic in clinical use, (iii) the reliance of the HSV-TK and CD-based gene therapy on ongoing tumor cell DNA replication, and (iv) the need for direct cell–cell contact to elicit an effective bystander cytotoxic response on tumor cells which fail to take up or express the transduced therapeutic genes such as in the case of HSV-TK.These considerations, with the findings that effective, strong clinical responses generally require combination chemotherapy, implies the need for development of alternate and complementary prodrug activation-based cancer gene therapies [33].

Generally, GDEPT systems like herpes simplex virus thymidine kinase/ganciclovir function intracellularly and this might limits the efficacy of the system and selection of the prodrug to membrane-permeable molecules. In a way to improve this situation, prokaryotic carboxypeptidase G2 displayed on the cell surface has been developed for GDEPT. However, the use of a non-human enzyme may encourage undesired immune responses, especially if multiple applications are required [3].

Herpes Simplex Virus Thymidine Kinase/Ganciclovir

The most prominent enzyme/prodrug strategy in cancer GDEPT approach is the HSV TK with the nucleoside analogue GCV [8, 24].

Ganciclovir and related agents which were developed as antiviral agents, are poor substrates for the mammalian nucleoside monophosphate kinase, however, they can be converted efficiently to the monophosphate by TK from HSV 1 (Figure 2) [8, 24].

Ganciclovir prodrugs were shown to be enzymatically converted to the corresponding monophosphates, which then underwent further conversion by other cellular enzymes to a number of toxic metabolites; the most active one is the triphosphates (Figure 2). When GCV-triphosphate competes with deoxyguanosine triphosphate, for incorporation into elongating DNA during cell division, it inhibits DNA synthesis leading to cells death. It should be worth noting, that prevention of the elongation of the newly synthesized DNA by DNA polymerase was inhibited by ACV, causing chain termination [8, 23, 24, 34].

The HSV TK/GCV combination is suitable for the eradication of rapidly dividing tumor cells invading non-proliferating tissue. The high cytotoxicity that was shown by GCV in HSV-TK transduced cells is due to its enhanced ability to be incorporated into DNA without inhibiting progression through the S-phase. [24] However, it is necessary that the target cells should be in active division at the time of the exposure, or that the prodrug should be continuously administered for allowing the cells to start DNA replication [8, 24].

Figure 2. Metabolism of the prodrug ganciclovir (GCV).

The presence of highly charged triphosphate in the HSV TK/GCV system makes it impermeable to lipid membranes resulting in diffusion difficulties of the drug, and cell-to-cell contact becomes necessary for bystander killing. In addition, many analogues of GCV that differ in lipophilicity from GCV have shown different bystander effects. However, the intercellular transport of these analogues depends on the presence of connexins in the tumor cells under treatment. Nevertheless, when 10% of the tumor cells expressed HSV TK, the tumor regression was achieved. This phenomenon was attributed to an activated GCV transfer through gap junctions, or an exchange of apoptotic vesicles [8, 23].

Cytosine Deaminase and 5-FC

The cytosine deaminase gene is considered the second widely used enzyme after HSV-TK. The system consisting of CD and 5-FC and is based on the production of a toxic nucleotide analogue. Cytosine deaminase catalyzes the hydrolytic deamination of cytosine to uracil; and thus converting 5-FC to 5-FU. The FDA has approved therapeutics within this approach for treating various cancers including prostate cancer [8, 9, 23].

The enzyme CD, encoded by this gene, is found in certain bacteria and fungi but there is no indication for its presence in mammalian cells. It can therefore catalyze the conversion of non-toxic 5-Fuorouracil (5-FU) prodrugs to 5-FU. 5-FU in further steps is transformed by cellular enzymes to potent pyrimidine antimetabolites, 5-FdUMP, 5-FdUTP and 5-FUTP (Figure 3). GDEPT therapy using CD has focused on one prodrug, the clinically used antifungal agent, 5-fluorocytosine. CD–GDEPT has been entered Phase I studies as a monotherapy for colon carcinoma of the liver or in combination with HSV-TK–GDEPT for local recurrent PC. Three pathways are involved in the induced cell death: thymidylate synthase inhibition, formation of 5-FU RNA complex and generation of 5-FUDNA complex. 5-FU is the drug of choice in the treatment of colorectal carcinoma and cancer chemotherapy. In vivo anti-tumor activity of the CD/5-FC combination has been demonstrated in several animal models, including gliomas, fibrosarcomas, carcinomas and metastatic formations of different origin [8, 23, 24].

Figure 3 illustrates the transformation of 5FC to 5FU and two active metabolites, 5-fluoro-2'-deoxyuridine 5'-monophosphate [5-FdUMP] and 5-fluorouridine 5'-triphosphate by bacterial or yeast CD (freely diffusible). It should be indicated, that both DNA and RNA are suspicious to damage by both active metabolites. The nuclear processing of ribosomal and messenger RNAs are inhibited by 5-FUTP which can be incorporated into RNA to replace UTP, whereas 5-FdUMP preventing DNA synthesis by irreversibly inhibition of thymidylate synthase. The rate-limiting step in the generation of 5-FdUMP and 5-FUTP is the formation of an intermediary metabolite, 5-fluorouridine monophosphate (5-FUMP) which may only be produced after a series of catalyzed enzymatic reactions [23].

Figure 3. Conversion of 5-FC to 5- FU by CD.

5-Fluorocytosine is a hydrophilic antifungal agent that has low toxicity in humans but a lack of endogenous enzymes makes its activation impossible. However, bacterial and yeast CD enzymes can convert 5-fluorocytosine efficiently to 5-fluorouracil (5-FU). Studies with tritiated-5-FC in a human glioblastoma cell line stably transfected with E. coli gene for CD showed slow entry of the drug into the cells by passive diffusion, and a rapid efflux. Therefore, the transport of this quite hydrophilic prodrug may be a limiting factor. The active form of 5-FC is quite polar but it is a diffusible species which makes it the most effective drug for colon cancer; being converted by cellular enzymes to ribosyl monophosphate 5-FdUMP, which is an irreversible inhibitor of thymidylate synthetase [24].

The strong bystander effect is one of the main advantages of CD/5-FC system because there is no need for cell-to cell contact, thus 5-FU can diffuse through cells by non-facilitated diffusion. In vitro experiments conducted by exposing mixed transfected and non- transfected populations to 5-FC showed that 1-30% of cells expressing CD could produce sufficient 5-FU in order to inhibit the growth of the neighbouring cells that do not express the enzyme, even when the cells were sparsely seeded. Significant amounts of 5-FU were found in the culture medium of treated CD-positive cells, and the transfer of the supernatant from transfectants exposed to 5-FC to non-transfected cells resulted in their death. Bystander effect was also observed in cells negative for gap junctions. Higher effect of bystander in vitro and cure rats in vivo compared to HSV TK/GCV or HSV TK/acyclovir indicates that CD/5-FC is the combination of choice for Epstein Barr virus-associated lymphomas, renal cell carcinomas, and thyroid carcinomas. On the other hand, anti-tumor effects and immunity to parental tumors induced by the HSV TK/GCV system were superior to those induced by CD/5-FC in a hepatocellular carcinoma model [8].

Immune-mediated distant bystander effect is associated with an infiltration of natural killer cells within the tumors induced by the CD/5-FC combination similar to the HSV TK/GCV. Immuno-competent mice pre-treated with CD/5-FC GDEPT exhibited significant resistance when re-challenged with wild type tumors, and the "vaccination effect" appeared to be dependent on the re-challenging tumor such as the eradication of CD expressing adenocarcinomas which conferred no protection against fibrosarcomas [8].

Regardless of the encouraging preclinical results, it becomes obvious that the treatment with a single GDEPT strategy had led to partial response. Accordingly, in order to increase the efficiency of gene therapy strategies, combinations of several strategies of treatment modalities were investigated [8].

Improved anti-tumor activity of CD/5-FC has been achieved by using co-transfecting cells along with genes for CD and uracil phosphoribosyl transferase. This combination was able to convert 5-FU to 5-FUM in a direct manner [8].

Unlike HSV-TK/GCV, the CD/5-FC system has a significant bystander effect that does not depend on gap junction intercellular communication, as 5-FU can readily move out of and into cells by non-facilitated diffusion. In vivo expression of CD alone is sufficient to cause an immune response and subsequent tumor regression [9, 24].

CD/5-FC therapy has been studied with E. coli enzymes, in a wide variety of cancers. When both 5-FC/CD and HSV-TK/GCV therapies were compared in a different in vivo models, both of them appeared to have similar efficacy in hepatocellular carcinoma [24].

Nitroreductase/CB 1954

The mustard prodrug CB1954 is a weak mono functional alkylating agent which can be activated into a potent DNA cross-linking agent. Since nitroreductases require NADH or NADPH as cofactors, activation of the prodrug can only take place intracellularly, limiting the use of the NTR/CB1954 combination for ADEPT [8].

Its application for GDEPT was demonstrated after cloning and insertion of E. coli NTR gene into retroviral, adenoviral and plasmid DNA vectors. NTR expression in several human and murine cells resulted in up to 2600-fold increase in sensitivity to CB1954, compared to the parental lines [8]

Enzymes that metabolize aromatic nitro groups are attractive to be utilized in the GDEPT approach due to large electronic changes that this process generates. The metabolism of a nitro group can lead to the corresponding hydroxylamine 4-electron reduction product as the major metabolite, or to an amine 6-electron reduction product, as minor [24]

Four classes of prodrugs for NTR have been studied: dinitroaziridinylbenzamides, dinitrobenzamide mustards, 4-nitrobenzylcarbamates and nitroindolines. However, most of the studies were performed with dinitroaziridinylbenzamides CB 1954 [24].

Dinitroaziridinylbenzamides CB 1954 is a relatively lipophilic prodrug that is efficiently reduced by NTR, where either the 4- or 2-nitro groups are reduced to the corresponding hydroxylamines at about equal rates. Molecular modeling studies have shown that the small aziridine residue allows the drug far enough into the binding pocket such that both the 2- and 4-nitro groups will have an access to the FMN. The 4- hydroxylamine is metabolized by cellular acetylation pathways to a cytotoxic DNA inter-strand crosslinking agent (Figure 4). It should be emphasized, that CB 1954 has demonstrated substantial bystander effects, because of the cell permeability of the hydroxylamine metabolite [24].

Figure 4. Bioactivation of the prodrug CB 1954 by nitroreductase (NTR).

Horseradish Peroxidase/ Indole-3-Acetic Acid

IAA is oxidized by HRP-compound I to a radical cation at neutral pH, which then undergoes scission of the exocyclic carbon-carbon bond to yield the carbon-centered skatolyl radical (Figure 5). The skatolyl radical rapidly forms a proxy radical in the presence of oxygen, which then decomposes to a number of products, the most important ones being indole-3-carbinol, oxindole-3-carbinol and 3-methylene-2-oxindole [8].

Figure 5. A possible mechanism involved in the toxicity of HRP/ IAA combination.

In anoxic solution, decarboxylation of the radical cation can take place and the carbon centered radical preferentially reacts with hydrogen donors. When activated by purified HRP, IAA inhibits colony formation in mammalian cells, while neither the enzyme nor the prodrug alone was cytotoxic at the concentration or times analyzed [8]. Furthermore, after oral administration of 100 mg/kg IAA, notoxicity was reported. The efficacy of the HRP/IAA system for GDEPT was evaluated in vitro. Prodrug activation was fast and efficient, since cytotoxicity could be evoked within a 2-hours exposure, and it was further increased after 24-hours incubation. This indicates a strong bystander effect induction. Moreover, cell contact for bystander killing was not required, as the cells were sparsely seeded at the time of prodrug incubation and the transfer of IAA- containing medium preconditioned by HRP+ cells to HRP- cells resulted in their death [8].

A novel cancer GDEPT approach may be provided by the delivery of the HRP gene to human tumors followed by treatment with IAA and analogues, with potential to target hypoxic cells, which are resistant to radiation and chemotherapy [8].

Prodrugs for HRP GDEPT

HRP is an iron-containing heme peroxidase that catalyzes the oxidation of a variety of phenols and amines, including indole-3-acetic acid, without the need of hydrogen peroxide as a cofactor. The oxidation mechanism by HRP has shown to involve a series of iron-contained free radical intermediates with a variety of oxidation levels [24, 35].

Indole-3-Acetic Acid (IAA)

Indole-3-acetic acid is considered a nontoxic agent to mammalian cells. It is oxidized by HRP, initially to a nitrogen centered radical-cation species that rapidly fragments via a carbon-centered benzyl radical; both radical species are short-lived, and unlikely to account for the observed bystander effects of IAA. The 3-methylene-2 oxindole, derived from the hydroperoxide of benzyl radical by an unclear pathway, has been suggested as the active diffusing species, able to react with DNA. This product has a half-life which is long enough to generate a bystander effect, and sufficiently lipophilic to be diffused rapidly by passive diffusion [24].

5-Fluoroindole-3-Acetic Acid (FIAA)

This prodrug is related to IAA. It is more cytotoxic than IAA for HRP-transfected human and rodent tumor cell lines, regardless of being less rapidly oxidized by HRP to the corresponding effector [24].

Cytochrome P450/Cyclophosphamide

The cyclophosphamide prodrug (CP) is activated by liver cytochrome P450 (CYP) metabolism via a 4-hydroxylation reaction (Figure 6). The 4-hydroxy intermediate breaks down to form the bifunctional alkylating toxin phosphoramide mustard, which then leads to DNA cross-linking, G2-M arrest and apoptosis in a cycle-independent fashion. The isomeric analogue isophosphamide (IP) is activated in the same way, and both CP and IP reactions require NADH and O2. CYP is a very complex enzymatic system, with a number of isoenzymes with different substrate specificity and activity against CP [8].

CYP2B6 and CYP3A4 are responsible for these processes in human liver, whereas CYP2B1 is the most active one. CYPs are present in the liver and in some human cancers, including colon, breast, lung, liver, kidney and prostate, and are known to express isoforms of the 3A and 1A subfamilies. The CP metabolite phosphoramide mustard does not diffuse efficiently across cell membranes, and this bystander effect is mainly due to diffusible precursors, such as 4-hydroxy-CP. Because of the short half-life of 4-hydroxy-CP, local conversion of CP is superior to its activation in the liver, thus affecting decomposition of the primary metabolite before it reaches the tumor [8]. In order to protect normal tissues, the administration of selective inhibitors of endogenous liver enzymes with the GDEPT system is necessary. Such enzymes are 2l, 2l-dichloro-progesterone and 3,5-dimethoxy- 2,6-dimethyl-4-ehyl-1,4-dihydropyridine, which are specific for liver [8].

Prodrugs for CYP Enzymes

Prodrugs for gene therapy that is activated by NADH cytochrome P450 (CYP) enzymes are compounds that are normally activated by one or more of CYP isozymes. Because many of these enzymes are expressed in liver much more than in tumor cells, it will be crucial to selectively increase the exposure of tumor cells to cytotoxic drug metabolites. This can be done by targeting expression of the enzymes to tumor cells by using gene vectors. There are only two prodrugs that utilize this approach: the alkylating agents cyclophosphamide and ifosfamide [24, 36].

Cyclophosphamide (CPA)

In conventional cancer chemotherapy, CPA is the most widely used alkylating agent.The mechanism by which this lipophilic alkylating agent exerts its activity is via initial hydroxylation to 4-hydroxycyclophosphamide (hydroxy-CPA) by CYP enzymes in the liver. Thus CPA has potential advantages over GCV and 5-FC which are cell cycle-specific agents, whereas the more lipophilic CPA metabolites do not require cell-cell contact for a bystander effect since they are distributed by passive diffusion [24].

Ifosfamide (IFO)

Ifosfamide is used as one of the conventional anticancer drug. It is related both chemically and mechanistically to cyclophosphamide. It has similar lipophilicity to cyclophosamide and releases the same ultimate metabolite, phosphoramide mustard [24].

Acetaminophen

The anti-inflammatory drug acetaminophen is oxidized by human CYP1A2 enzyme to form the cytotoxic metabolite N-acetylbenzoquinoneimine, which is the major source of toxicity of this drug. Transfection of H1A2 MZ cells with human CYP1A2 sensitized them for the treatment with acetaminophen, because of the generation of a substantial bystander effect. Acetaminophen is a possible prodrug for GDEPT when it is conjugated with CYP1A2 [24].

Carboxypeptidase G2/CMDA

The prodrug is converted to an intermediate metabolite, and in order to form the active drug this requires catalysis by cellular enzymes. In the case that there is a lack or a decrease in the expression of these enzymes in the target cells tumor resistance might be imminent [8].

The bacterial enzyme carboxypeptidase G2 (CPG2), which has no mammalian counterpart, has the ability to cleave the glutamic acid moiety from the prodrug containing it (CMDA), and as a result DNA-cross-linking mustard drug, 4-[(2-chloroethyl)(2-mesyloxyethyl amino]benzoic acid, is released without any further catalysis [8].

The GDEPT enzyme carboxypeptidase G2 (CPG2) has the ability to convert alkylating agent mustard prodrugs into potent cytotoxic drugs that induce apoptosis. CPG2 is used in model non-targeted GDEPT protocols when is transfected and expressed as a surface-tethered enzyme [37, 38].

Prodrugs for Carboxypeptidases (CP)

Carboxypeptidases have been investigated for use in gene therapy because of their ability to cleave glutamate moieties. They generate this enzyme from various species of Pseudomonas bacteria; no mammalian counterpart exists [39]. These enzymes have been used primarily in ADEPT protocols, because the substrates for this type of enzymes are di-acids, where cell exclusion of very polar prodrugs up to activation is beneficial. Moreover,they have been adapted for use in GDEPT by being engineered for surface expression on cells (Figure 6) [24, 40].

Figure 6. Pathways for catalyzed-cyclophosphamide (CP) by cytochrome P450 (CYP 450).

4-[(2-Chloroethyl) (2-Methyloxyethyl) Amino] Benzoyl-L-Glutamicacid (CMDA)

Figure 7. Conversion of the prodrug CMDA into cytotoxin.

The too polar mixed mustard CMDA is a prodrug for ADEPT in combination with the enzyme carboxypeptidase G2 (CPG2), which cleaves glutamate to generate active carboxylic acid species. However, studies in human adenocarcinoma cell lines and human colon carcinoma cell lines, that internally expressed CPG2, showed enhanced sensitivity to CMDA. This indicates that these di-acids do enter cells (Figure 7) [24, 39, 40].

Cell killing was completed and achieved in 4-12% of cells that expressed the enzyme, indicating a substantial bystander effect over the much more lipophilic released aniline mustard effector. Nonetheless, the requirement for cell killing with surface tethered compared to internally-expressed CPG2 requires lower levels of enzyme and shorter exposures to prodrug [24, 39, 40].

Anthracycline Glutamates

Prodrugs of anthracycline topoisomerase inhibitors, such as doxorubin with glutamate residues directly attached to the glycoside nitrogen, were not found to be good substrates for CPG2. Therefore, analogues prodrugs with a 4-benzylcarbamate spacer group were investigated. These prodrugs have shown to undergo 1,6-elimination followed by glutamate cleavage by CPG2 releasing the active doxorubicin [24].

Methotrexateα-Peptides (MTX-Phe)

Methotrexate-α-peptides are prodrugs of methotrexate (MTX), a potent inhibitor of dihydrofolate reductase, and a widely used anticancer drug. The prodrugs of methotrexate are poor substrates for the reduced folate carrier. Unlike MTX, these prodrugs cannot be taken by the cell, but they can be cleaved to methotrexate by carboxypeptidase A1 (CPGA) [24, 41].

Summary and Conclusion

Gene therapy is a promising approach. Some major obstacles remain to be solved before these new strategies become routinely adopted in the clinic. One of the main challenges remaining is improvement of gene delivery, and thus therapeutic efficacy. Several clinically successful prodrugs have been developed. Clinical trials have classified the issues of safety and toxicity, and it can be anticipated that the results obtained in the preclinical studies will be quickly translated into the clinic.

In this chapter, we have reviewed the various GDEPT systems studied for treating cancer tumors. Although numerous GDEPTs have been developed and evaluated, careful consideration of the properties of these systems such as enzymes, prodrugs and toxic metabolites should be considered when determining the optimal system/s (either alone or in combination) for treating cancers. Researchers have continuously designed new prodrugs with improved stability and increased efficacy.

In the selection of prodrugs, there are many factors to be considered for each particular activating enzyme such as the high turnover by the enzyme and the large differential cytotoxicity between the prodrug and its activated form.

Finally, all approaches should be considered for testing in order to achieve complete cure for this challenging disease. Synergies between different GDEPTs and other modalities are to be explored for maximizing therapeutic benefit with a minimal toxicity.

References

[1] Weyel, D.; Sedlacek, H. Müller, R. & Brüsselbach, S. (2000) Secreted human b-glucuronidase: a novel tool for gene-directed enzyme prodrug therapy.*Macmillan Publishers Limited.* 7, 224–231.

[2] Azrak; R.G.; Cao, S.; Slocum, HK.; Tóth, K.; Durrani, FA.; Yin, MB.; Pendyala, L.; Zhang, W.; McLeod, HL & Rustum, YM. (2004) Therapeutic Synergy Between Irinotecan and 5-Fluorouracil against Human Tumor Xenografts. *Clinical Cancer Research.* 10, 1121-1129.

[3] Heine, D.; Muller, R. & Brusselbach, S. (2001) Cell surface display of a lysosomal enzyme for extracellular gene-directed enzyme prodrug therapy. *Nature Publishing Group* 8, 1005-1010

[4] Niculescu-Duvaz, C. I. (2002) Approaches to Gene-Directed Enzyme Prodrug Therapy (GDEPT), in Cancer Gene Therapy. *Springer US.* 403-409.

[5] Both, GW. (2009) Recent progress in gene-directed enzyme prodrug therapy: an emerging cancer treatment. *Curr Opin Mol Ther* 11, 421-432.

[6] Bhaumik, S.; Sekar, T.; Depuy, J.; Klimash, J. & Paulmurugan, R. (2012) Noninvasive optical imaging of nitroreductase gene-directed enzyme prodrug therapy system in living animals. *Macmillan Publishers Limited.* 19, 295-302.

[7] Hlavaty, J.; Petznek, H.; Holzmüller, H.; Url, A.; Jandl, G.; Berger, A.; Salmons, B.; Günzburg, W. & Renner, M. (2012) Evaluation of a Gene-Directed Enzyme-Product Therapy GDEPT) in Human Pancreatic Tumor Cells and Their Use s In Vivo Models for Pancreatic Cancer. *Hlavaty Plos ONE.* 7, p1

[8] Greco, O.; Dachs, G.U.; (2001) Gene directed enzyme/prodrug therapy of cancer: Historical appraisal and future prospectives. *Journal of Cellular Physiology.* 187, 22-36.

[9] Dachs, G.U.; Michelle, A.; Hunt, Sophie Syddall, Dean, C & Singleton, A.V. (2009) Bystander or no bystander for gene directed enzyme prodrug therapy. *Molecules.* 14, 4517-45.

[10] Niculescu-Duvaz, I. & Springer, C. (2005) Introduction to the background, principles, and state of the art in suicide gene therapy. *Molecular Biotechnology.* 30, 71-88.

[11] Klein, R.; Ruttkowski, B.; Schwab, S.; Peterbauer, T.; Salmons, B.; Walter, H. & Hohenadl. C. (2008) Mouse mammary tumor virus promoter-containing retroviral promoter conversion vectors for gene-directed enzyme prodrug therapy are functional in vitro and in vivo. *J Biomed Biotechnol.* p. 683505.

[12] Niculescu-Duvaz, I. & Springer, C.J. (1997) Gene-directed enzyme prodrug therapy: a review of enzyme/prodrug combinations. *Expert Opinion on Investigational Drugs.* 6, 685-703.

[13] Tupper, J.; Tozer, G.M.& Dachs, G.U. (2004) Use of horseradish peroxidase for gene-directed enzyme prodrug therapy with paracetamol. *British Journal of Cancer.* 90, 1858 − 1862.

[14] Seo, G.-M.; Rachakatla, R.; Balivada, .; Pyle, M.; Shrestha, T.B.; Matthew, T. B.; Myers, C.; Wang, H.; Tamura, M.; . Bossmann, S.H. & Troyer, D.L. (2012) A self-contained enzyme activating prodrug cytotherapy for preclinical melanoma. *Molecular Biology Reports.* 39, 157-165.

[15] Rooseboom, M.; Commandeur, J.N.M.& Vermeulen, N.P.E.(2004) Enzyme-Catalyzed Activation of Anticancer Prodrugs. *Pharmacological Reviews.* 56, 53-102.

[16] Mitchell, D.J.& Minchin, R.F. (2008) E. coli nitroreductase/CB1954 gene-directed enzyme prodrug therapy: role of arylamine N-acetlytransferase 2. *Nature Publishing Group.* 15, 758-764.

[17] Gadi, V. K.; Alexander, S. D.; Kudlow, J. E.; Allan, P.; Parker, W. B.& Sorscher, E .J. (2000) In vivo sensitization of ovarian tumors to chemotherapy by expression of E. coli purine nucleoside phosphorylase in a small fraction of cells. *Gene Ther.* 7,1738 - 1743.

[18] ALBERT, A. (1958) Chemical aspects of selective toxicity. *Nature.* p. 421-422.

[19] Dahan, A.; Khamis, M.; Agbaria, R. & Karaman, R. (2012) Targeted prodrugs in oral delivery: the modern molecular biopharmaceutical approach. *Expert Opinion on Drug Delivery9*, 1001–1013.

[20] Karaman, R.; Fattash B. & Qtait A. (2013) The future of prodrugs – design by quantum mechanics methods. *Expert Opinion on Drug Delivery10*, 713–729.

[21] Karaman R. (2013) Prodrugs design based on inter- and intramolecular processes. *Chem. Biol. Drug.Des.* 82, 643–668.

[22] Jolanta, B.; Zawilska, Wojcieszak, J.; Agnieszka, B. & Olejniczak, (2013) Prodrugs: A challenge for the drug development. *Institute of Pharmacology Polish Academy of Sciences.* 65, 1-14.

[23] Russell, P.J.& Khatri, A. (2006) Novel gene-directed enzyme prodrug therapies against prostate cancer. *Expert Opinion on Investigational Drugs.* 15, 947-961.

[24] Denny, W.A. (2003) Prodrugs for Gene-Directed Enzyme-Prodrug Therapy (Suicide Gene Therapy). *Journal of Biomedicine and Biotechnology.*1, p. 48-70.

[25] Karaman, R. (2013) The Prodrug Naming Dilemma. *OMICS Publishing Group.* 2

[26] Perry, M.J.; Todryk, S.M.& Dalgleish, A.G. (1999) The role of herpes simplex virus thymidine kinase in the treatment of solid tumours. *Informa Healthcare.* 8, 777-785.

[27] Xu, G. & McLeod, H.L. (2001) Strategies for Enzyme/Prodrug Cancer Therapy. *Clinical Cancer Research.* 7, 3314-3324.

[28] Culver, KW.; Ram, Z.; Wallbridge, S.; Ishii, H.; Oldfield, EH. & Blaese, RM. (1992) In vivo gene transfer with retroviral vector-producer cells for treatment of experimental brain tumors. *Science.* 256, 1550-1552.

[29] Freeman, S.M.; Ramesh, R. & Marrogi, A.J. (1997) Immune system in suicide-gene therapy. *The Lancet.* 349, 2-3.

[30] Elshami, AA.; Saavedra, A.; Zhang, H.; Kucharczuk, JC.; Spray, DC.; Fishman, GI.; Amin, KM.; Kaiser, LR. & Albelda, SM. (1996) Gap junctions play a role in the ``bystander effect" of the herpes simplex virus thymidine kinase ganciclovir system in vitro. *Gene Ther.* 3, 85-92.

[31] Freeman, S. M.; Abboud, C. N.& Whartenby, K. A. (1993) The "Bystander Effect": Tumor Regression When a Fraction of the Tumor Mass Is Genetically Modified. *Cancer Research.* 53, 5274-5283.

[32] Huber, B.E.; Austin, E.A.; Richards, C.A. & Davis, S.T. (1994) Good SS.Metabolism of 5-fuorocytosine to 5-fuorouracil in human colorectal tumor cells transduced with the cytosine deaminase gene: significant antitumor effects when only a small percentage of tumor cellsexpress cytosine deaminase. *Proc. Nati. Acad. Sci. USA.* 91, 8302- 8306.

[33] WAXMAN, D.J.; Chen, L.; Hecht, J.E. & Jounaidi, Y. (1999) CYTOCHROME P450-BASED CANCER GENE THERAPY: RECENT ADVANCES AND FUTURE PROSPECTS. *Drug Metabolism Reviews.* 31, 503-522.

[34] Mesnil, M. & Yamasaki, H. (2000) Bystander Effect in Herpes Simplex Virus-Thymidine Kinase/Ganciclovir Cancer Gene Therapy: Role of Gap-junctional Intercellular Communication1. *Cancer Research.* 60, 3989-3999.

[35] Wardman, P.(2002) Indole-3-acetic acids and horseradish peroxidase: a new prodrug/enzyme combination for targeted cancer therapy. *Curr Pharm Des*. 8, 1363-1374.

[36] Waxman, DJ.; Chen, L.; Hecht, JE. & Jounaidi, Y. (1999) Cytochrome P450-based cancer gene therapy: recent advances and future prospects. *Drug Metab Rev*. 31, 503-522.

[37] Schepelmann, S.; Hallenbeck, P.; Ogilvie, L. M.; Hedley, D.; Friedlos, F.; Martin, J.; Scanlon, I.; Hay, C.; Hawkins, L. K.; Marais, R. & Springer, C. J. (2005) Systemic Gene-Directed Enzyme Prodrug Therapy of Hepatocellular Carcinoma Using a Targeted Adenovirus Armed with Carboxypeptidase G2. *Cancer Research*. 65, 5003-5008.

[38] Friedlos, F.; Davies, L. & Scanlon, I. (2002) Three new prodrugs for suicide gene therapy using carboxypeptidase G2 elicit bystander efficacy in two xenograft models. *Cancer Res*. 62, 1724-1749.

[39] Caroline, J.; Antoniw, P.; Kenneth, D.; Searle, F. & Jarman, M. (1990) Novel prodrugs which are activated to cytotoxic alkylating agents by carboxypeptidase G2. *J Med Chem. British journal of cancer*. 33, 677–681.

[40] Marais, R.; Spooner, R. A.& Light, Y. (1996) Gene-directed Enzyme Prodrug Therapy with a Mustard Prodrug/Carboxypeptidase G2 Combination. *Cancer Research*. 56, 4735-4742.

[41] Niculescu-Duvaz, I.; Niculescu-Duvaz, D. & Friedlos, F. (1999) Self-immolative anthracycline prodrugs for suicide gene therapy. *Journal of clinical investigation*. 13, 2485-2489.

In: Prodrugs Design – A New Era
Editor: Rafik Karaman

ISBN: 978-1-63117-701-9
© 2014 Nova Science Publishers, Inc.

Chapter VII

Antibody Directed Enzyme Prodrug Therapy (ADEPT): A Promising Cancer Therapy Approach

*Wajd Amly[1] and Rafik Karaman[1,2]**

[1]Pharmaceutical Sciences Department, Faculty of Pharmacy
Al-Quds University, Jerusalem, Palestine
[2]Department of Science, University of Basilicata, Potenza, Italy

Abstract

The conventional old treatment method for cancer therapy is associated with severe side effects along with several limitations. Therefore, searching and developing new methods for cancer became crucial. This chapter focuses on a relatively new method for cancer treatment named antibody directed enzyme prodrug therapy (ADEPT). This approach consists of two steps by which the first step involves an administration of antibody-drug activating enzyme conjugate (AEC) to target the tumor and to be accumulated predominantly at the tumor cells that have the wanted tumor associated antigen, and to be allowed to localize and clear the unbounded conjugate from the plasma. The second step involves a nontoxic prodrug which is injected systemically and is converted to its corresponding active form with high tumor concentration by the localized enzyme.

The chapter describes in details the most used enzyme-antibody systems, their advantages and disadvantages.

Keywords: Antibody directed enzyme prodrug therapy (ADEPT), cancer therapy, enzyme-antibody conjugate, solid tumor, monoclonal antibody, tumor antigen, fusion protein, physiologically based pharmacokinetic model (PBPK)

---

* Corresponding author: Rafik Karaman, e-mail: dr_karaman@yahoo.com; Tel and Fax +972-2-2790413.

List of Abbreviations

ADEPT	Antibody directed enzyme prodrug therapy
AEC	Antibody- enzyme conjugates
VDEPT	Virus directed enzyme prodrug therapy
GDEPT	Gene directed enzyme prodrug therapy
scFv	Single chain variable fragment
CEA	Carcino- embryonic antigen
mAb	Monoclonal antibody
CPG2	Carboxypeptidase G2
CD	Cytosine deaminase
βL	β- lactamase
PGA	Penicillin G amidase
PVA	Penicillin V amidase
AP	Alkaline phosphatase
5-FC	5- Fluorocytocine
5-FU	5- Fluorouracil
NR	Nitroreductase
UDPGT	Uridinediphosphateglucuronyl transferase
MTX	Methotrexate
TSA	Transition state analogue
HER-2	Human epidermal growth factor receptor- 2
ACE	Angiotensin-converting-enzyme
MHC II	Major histocompatibility complex class II
PBPK	Physiologically based pharmacokinetic model
FcRn	Neonatal Fc-receptor
GA	Geldanamycin
DP2	Dynamic programming for Deimmunizing protein
E_{max}, prodrug	Maximum rate constant for converting prodrug to active drug by AEC (1/min).
EC_{50} prodrug	EC50 for converting prodrug to active drug by AEC (mol/ml).
P	Effective permeability coefficient
Clint	Liver intrinsic clearance
PS	Permeability-area product
f_{up}	Unbound free fractions in plasma
IC50	half maximal inhibitory concentration
AUC	Area under the curve
Mwt	molecular weight

Introduction

Chemotherapy plays a crucial role in treatment strategies for cancer, but it has several disadvantages that limits its use including lack of selectivity for tumor versus normal cells, systemic toxicity, and inadequate tumor concentration of the drug and the possibility of drug resistant tumor cells [1]. During the past 40 years, an intensive search for compounds that selectively attack the cancer cells without causing severe damage to normal tissues has been commenced, where a number of agents have been clinically tested and some have shown considerable efficacy, nevertheless, their effects on normal tissues have usually been dose limiting [2]. In addition, cancer cells biological versatility resulted in withstand exposure to cancer agents which is the main cause for drug resistance [2]. To overcome this obstacle, several strategies have been carried out including alternative formulations (e.g., liposomes), resistance modulation (e.g., PSC833), antidotes/toxicity modifiers (e.g., ICRF-187) and gene therapy [1]. On the other hand, tumor antigens have been defined and the notion of selectively targeting cancer cells via antibodies, first mentioned in the early 1900s, has translated into various forms of selective delivery [2]. The antigen itself could be intracellular, membrane bound or secreted into the extracellular fluid compartment, where an intracellular location of the antigen poses the problem of being difficult to be accessed by antibody vectors [3].

It seems that the more important factor to be considered in this approach is not whether the target (antigen) is membrane bound or secreted but it is the density of the antigen because this could be the factor for determining the number of antibody molecules retained at target sites and the steric effects that might operate at cell membranes [3].

A phenomenon of modulation and capping in the presence of specific bivalent antibody occurs with membrane bound antigens, and it has been demonstrated to be largely restricted to lymphoid cells and polymorphonuclear leukocytes and it is uncertain in solid tumors [3]. Inhibition of the capping and modulation has been achieved by microtubule acting agents including colchicine, vinblastine and neocarcinostatin, and by the use of univalent antibodies (IgG-Fab/c). However, if endocytosis of the antibody-toxin complex is required in order to achieve cytotoxicity, then it is useful to maintain modulation [3].

As mentioned above, the notion of using antibodies against a malignant cells antigen is not new and the history of antibody conjugates is marked by difficulties that have been identified and solved [4]. A variety of cell killing agents have been covalently attached to antibody or antibody fragment directed against a tumor antigens like cytotoxic drugs, biotoxins and radioisotopes, and the limitations of each approach have been identified [3, 4]. The advantages of using antibody conjugates is that it allows for specificity and potency enhancement by utilizing the antibodies that are specific to cell surface proteins, despite some limitations that have been encountered using this approach, especially for the treatment of solid tumors including the difficulty associated with macromolecule delivery to solid tumors, antigen tumor surface expression heterogeneity and expression of the antigen by normal tissues [4]. Table 1 summarizes some of the advantages and disadvantages of the antibody conjugate approach [4].

Monoclonal antibodies to deliver chemotherapeutic drugs, bacterial and plant toxins and radionuclides to tumor cells have been used, however, the currently available intact antibodies (molecular mass-140-160 kDa) and the small-sized antigen binding fragments (molecular mass ~25 kDa) are much larger than the classical anti-cancer drugs (molecular mass 250-500 Da) resulting in difficulties to deliver a tumor-sterilizing dose [5, 6]. Therefore, monoclonal antibodies were replaced by a more potent toxins such as diphtheria, ricin and abrin where a single toxin was introduced into a cell by an internalizing antibody that is capable of destroying it by inactivating ribosomes and thereby inhibiting protein synthesis [2]. Ribonuclease − antibody conjugate has similar potency and may in addition avoid the immunogenicity problem of the biotoxins [2]. The immune-toxins have faced three major problems: the antibody-toxin conjugate immunogenicity; their effect on human vasculature resulting in vascular leak syndrome and the heterogeneity of antigen expression, therefore, many clonogenic antigen negative cells fail to internalize the toxin [2]. On the other hand, using the short-range radioisotopes attached to antibodies helped to overcome this problem by binding to antigen-positive cells and killing these along with 'bystander' cells that may be marker negative [2, 7].

Table 1. Advantages and disadvantages of antibody conjugate

Advantages	Disadvantages
- Selective target to the antigen. - Stable conjugate resulting in prolonged half-life. - Possibility of using highly potent agent that selectively delivered. - Wide therapeutic range. - Reduction in toxicity and side effects.	- Tumor has to be tested for expression of the antigen. - Possibility of toxicity as some of the targets may be expressed by normal tissues. - Toxic payload may have some premature release. - Achievement of insufficient lethal concentration due to the inability of enough conjugate to reach the target cell. - Heterogeneity of antigen expression especially in solid tumors.

The disadvantage of this approach is that only a small proportion of the administered antibody is localized into the tumor, and the rate of localization is slow; therefore, the radiation dose which is administered to the tumor is not larger than that was administered to normal tissues, hence, it is dose limiting. Nevertheless, this therapy has proved effectiveness in the most radiosensitive tumors such as lymphomas [2].

When antibodies or antibody conjugates are given intravenously (i.v.), they penetrate normal tissues more rapidly than tumor tissues due to the nature of the cancer tissues which are relatively avascular compared to normal tissues [2]. Due to the fact that antibodies bind to specific targets on cancer cells, the concentration of antibody increases with time, whereas it falls in normal tissues that do not bind antibodies. Therefore, it would be beneficial to obtain the desired cytotoxic drug activation when the most favorable ratio of tumor to normal tissue antibody had been achieved [2].

Selective expression of the target antigen by tumor cells is desired for obtaining a successful form of antibody-mediated targeting [7].

In general, antibodies directed at secreted antigens are unsuitable for cytotoxins that require an intracellular site of action because they are unlikely to be endocytosed; in contrast to those directed at membrane bound antigens which can be endocytosed. Nevertheless, secreted antigens are suitable targets for radiation carrying antibodies [3, 7]. On the other hand, heterogeneity in antigens distribution within tumor cell populations, where some cells express the antigen and so called antigen positive and others fail to express it and called antigen negative, is considered a major problem because cells that don't express the targeted antigen would fail to bind and internalize the antibody-drug conjugate [8]. It is to be taken into consideration that when a drug or toxin is bound to antibody only a fraction of the cells constitute targets is able to internalize the cytotoxin. This can be resolved by the use of antibody "cocktails" in which a mixture of antibodies aimed at two or more discrete antigens used in noncompetitive combination [3, 7]. If the expression of antigen is cell cycle related then it would be expected that repeated treatments would provide a greater fraction access to the cancer cell population [3].

The notion of generating cytotoxic drug from a non-toxic drug utilizing enzymes present in tumor tissues or specific tumor cells has been investigated in 1960s [2]. Philpott and coworkers was the group advocated the idea of using antibodies to carry a specific enzyme to cancers, and the concept known as antibody directed enzyme prodrug therapy (ADEPT) was then proposed [9].

Antibody Directed Enzyme Prodrug Therapy (ADEPT)

Realizing that a delivery and effector functions of a selective pharmaceutical agent have different characteristics had led to the concept of component delivery [3]. Moreover, the desire to localize a drug cytotoxic action on tumor sites, and to reduce the shortcomings associated with systemic chemotherapy, such as a lack of tumor selectivity and drug resistance has become crucial to search for new methods to deliver anti-cancer agents specifically to cancer sites [10, 11].

In order to localize the cytotoxic drug action only to the desired tumor cells, few requirements need to be met: a generation of the cytotoxic agent exclusively at the tumor location, and a retention of the anticancer agent inside those cells with a potential that its activity will be demolished once leaving the tumor site [11].

The concept of antibody directed enzyme prodrug therapy (ADEPT) consists of two steps, where in the first step, an antibody-drug activating enzyme conjugate (AEC) is targeted to the tumor and accumulates predominantly at the tumor cells that have the desired tumor associated antigen; given an adequate time to be localized and cleared. In the second step a non-toxic prodrug is injected systemically that is converted to its corresponding active form with high tumor concentration by the localized enzyme (Figure 1) [7, 11-13]. Consequently, optimizing the interval between the enzyme and prodrug administrations is crucial to guarantee an accumulation of the drug at the tumor site rather than in normal tissue, and hence, decreasing the systemic toxicity [1].

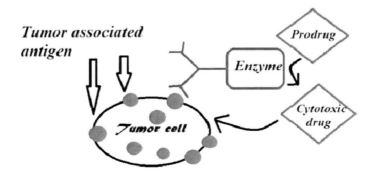

Figure 1. A schematic diagram showing the mechanism of the ADEPT approach.

It should be indicated, that after an administration of F(ab')2 antibody-enzyme conjugate, much of the dose remains for several days in the vascular compartment allowing for the enzymatic activity at tumor and plasma to subside [3]. The conjugate is cleared quickly when the corresponding antigen is present in plasma and immune conjugates are formed [3]. It is crucial to wait until plasma enzyme levels fall to very low values or to be cleared before giving the prodrug.

Techniques used to enhance AEC clearance are discussed in separate sections of this chapter.

Advantages of Adept

A number of advantages are associated with ADEPT system. Firstly, separation of the antibody- enzyme conjugate (AEC) and prodrug administrations provides sufficient time to allow the conjugate to localize within the tumors and cleared from the plasma, and secondly, amplification effect; where many hundreds of non-toxic prodrug molecules can be activated by a single enzyme molecule [2, 7, 14]. In addition, tumor penetration is easier and is facilitated in high extent by small-sized active drugs [2, 14]. Further, the active drug is generated extracellularly, and if it has a good lipophilic properties it can diffuse into the cancer tissues to attack cells which do not express the target's antigen; a concept known as bystander effect [2, 13]. Another advantage is that the risk of second therapy-induced cancers, a common problem associated with conventional therapy, is hindered or reduced, as the active cytotoxic agent can be reserved to tumor sites [2, 13]. Further, the delivery of the cytotoxic drug via targeting cancer-specific antigens concentrates the drug at the cancer site, which aids in better diagnostic imaging and treatment of cancers. For instance, overexpressing cancer cell surface has ~ 2,000,000 HER-2 receptors, whereas a non-overexpressing normal cell has 10,000 − 20,000 molecules which demonstrates about a 100-fold higher drug concentrations delivered to cancer cells than normal cells [15]. A particular advantage is the possibility to use extremely potent agents such as nitrogen mustards and palytoxin that are too toxic to be readily used in conventional chemotherapy [7].

Potential Problems of Adept

Despite the respected number of advantages, ADEPT has showed some problems that need to be solved. Such problems are: (i) finding a substantial resources for the antibody, antibody-fragment production, conjugation chemistry and recombinant approach for AEC production, (ii) the importance of developing an accelerated blood clearance technique for the residual AEC, (iii) the need of identifying appropriate enzymes and (iv) the ability to generate a relatively inert prodrug that is activated only by an appropriate enzyme to yield a highly cytotoxic agent having a short plasma half-life at the tumor site [2]. In addition, there is a potential for AEC to have the following: (a) a poor tumor penetration and poor uptake, (b) in vivo disintegration, (c) inhibition of tumor localization due to a presence of blood antigen, (d) immunogenicity associated with the use of non-human enzyme, (e) lack of specificity when using a human enzyme, (f) high cost associated with the production process and (g) inadequate clearance of the unbound AEC [2, 14, 16, 17]. Another important disadvantage is that the systems under study constitute single-agent therapy that may be ineffective and/or may promote development of drug resistance [18].

Approaches to Deliver Prodrug- Activating Enzyme into Tumor Cells

ADEPT is a three-component system consisting of a drug-activating enzyme, a prodrug, and a targeting antibody, where the enzyme and prodrug components of the strategy count for serious challenges to the practical application of this approach [19]. For a successful therapy, the prodrug has to achieve a number of requirements; it should display low systemic toxicity, low cell intake and good hydrophobicity [20]. It also has to be designed in a way that allows only for the enzyme–antibody conjugate to be localized at the tumor site to catalytically convert the prodrug to its active form.

Consequently, the active drug should be easily released by an exogenous enzyme and penetrate the cancer cells with a short half- life to prevent toxicity to normal cells [8, 20]. Furthermore, the AEC should display binding specificity to tumor antigen, low immunogenicity, capable of processing a wide variety of drugs and not to be inhibited by either the prodrug or the drug and have a high intrinsic activity [19-21].

Endogenous human enzymes cannot be used for ADEPT, since expression of the endogenous enzyme could generate cytotoxic compounds that might lead to systemic toxicity. In order to prevent a prodrug from being activated by human endogenous enzyme, bacterial enzymes have been alternatively used; still, the usage of exogenous non-human proteins in human therapy raises the issue of the immunogenicity as it elicits a vigorous antibody response that limits repeated administration of the protein [19].

Important Factors for Adept

1. Antibodies in Adept

Antibodies have received a great attention as potential tool for anticancer therapy and they have become a prompt expanding class of pharmaceuticals for treating cancer. Antibodies are engineered in such a way that allows them to adapt their unique biological properties. [22].

Despite chemists effort to develop novel cytotoxic agents with unique mechanisms of action, many of these compounds still suffer from tumor selectivity shortage and have not been therapeutically useful, therefore, antibodies are a key component in ADEPT that can bind tumor-associated antigens because they ensure selective prodrug activation [23, 24]. Very few monoclonal antibodies are therapeutically in use despite their high selectivity because they only display modest cell killing activity.

Monoclonal antibodies linked to highly cytotoxic drugs can be regarded as either conferring higher tumor selectivity to cytotoxic drugs, that are too toxic to be used on their own, or conferring cell killing influence to monoclonal antibodies that are tumor-specific but not sufficiently cytotoxic [24]. Different important requirements of Ab-conjugates used in ADEPT are the localization at the tumor site, ideally with high affinity, having a minimum binding to normal sites, rapid clearance from plasma compartments and covalent binding with enzyme must not destroy the antibody ability to bind to its associated antigen, nor should it alter the enzyme activity. In addition, the conjugate linkage has to be stable for more than 72 hours in order to allow separated administrations of the conjugate and the prodrug [7, 23].

Two contradicted factors are involved in the penetration of tumors by AEC: the tumors blood vessels and interstitium which are leakier than those of normal tissues; it is an advantage for macromolecules localization which leads to poor macromolecules uptake [23].

In an attempt to overcome this limitation, an Ab fragments were used e.g., F (ab')2, F(ab') and single-chain variable fragments (scFv), to improve the interstitial rate of transport, and these fragments have shown better penetration properties and more rapid clearance compared to the intact Ab [23]. Studies performed using AEC containing antibody directed against carcino-embryonic antigen (anti-CEA), F(ab') 2 fragments (Figure 2) showed superiority vs. the intact monoclonal antibody (mAb) or Fab antibody fragment in terms of concentration and persistence at the tumor site and tumor to blood ratio [2].

Dwell time in the tumor is also vital, and bivalent antibodies may have more extended dwell times [2].

Examples of antibodies that were considered for use in ADEPT and directed at the antigens are listed in Table 2. Taking into consideration the size of Ab make IgM antibodies, less preference is given to large sized antibodies since their bulkiness contributes to a slower escape from the vascular compartment and a slow penetration into the tumors [2].

Table 2. Antibodies and antigen used in reported ADEPT systems

Target tumor	Antigen	Antibody	Ref.
Choriocarcinoma CC3	Human chorionic gonadotropin β	W.14, SB10	[25]
Adenocarcinoma colon LS154T	Carcino-embryonic antigen	A5B7	[7, 23]
Adenocarcinoma ovary Colon (H3347) & lung	Carcino-embryonic antigen	A5B7	[26]
(H2981) carcinomas	Not specified	L6	[7, 27, 28]
B cell lymphomas	CD20	1F5	[27, 28]
Melanoma 3677	Not specified	96.5	[29]
Breast, MDA, Mb361	c-ErbB2 p185	ICR 12	[30]

2. Enzymes in Adept

Enzyme selection is very crucial because appropriate prodrugs can be designed for almost any enzyme [31]. The major contemplations for choosing the enzyme is the ability of the latter to alter the prodrug to its active form in high efficiency and preferably to be a non-mammalian origin, although mammalian enzymes with no human analogue may be practical, nevertheless, microorganisms are more likely to be a better choice [3, 7, 31, 32]. It should be worth noting that hydrolyzing enzymes that do not require cofactors is the best among other enzymes to be used in ADEPT studies [15].

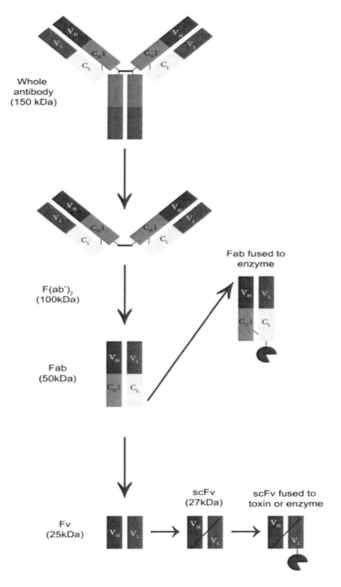

Figure 2. A Diagram represents an intact antibody, antibody fragments and antibody- enzyme conjugates.

Aspects affecting the selection of enzyme comprise low immunogenicity, optimum pH, small size, in vivo high stability and no appearance in human tissues, or at least lack from extracellular fluids [2]. As for human enzymes, they have the benefit of being low immunogenic, nevertheless they lack specificity, in contrary to bacterial enzymes which offer specificity, but having an immunological problem; however, if the immunogenicity is controllable, then the overriding consideration is specificity [2, 31].

If a human enzyme is chosen for the development of a non-immunogenic conjugate, it is preferred to be an intracellular enzyme because endogenous enzymes if used might raise the possibility of prodrug activation in the blood [7].

Categories of Used Enzymes

1. Class I: Enzymes of Non-Mammalian Origin

These enzymes have no mammalian homologue; such enzymes are carboxypeptidase G2 (CPG2), cytosine deaminase (CD), β-lactamase (βL), penicillin G amidase (PGA), penicillin V amidase (PVA).

Bacterial enzymes have a number of advantageous that make them an attractive choice for ADEPT systems; they tend to be stable, possess high catalytic rates, readily available on a large scale owing to their lack of post-translational modification. In addition, they have good kinetic parameters, generally easier to manufacture than mammalian enzymes [23, 33].

One of the most interesting enzymes to work with is- β-lactamase, which has been reported to be able to activate a variety of prodrugs to release the commonly used cancer drugs, such as doxorubicin, vinblastine, taxol, paclitaxel, and melphalan. These enzymes are relatively small single domain proteins that tend to be very stable and easily purified [33]. The disadvantage of using this class of enzymes is the immunogenicity.

2. Class II: Enzymes of Non-Mammalian Origin with a Mammalian Homologue

As revealed earlier, the enzymes should be selected such that they should have a low levels of their endogenous equivalents present in the blood [5]. Examples of Class II enzymes consist of - β- glucuronidase and nitroreductase. One of the benefits provided by bacterial - β-glucuronidase over its human equivalents is that it has a higher turnover rate and a pH optimum of 6.8, instead of 5.4 [5, 23]. Like Class I enzymes, immunogenicity is a drawback.

3. Class III: Enzymes of Mammalian Origin

Alkaline phosphatase (AP), carboxypeptidase A and β-glucuronidase are examples of this class of enzymes. It is expected that these enzymes will offer less immunogenic response than enzymes derived from bacterial or fungal origin; this allows for repeated rounds of therapy, however, these endogenous enzymes can lead to non-specific drug activation [5].

In prodrug design, a number of firm structural necessities imposed by the enzyme should be met. Enzymes, such as β- lactamase has a substrate recognition which depends mainly on one region of the substrate and is independent on the rest of it; thus providing great flexibility as they can catalyze the conversion of variety of prodrugs having different chemical structures [23].

To utilize human enzymes in ADEPT system, two requirements should be met: (1) to exploit any appropriate enzyme that is overexpressed at the tumor site and if such enzyme is found, then it becomes unnecessary to target the enzyme to the tumor and (2) if a human enzyme is found and having the appropriate kinetic characteristics towards the designed prodrug and is expressed only at a very low concentration in normal tissues [11].

4. Fusion Protein

The fusion of the gene encoding an enzyme along with that encoding an antibody, and overexpressing the product in an appropriate expression system is known as the fusion protein concept [11]. scFv antibody is a fusion protein and its development is a useful step to minimize the inherent variability in chemical conjugation of antibodies to enzymes, and it is the first fusion protein developed specifically for an ADEPT application; it is composed of human β-glucuronidase fused to the CH domain of BW431; a high-avidity anti-CEA antibody [7, 11].

Another product integrates scFv anti- CEA antibody (MFE) with CPG2 to yield MFE23-CPG2 fusion protein was produced and expressed at first in E. coli, but the low amount yielded and the suboptimal pharmacokinetics discouraged a distinct enhancement. However, it has alternatively expressed in the yeast Pichia pastoris (MFE- CP) in large scale and stable glycosylated products. The advantages provided by glycosylation are better pharmacokinetics profile and tumor localization, and the fusion protein can be used for an activation of a wide range of alkylating prodrugs [11].

Glycosylation can be used to modify tumor/blood ratio, and the E. coli expressed fusion protein, MFE23- CPG2, gave tumor: blood ratio of 19:1 at 48 hours, whereas the glycosylated form gave a value of 185:1 at 6 hours after administration. This allows the prodrug to be given 6 hours prior the fusion protein [11].

Fusion proteins have provided some potential benefits which include the possibility to modify them to match necessities. The relatively small size of fusion proteins favors their tumor penetration and rapid clearance from normal cells and plasma, yet, the retention time at tumor site might be shorter than the retention time obtained with chemical conjugates [11].

Specific Design of Adept System

1. β- Lactamase (β-L)

βL is a highly specific enzyme for β-lactams and is not endogenous to the mammalian system and therefore, it is subjected to minimal interference of enzyme substrates and endogenous enzyme systems. βL enzymes have brought a substantial thoughtfulness towards the use of βL for prodrug activation [5, 7, 34]. The Desire to develop a 'dual-action cephalosporin' antibiotics that intended to expel potent antibacterial agents when acted upon by βL producing bacterial strains set the phase for designing cephalosporin-containing anticancer prodrugs [5]. Cephalosporin nitrogen mustard derivatives are an example of one of the first reported cephalosporin-based anticancer prodrug that is activated by broad scale βL enzymes from Enterbacter cloacae. Extension of this work includes prodrugs of other nitrogen mustards, doxorubicin, mitomycin C, vinca alkaloid, and paclitaxel and carboplatinum analogues. A diverse array of βL enzymes from E. cloacae, E. coli, and B. cereus were used to activate these prodrugs [5, 7]. The chemical structures of some of the prodrugs activated by βL enzymes are shown in Figure 3.

One of the first reported in vivo activities of mAb- βL system was cephalosporine- vinca alkaloid prodrug using a βL enzyme from E. cloacae; the prodrug was linked to mAb Fab' fragment such that recognition of CEA, TAG-72 and KS1/4 antigens on tumor tissues was observed. Therapeutic effects of mAb- enzyme conjugate in combination with vinca prodrug were studied in models of human colorectal carcinoma in nude mouse and it was found in all cases to be superior to naked drug therapy [5].

In related studies, doxorubicin and phenylenediamine mustard prodrugs were evaluated in combination with an anti-melanoma mAb– βL conjugate, by which βL enzyme is linked to the Fab' fragment of the 96.5 mAb, which recognizes the melanotransferrin antigen occurs on most melanomas and several carcinomas. The in vitro cytotoxicity results revealed that doxorubicin prodrug, C-Dox, was less toxic than doxorubicin by about nine-fold, whereas the nitrogen mustard prodrug, CCM, was 26 times less toxic than phenylenediamine mustard [5, 34]. Doxorubicin administered systemically at the maximum tolerated dose had negligible activity, whereas the effect of 96.5- βL with CCM was much more noticeable than in those obtained with C-Dox. Regressions in 100% of the treated mice at doses that caused no apparent toxicity were detected [5].

The preparation of the conjugates used in these studies was achieved by linking maleimide-substituted βL to cysteine on the mAb–Fab' fragments which provided a reasonable high tumor to blood ratio nearly 3 days post-administration of the prodrug treatment [5]. A more uniform chemical conjugation strategy to prepare mAb–Fab'– βL conjugates was oxidation of βL threonine with periodate to form an aldehyde which was coupled to βL via a bifunctional cross-linking reagent. Using this approach the conjugate yield was three times higher, and was cleared from the blood more rapidly than with the so called "random chemistry".

Recombinant technology is a sophisticated method for mAb– βL production, and a fusion between the gene encoding variable regions of the anti-carcinoma mAb L6 and the gene encoding B. cereus β L had been achieved, and the corresponding protein was expressed in E. coli and was purified by affinity chromatography and the resulted fusion protein retained enzymatic activity and was able to show in vitro prodrug activation [5]. On the other hand, another related study had used disulfide-stabilized-Fv– βL fusion proteins which were produced in E. coli, by which the mAb fragments used were from a humanized mAb of murine origin, and were fused to RTEM-1 class A βL enzyme, and this fusion protein recognizes p185 (HER2) antigen present in many breast and ovarian carcinomas [5].

The anti-melanotransferrin L49–scFv– βL conjugate consists of mAb binding regions of L49 fused to E. cloacae is one of the most widely studied fusion proteins for prodrug activation. The L49 mAb binds to most human melanomas and to several carcinomas like the 96.5 mAb that was mentioned earlier in this chapter [5]. Studies revealed that L49–scFv– βL retained the antigen binding capability of monovalent L49 as well as the enzymatic activity of βL, and was able to activate CCM in an immunologically specific manner [5]. Interestingly, the fusion protein demonstrated very high tumor to blood ratios after few hours of administration and ratios of 13, 66 and 105 were obtained with 4, 12, and 24 hours post L49–

scFv– βL injections, respectively. In addition, it was possible to effectively administer CCM within 12 hours of the fusion protein because of the rapid kinetics of intratumoral uptake and systemic clearance [5].

Figure 3. Chemical structures of CCM and C-mel prodrugs that are activated by βL enzymes.

The therapeutic effects of both L49–scFv– βL and L49–Fab′– βL in combination with CCM, were compared in two models of human renal carcinoma, and despite the fact that both conjugate/prodrug combinations were very active, L49–scFv– βL showed superiority in both tumor models and used much lower prodrug doses. The differences between the two conjugates become apparent; a high activity is sustained with L49–scFv– βL, but it was lost in the case of L49–Fab′– βL. Hence, the fusion protein is uniform in composition, having an ideal pharmacokinetic profile for prodrug activation, and can lead to noticeable antitumor activities if given in combination with antitumor prodrugs [5].

2. Cytosine Deaminase (CDase, CD)

CDase is present in several bacteria and fungi but not in mammalian cells, because of this reason CDase is currently investigated for use in ADEPT and GDEPT prodrug approaches. ADEPT system is significantly dependent on accomplishing high tumor to non-tumor conjugate ratios at the time of a prodrug administration, and this is further illustrated with the enzyme CDase, a protein that converts the noncytotoxic antifungal drug, 5-fluorocytosine (5FC), to the approved anticancer agent 5-fluorouracil (5FU). Importantly, CDase activity is absent in humans, explaining the tolerability of high doses of 5FC when treating fungal infections [5, 7, 32, 34].

Chemical conjugation between CDase from yeast and L6 mAb (H2981- specific) was designed, where the L6-CDase conjugate showed a full binding and enzymatic activities and was able to localize in human tumor xenografts in nude mice, nonetheless, clearance from the blood was extremely slow, and it took a prolonged time to obtain low tumor to blood ratios [5].

3. Carboxypeptidase G2 (CPG2)

The bacterial enzyme CPG2 was one of the earliest reported enzymes for anticancer prodrug activation; it is an exoprotease that cleaves terminal glutamic acid amides.

Prodrug **1**, 4[(2- chloroethyl) (2-mesyloxyethyl) amino] benzoyl-L-glutamate, after enzymatic hydrolysis gives the glutamic acid nitrogen mustard **2**. Preliminary studies in nude mice with subcutaneous human choriocarcinoma xenografts using a combination of mAb–CPG2 conjugates with prodrug **1** showed a respected in vivo effects, and the combination of prodrug **1** with Fab'2 fragment of the anti-human chorionic gonadotrophin Ab–W14 conjugated to CPG2 resulted in curing of established tumors after one course of therapy [5, 7, 25, 34].

The first pilot scale clinical trial of ADEPT was commenced between 1991 and 1993 using prodrug **1** in combination with CPG2 and Fab'2 fragment of the anti-CEA mAb A5B7 conjugate in patients with advanced colorectal cancer. This study was carried out after an extensive studies in nude mice with different human xenografts, and evaluation of the prodrug was attained during the initial study stage in order to govern its safety and toxicity [5, 11, 34].

Gamma camera scan showed that radio-labeled conjugate was localized at the tumor site, however, some of the resulted toxicity was thought to be due to the drug solubilization with dimethyl sulfoxide [11].

On the other hand, a new study on the use of triazenes; compounds that belong to a group of alkylating agents which exert their effect by DNA methylation, mediated by methyldiazonium ion, a highly reactive metabolite of triazenes showed a respected anti-cancer effect. Among these compounds is dacarbazine (DTIC), **3** which remains the reference drug in the treatment of metastatic melanoma [35].

Antibody Directed Enzyme Prodrug Therapy (ADEPT)

Figure 4. Conversion of triazine prodrug into the alkylating agent MMT and L- glutamic acid by CPG2.

The biological action of DTIC is as a result of its DNA and RNA alkylation capability. This alkylation is occurred via monomethyltriazene **4** followed by metabolic oxidation by cytochrome P450 enzymes. Since monomethyltriazenes are good leaving groups, coupling these entities to carboxypeptidase substrates was considered to be suitable for prodrugs such as **5,** capable of regenerating the alkylating metabolite **4** via the pathway depicted in Figure 4. Furthermore, triazenes are small molecules with adequate lipophilicity, therefore, they will be free to diffuse throughout the tumor sites [35].

4. Nintroresuctase (NR)

Nitroreductase has been isolated from E. coli, and it uses NADH or NADPH as a cofactor, and is inhibited by the DT-diaphorase inhibitor dicoumarol [34].This enzyme catalyzes the activation of the antitumor prodrug CB1954 to the cytotoxic metabolite 5-aziridin-1-yl-4-hydroxylamino-2-nitrobenzamide, and it has been shown that NR- CB 1954 conjugation was cytotoxic to V 79 cells that were only insensitive toward CB 1954 [7, 34, 36].

5. Purine- Nucloside Phosphorylase

The phosphorylase enzyme is found in bacteria, such as E. coli, and mammals where it is located especially in liver, brain, thyroid, kidney, and spleen and the highest concentrations found in the kidney, peripheral lymphocytes and granulocytes. This enzyme can be used in ADEPT, GDEPT, and VDEPT approaches that utilize prodrugs which cannot be activated by human purine-nucleoside phosphorylases due to large differences in the specificity of E. coli and human purine-nucleoside phosphorylases [34].

9-(-β-2-deoxy-erythropentofuranosyl)-6-methylpurine (MeP-dR) prodrug is activated by E. coli purine-nucleoside phosphorylase to its active metabolite, 6-methylpurine, and it has showed 20-fold less cytotoxicity to Hep-2 cells than 6-methylpurine, however, the corresponding mammalian enzymes cannot catalyze this conversion. This is the reason why ADEPT/GDEPT approaches were developed and have shown success in the treatment of human colon carcinoma, melanoma, breast and prostate cancer [34].

6. Alkaline Phosphatase (AP)

AP is widely distributed, therefore, it cannot be used for local prodrugs activation except by using ADEPT, GDEPT, or VDEPT approaches.

Using the ADEPT strategy which involves the L6-AP conjugate the activation of the prodrugs mitomycin C phosphate, p-[N,N-bis(2-chloroethyl)amino]phenyl phosphate and p-[N,N-bis(2-chloroethyl)amino]phenol and N-(4-phosphonooxy) phenylacetyl)-doxorubicin was studied. The study revealed that the cytotoxicity of these prodrugs was largely enhanced after being activated by AP [7, 32, 34, 37].

7. β - Glucuronidase

β-Glucuronidase prodrugs problems include their rapid clearance, predominant activation in inflammatory necrotic tumor areas, and their very poor cell uptake. These had led to a lack of intracellular activation, therefore, ADEPT and GDEPT approaches have been developed in an attempt to overcome these obstacles [34, 38].

Example for such approach is mAb–β-glucuronidase (mAb–GUS) fusion protein for the doxorubicin glucuronide prodrug activation, where the fusion protein consists of a Fab' fragment of the anti-CEA mAb BW431 linked to human placental GUS [5].

In vivo experiments were conducted in nude mice with subcutaneous human colorectal carcinoma xenografts by injecting the fusion protein, followed by an administration of doxorubicin glucuronide prodrug at 1/6 the maximum tolerated dose. 7 days later, interestingly, significant therapeutic effects were acquired and were greater than those accomplished by systemic doxorubicin treatment, and the conjugate was localized in the tumors, but blood and normal tissue clearance time was almost 7 days due to the conjugate high molecular weight (greater than 250 kDa) [5, 11]. It was proven by pharmacokinetic studies that BW431–GUS/prodrug conjugate led to higher intratumoral and lower normal tissue doxorubicin levels than the treatment with doxorubicin. More importantly, this work had exposed some degree of prodrug own selectivity against tumors, owing to a release of lysosomal GUS from necrotic sites within solid tumors. Therefore, doxorubicin glucuronide prodrug is considered for development in the untargeted form as a tumor-selective prodrug [5].

Site-directed mutagenesis to form enzymes that hydrolyze biologically stable prodrugs is one of the most sophisticated approaches towards the use of human enzymes for anticancer prodrug activation, and for that a sequence of methotrexate amides were assessed for stability towards human pancreatic extracts; a major source for carboxypeptidase A1 (hCPA1), where methotrexate-phenylalanine was found to be rapidly hydrolyzed, whereas some of the hindered derivatives, specifically methotrexate-α-3-cyclobutylphenylalanine and methotrexate-α-3-cyclopentyltyrosine were stable [5].

8. Penicilline Amidase

This enzyme is present in different bacteria such as E. coli and it is not in humans. Different prodrugs were tested in conjugation with this enzyme, Doxorubicin-N-p-hydroxyphenoxyacetamide (DPO) is one example of such prodrugs; it was synthesized as a prodrug for doxorubicin which is activated by bacterial penicillin V amidase (PVA). This prodrug was found to be 20 to 80-fold less cytotoxic than its corresponding drug. Pretreatment of lung carcinoma cell line and B-cell lymphoma cell line with the enzyme immunoconjugate resulted in a 12.5-fold and 7.5-fold enhancement in the cytotoxicity in comparison with the treatment with the prodrug alone. Cytotoxicity using this approach was lower than after treatment with doxorubicin alone, demonstrating partial prodrug activation [34, 39].

9. Carboxylesterase

Carboxylesterases are widely distributed, as a result they cannot be used to activate prodrugs locally, yet, they can be used with ADEPT or GDEPT approaches, and carboxylesterase prodrugs have been developed mainly to increase the bioavailability of cytostatic drugs [34].

Example of clinically used prodrug is camptothecin analog, 7-ethyl-10-[4-(1-piperidino)-1-piperidino] carbonyloxycamptothecin (CPT-11, irinotecan). It is activated by carboxylesterase enzymes to a potent DNA topoisomerase I inhibitor 7-ethyl-10-hydroxycamptothecin (SN-38). Details on this approach will be discussed later on this chapter [34, 40].

10. Prodrugs in Adept

A matching pair of enzyme and prodrug is required for the ADEPT approach. Tumors with poor vascularization are considered a major problem for cancer therapy in general [23].Tremendously important for efficacy are the delivery and penetration of molecules across the physiological barriers of the tumor. Two important factors control the compound uptake into the tumor and they are: the extraction coefficient by the tumor and the blood flow [23]. Chemical structure of the prodrug (such as lipophilicity) and the properties of the physiological barrier are determinant for the prodrug extracted portion from the blood flow by the tumor, therefore perceptibly, a prodrug can be designed to meet the optimum lipophilicity, on the other hand, the blood flow is a tissue related concern [23]. Other factors to be considered are the pharmacokinetic properties of the prodrug and the likelihood for leak-back of the drug from the tumor site [23].

In order to design effective prodrugs, a number of requirements need to be met: the prodrug must be noticeably less toxic than the active drug, and the selection of the linkage of the cytotoxic agent should be taken into consideration in the design phase. The drug's functional group critical for cytotoxicity should be attached to the enzyme's substrate moiety, and the latter should have good binding affinity to the enzyme and be converted only by the target antibody-enzyme conjugate, and not by the host enzymes [2, 9, 17, 32]. Additionally, the prodrug needs to be activated and retain activity at the cancer sites only. This means that the active drug should initiate its cytotoxic effect on DNA as soon as it reaches it. Hence, antimetabolites are not good candidates due to the extended period of time needed to cause blocking of DNA synthesis. Moreover, optimum half- life is required in which long half-life would allow back diffusion to the blood whereas short half-life might not be long enough to take advantage of the drug's diffusibility [11]. It is also desirable to have the active drug behaves in a dose dependent manner, and the prodrug should neither be excreted from the body fast enough nor enter cells randomly, and for both reasons the prodrug should possess suitable polarity [11, 17].

Cytotoxic drugs are potential candidates for this approach. Agents have been chosen based on their ability to show some selectivity and cytotoxicity, however, the active drug should be much more cytotoxic than its prodrug [3].

Drugs released by various targeted enzymes can be clinically approved, such as etoposide, doxorubicin, paclitaxel and methotrexate. Furthermore, compounds with similar structural features to approved anticancer medications, such as nitrogen mustards, platinum derivatives and vinca derivatives, drugs that are too toxic to be administered systemically, such as palytoxin, potent nitrogen mustards, cyanide and enediynes, and prodrugs of clinically approved anticancer agents have a potential to obtain an anticipated activities and toxicities using the ADEPT approach (Table 3) [5].

Table 3. Enzymes and related drugs for ADEPT

Enzyme	Active drug released	Ref.
Alkaline phosphatase	Doxorubicin	[7, 38]
	Etoposide	[7, 27]
	Mitomycin	[7, 28]
	Phenol mustard	[37]
Carboxypeptidase A	Methotrexate	[7, 41]
Carboxypeptidase G2	Nitrogen mustard	[23, 25]
Cytosine deaminase	5- Fluorouracil	[7]
α- Galactosidase	Doxorubicin	[42]
β- Galactosidase	Anthracyclin derivatives	[43]
	5- Fluorouracil	[44]
β- Glucuronidase	Doxorubicin	[45]
	Phenol mustard	[46]
β- Lactamase	Nitrogen mustard	[47]
	Doxorubicin	[48]
	Mitomycin	[49]
	Vinca derivatives	[50]
	Palitaxel	[51]
Nitroreductase	Mitomycin C	[52]
	Doxorubicin	[52]
	Nitrogen mustard derivatives	[52]
Penicillin amidase	Doxorubicin	[7, 53]
	Melphalan	[7, 53]
	Palytoxin	[7, 54]

Prodrugs Established for Adept

1. Alkylating Agent's Prodrugs

Prodrugs [55-57] derived from alkylating agents are widely used in many ADEPT approaches with a variety of activating enzymes (e.g., CPG2, AP, β-L, β-G). There are a number of reasons encouraging the use of alkylating agents because the active cytotoxic moieties released by these agents have shown cell cycle-independent activity, a good diffusion properties in tissues, equal toxic to well oxygenated and hypoxic cells, dose dependent and effective against quiescent cells and induce less acquired resistance than other chemotherapeutic agents; thus, they are likely to be fatal to all cells at high concentrations [3, 7, 23].

Variations of more than 100-fold in the chemical reactivity of the prodrug and its active drug have been measured, and prodrugs that have the capability to release their active drugs with very short half-lives have been designed [23].

The bacterial activating enzyme, CPG2, was used in the early ADEPT approach and a cleavable amide bond that linked between an aromatic ring and a glutamic acid moiety was used in order to enable conversion of the nitrogen mustard drugs into the designed prodrugs and to be activated in later stages by CPG2 [2, 23].

The enzymatic cleavage of prodrug **6**, 4[(2-chloroethyl) (2 mesyloxyethyl) amino] benzoyl-l-glutamate, CMDA (Figure 5) releases the active drug **7** which is more reactive than **6**. Studies on ADEPT for this system demonstrated the ability to achieve both the ablation of growth delays of OvCar-433 ovarian human tumor xenografts (using an anti-carcino-embryonic antigen (CEA) Ab-A5B7 linked to CPG2) and chemo-resistant choriocarcinoma human tumor CC3 xenografts in nude mice with one course of treatment (using anti-human chorionic gonadotrophin Ab, W14, conjugated to CPG2) [23, 58].

A CPG2 and ICR12 monoclonal antibody conjugation with prodrug **1** was used in ADEPT study in mice bearing MDA MB 361 tumors. The study showed prompt sustained dose-dependent deteriorations and stasis which persevered for up to 90 days after only one course of treatment, whereas ineffectiveness was shown with a control chemotherapy in the same tumor model with conventional drugs at maximum endured doses [23].

Figure 5. Enzymatic cleavage of prodrug **6** to **7**.

As we mentioned earlier, a pilot scale clinical trial in patients with colorectal carcinoma using CMDA was conducted, and the study results have verified the ADEPT viability, however, myelosuppression occurred as a side effect due to long half-life of the activated drug which diffused back to the bloodstream and caused this kind of toxicity [59]. Therefore, additional studies concerning the design of prodrug systems activated by CPG2 were initiated and aimed to prevent active drug leakback from the tumor [23].

Recently, a new bisiodophenol mustard compound, 4[bis(2-iodoethyl)amino-phenyl]oxycarbonyl-L-glutamic acid, named ZD2767P, found to be a good substrate for CPG2 and has shown a release of the active drug ZD2767D, a nitrogen mustard that is very potent against tumor cells (IC50= 0.33 μM) with very short half- life thus preventing a leak back from the tumor (Figure 6) [15, 23]. ZD2767 has replaced CMDA because of its decreased half- life (2 minutes) and increased potency, and CPG2- anti- CEA conjugate combination with ZD2767P has been reported to cause improvement in antitumor activity in a colorectal tumor xenograft model [58]. The drug was able to kill both quiescent and proliferating LoVo cells, and it was at least 300- fold more potent than the original benzoic acid mustard drug used in the early ADEPT experiments [60].

Figure 6. Chemical structures of ZD2767P and ZD2767D.

Alkaline phosphate enzyme (AP) and prodrugs that are cleaved by this enzyme were also used in some of the early ADEPT systems. Several AP conjugates with antibodies: L6, 1F5 (directed against antigen on human carcinomas) and BW 431/26 (an anti-CEA antibody) were used to convert prodrugs to their active drugs; phenol mustard phosphate (POMP) **8** was one of those prodrugs that were examined using the ADEPT system.

-Gβ-G, despite being of mammalian origin, was received a good attention as it was anticipated to have advantages over other enzymes in ADEPT. For instance, β-G has a high specificity for the glucuronyl residue and little recognition for the aglycone, and its human serum concentration is very low. Additionally, some studies proposed that retransformation of activated prodrug that was not taken up by tumor cells to the corresponding inactive glucuronide in organs possessing high levels of UDPGT could occur, thus, a number of prodrugs were developed to be activated by β-G such as the alkylating agent prodrug, 4-[bis(2-chloroethyl)aminophenyl]-b-glucopyranosyl-uronicacidtetra-N-butyl ammonium salt, **9**, (BHAMG) which was shown to be cleaved by β-G to release the corresponding nitrogen mustard **10** (HAM), where the prodrug: drug cytotoxicity ratio in colorectal carcinoma cell line was 56: 1 (IC50 for **10** = 34 μM and IC50 for **9**= 1890 μM) [23].

Another activating enzyme that has been utilized in ADEPT is NR from E. coli, used in conjunction with alkylating agent prodrugs, wherein the exceptional activity of the prodrug CB 1954, **11,** was identified against the rat Walker carcinosarcoma. Studies have proved that CB 1954 is converted specifically by the rat DT-diaphorase present in the Walker tumor, to a potent difunctional agent, **12,** that has the ability to cause DNA-DNA interstrand crosslink, however, the associated disadvantage with this approach is the requirement of an additional reducing co-substrate for cytotoxic activation since NADH or NAD(P)H is required. However, to overcome this problem, enzyme-selective co-substrates with longer biological half-lives than NADH or NAD(P)H have been developed [23, 34].

Another evaluated enzyme in an ADEPT system which utilizes alkylating agent prodrugs was PVA. PVA has the advantage of being readily available as it is involved in industrial manufacturing of the penicillanic acid. A number of nitrogen mustard prodrugs were synthesized and were inactivated by acetylation of their amino functions. An example for such approach is the 4-hydroxyphenyloxyacetamide derivative of melphalan (**13,** MelPO), the prodrug was approximately 10^2 less toxic than its parent drug [23, 34, 39].

2. Prodrugs Developed from Enediynes

The enediynes represent a class of extremely toxic anticancer antibiotics (e.g., esperamycin, IC50 =30 pM against L1210 cells), and potent synthetic analogues have been synthesized in which after activation they undergo internal cyclization leading to benzene-1,4 di-radicals that has the ability to simultaneously extracting protons from ribose moieties on each DNA chain, generating double-strand breaks [23].

3. Prodrugs Developed from Anti Metabolites

Prodrugs Developed from MTX

Methotrexate-L- α-L- alanine (**14**, MTX- α-ala) was used with the enzyme CPA in the early ADEPT system, and the reason behind this is the fact that derivatization of MTX carboxyl group by an amide or an ester greatly impaired the internalization of MTX by active transport, that's why it was suggested that MTX- α-peptides could be enzymatically hydrolyzed by Ab-CPA conjugates, liberating MTX, **15** [23].

Studies revealed a toxicity enhancement of compound **14** against L1210 mouse leukemia cells when CPA was added to the system (from IC50=2.0 MμM to IC50 = 0.085MμM) whilst compound **15** alone was more cytotoxic (IC50 = 0.024MμM) [23].

Prodrugs Developed from 5- Fluorouracil

This system was considered to take advantage of the transformation of the antifungal agent 5-fluorocytosine (**16**, 5-FC) into the well-known anticancer agent, 5-fluorouracil (**17, 5-FU**), and to be used in human colon cancer which is refractory to many other chemotherapeutic approaches. The cytotoxicity was measured in H2981 human lung adenocarcinoma cells for both the prodrug and the drug. The IC50 for 5-FU was 20 M μM whereas 5-FC proved to be non-cytotoxic, however, the L6-CD (L6 binds H2981cells) conjugate with 5-FC was as cytotoxic as 5-FU alone [23].

Further studies demonstrated that a clearing step using L6-anti-idiotypic 13B clearing Ab given 24 hours after L6-CD conjugate increased the tumor: blood ratio from 1.3:1 to 42:1, and as a result more than 800 mg/kg of 5-FC could be administered, while the maximum tolerated dose of 5-FU was only 90 mg/ kg [23].

4. Prodrugs Developed from Natural Anti-Cancer

Prodrugs Developed from Anthracyclin and Other Anti Cancer Antibiotics

Due to the potent antineoplastic activity of the anthracyclin antibiotics they were the main compounds chosen for ADEPT. Several systems were developed, and one of the early ones used was AP in combination with a doxorubicin-phosphate (DOX-P), prodrug **18**, which has a cytotoxicity less than that of doxorubicin which was increased by the L6-AP conjugate addition [23].

Prodrugs Developed from Antimitotic Compounds

Anticancer compounds that can be cleaved by AP enzyme were used in order to convert etoposide phosphate, **19** (EP) to its parent drug. Prodrug **19** (EP) was selected due to its vulnerability to be cleaved by AP enzyme and because it has IC50 of 100 times lower than that of its parent drug [23]. For etoposide, the IC50 =1 M µM in H3347 50 metastatic human colon carcinoma cells was determined, compared to only 35% inhibition at 100 M µM for EP in the same system [23].

Other studies aimed to prove that combination of prodrugs activated by a single enzyme, with increased tumor specificity and antitumor efficacy as well as, possibly, avoidance or delay of drug resistance development are the prodrug irinotecan (CPT-**11**) and a novel dipiperidinyl derivative of etoposide [1,4'-dipiperidine-1'-carboxylate-etoposide (dp-VP16)]. The rabbit carboxylesterase (rCE) enzyme was shown to efficiently activate both prodrugs [18].

dp-VP 16

Another class of compounds which is a good candidate to be utilized in ADEPT is vinca alkaloids, such as 4-desacetylvinblastinehydrazide, DAVLBH, due to their cytotoxic potency (IC50=M 10^{-2} μM) Several types of cephalosporin-DAVLH derivatives were synthesized and studied, such as cephem-sulfoxide **20** which was chosen for advance investigation. The study on **20** and its parent drug showed a cytotoxicity difference of 5- fold between the prodrug and its active drug, DAVLBH [23].

20

5. Prodrugs Developed from Toxines

PGA enzyme cleaves the acetamido bond of substrates. Palytoxin (PTX) a compound isolated from the Hawaiian tropical coelenterate; palythoatuberculosa, kills cells that express the Na-K-ATPase-associated receptors. PYX possess one of the most potent cytotoxic substances known (IC50= 3.10^{-6} μM in H2981 cells), and its corresponding 4-

hydroxyphenyloxyacetamide (NHPAP) proved to be 10^3-fold less toxic than PTX with an IC50 $>10^{-2}$ μM in H2981 cells, and when cells were pretreated with PGA, then by NHPAP, the cytotoxicity of the prodrug equaled that of PTX (IC50 = 4×10^{-6} μM) [23].

6. Duocarmycins and Antibiotic cc-1065 Based Prodrugs

Early investigations using prodrug **21** in the presence of the antibody–β-glucosidase conjugate showed no therapeutic effect. Since then, new suggestions and modifications to yield an effective cytotoxic agent have initiated, and it was proposed that for a successful cancer therapy, the IC50 value of the cytotoxic agent derived from the prodrug should be less than 10 nM. In addition, the cytotoxicity ratio between the prodrug and the corresponding drug should exceed 1000 (Figure 7) [20, 61].

Figure 7. Activation of the acetal glycoside BE-1. 21 a first generation prodrug by an antibody- B-glycosidase conjugate to give the alkylating agent 22 as the active drug.

CC-1065 antibiotic is a good target to pursue because it acquires a high cytotoxicity with an IC50 of about 0.03 nM. It contains a spirocyclopropyl-cyclohexadienone moiety that is able to alkylate N3 of adenine in AT-rich parts of the DNA minor groove [14, 61].

One study that investigated the enzyme-immuno conjugate of the seco-CBI-Q-galactoside, **23** having the group ind2, showed promising results; presence of - β-D-galactosidase led to the highly cytotoxic CBI, **24**. Further, the study showed that prodrug **23** is nontoxic to normal organs and blood parameters of SCID mice using therapeutic doses. The study indicated that prodrug **23** was not converted into **24** by the enzymes expressed by the SCID mice. The study concluded that prodrug **23** showed high potency, excellent selectivity, low systemic toxicity, water solubility due to the presence of sugar moiety and cell membrane impermeability, which allows for cellular human galactosidase to be used for activation [14, 61].

The newly synthesized third-generation compounds revealed an excellent characteristics, QIC50 values of up to 4800 and a very high cytotoxicity of the corresponding drugs (e.g., IC50 = 4.5 pM), and the most promising candidates for clinical studies were prodrugs **26** and **27**, that are currently under investigation by pharmaceutical companies [20]. These prodrugs are analogs of the highly cytotoxic natural antibiotics CC-1065 and the duocarmycins, and exert their cytotoxic action presumably through a sequence-selective alkylation of double-stranded DNA [20].

7. Prodrugs for Reductive Activation

Beside the previously described prodrugs, new techniques concerning the incorporation of prodrugs that are reductively activated have been designed to target hypoxic tumor tissues that are known to overexpress several endogenous reductive enzymes.

As known, hypoxia is a common feature of most solid tumors occurring from ineffective microvascular systems associated with rapid tumor growth, which creates a leaky vasculature and lethargic blood flow that leads to increased pressure and low pO2 within all of the tumors except for the periphery and hypoxic tumor cells. This allow for radiotherapy and chemotherapy resistance and cause for huge challenge to cancer therapy due to the following reasons: (i) the remoteness of hypoxic cells from blood vessels and anticancer drugs usually cannot reach these hypoxic tumor cells, (ii) the possibility of re-oxygenation and growing of hypoxic cells once using a treatment that kills better-oxygenated cells making a significant contribution to repopulation of the tumors, (iii) persistence of tumor cells in the hypoxic environment that might encourage the growth of more malignant tumor cells and (iv) up-regulation of genes associated in drug resistance including genes encoding p-glycoprotein by tumor cells adapted to hypoxia [6, 17, 62-64].

Alternatively, hypoxia represents new opportunities for selective cancer treatment as it differentiates tumor cells, particularly solid tumor cells from normal cells, and the advantages of having limited side effect due to the limited effect of the prodrug on hypoxic tumor region after activation since the release of the active drug achieved upon reduction under hypoxic environment [62].

Several anticancer prodrugs have been designed to use both the endogenous and exogenous reductive enzymes that are either one- or two-electron reducing systems, such as NADPH-cytochrome P450 reductase, DT-diaphorase, xanthine oxidase/xanthine dehydrogenase, and cytochrome b5 reductase, for selective activation, and four major classes of anticancer prodrugs have been explored for reductive activation: quinones, nitroaromatics, N-oxides, and metal complexes [62, 64].

A- Quinones

Quinine containing compounds are important class of biologically active agents because they have strong inclination to form a fully aromatic system, and the first clinically used quinone-containing drug documented as a bioreductive and hypoxia-selective alkylating agent is Mitomycin C (MMC, **28**). Its mechanism of action is via a reductive metabolism followed by well-defined fragmentation to bifunctional alkylating species that crosslink DNA through guanine–guanine in the major groove [62].

Other examples are EO9 (**29**) and AZQ (**30**) which are two principal aziridinyl-quinones, analogues of MMC developed as hypoxia selective agents, and they were shown to be potent alkylating agents once they are reduced to the corresponding aziridinyl hydroquinone. The reduction step results in an increase of the aziridine nitrogen efficiently for protonation and activation. It should be mentioned that EO9 is in clinical trial for bladder tumor [62].

Anticancer drugs can also be released from benzoquinone conjugates; one example is the conjugate **31** of the nitrogen mustard which under hypoxic conditions is activated to produce 4-[bis(2-chloroethyl)amino]benzoic acid and under physiological pH, the anionic nature of the carboxylate increases the electron density of the aromatic ring which favors the formation of the aziridinium species that have the ability to alkylate DNA [62].

B. Nitroaromatics

A number of flavoprotein enzymes can reduce nitroaromatic compounds in cells via stepwise addition of up to six electrons; still, the major enzymatic metabolite is usually hydroxylamine, and RSU1069, **32**, was the first agent displaying a significant enhancement in hypoxia selectivity which is functioning as a bifunctional alkylating agent upon reduction [62].

C. N- Oxides

N-oxides containing compounds were defined as cytotoxic agents as early as the 1960s and because of their potential to be selectively reduced under hypoxic conditions or by certain reducing enzymes; they have received attention as bioreductively activated prodrugs. Examples of such class are tirapazamine (TPZ, **33**); investigated for uterine cervix tumor, and AQ4N (**34**) studied for brain tumor, chronic lymphocytic leukemia and non- Hodgkin lymphoma. Both prodrugs were advanced into clinical trials and have shown promising results in combination with radiotherapy and other chemotherapies [62].

D. Metal Complexes as Prodrugs

Metal complexes, especially those of cobalt, have been exploited as potential prodrugs to target tumor hypoxia due to the fact that metal complexes with cytotoxic ligands at high oxidation state would either stabilize the active cytotoxic agents or protect them from rapid metabolism and that the complexes once reduced would become unstable somewhat at the lower oxidation state releasing the corresponding cytotoxic ligands. Therefore, a design requirement for such prodrug is a metal ion of two accessible oxidation states and a large stability difference between the complexes of the different oxidation states for an efficient release of the active cytotoxic agent [62].

E. Miscellaneous Prodrugs

Disulfide and azido functional groups have been used in the design of prodrugs to selectively target hypoxic tumor cells. For example, several prodrugs of paclitaxel; one of the most extensively used anticancer agents and is effective in many types of cancer, have been designed in an attempt to overcome the problems associated with their parent drug, such as low aqueous solubility, dose-limiting toxicity, and drug resistance. The ACE inhibitor, captopril, having anti-angiogenic effects, was attached to paclitaxel at 20-OH through a 2, 2-dimethyl-4-mercaptobutyricacid linker to give the conjugate **35**. This was done in order to achieve reductive activation in hypoxic tumor tissues and to improve solubility. The study revealed that conjugate **35** underwent cyclization with a half-life of 25 minutes upon reduction by DTT, and it was found to have superior in-vivo anticancer activity compared to paclitaxel [62].

Decreasing Enzyme Activity in Blood by Enhancing AEC Clearance

Most of the administered enzymes present in normal tissues hours-days after the administration of a conjugate. Furthermore, human normal tissues constitute a 50-500-fold greater volume than tumor tissues, therefore, it is expected that a prodrug will be transformed to its active drug in normal tissues in larger extent than in tumor tissues. Hence, a clearance method of enzymes from the blood before an administration of a prodrug is a crucial step in utilizing the ADEPT system [2, 11].

Clearance of AEC conjugate from plasma can be speeded up by the use of a three-phase system, in which a galactosylated anti-enzyme antibody is used to inactivate and clear the circulating enzyme antibodies directed at any part of the AEC conjugate via the galactose receptors on hepatocytes. An example of this method is SB43, a monoclonal antibody directed against and inactivates the enzyme CPG2. In a clinical trial of ADEPT using A5B7-F(ab')2- CPG2 conjugate and the galactosylated SB43 clearing antibody, the tumor: blood ratio exceeded 10000: 1 [11, 65]. Despite these promising results, the use of a clearing antibody might augment the complexity of a third treatment stage for ADEPT. Therefore, new investigations on whether glycosylation of the antibody-enzyme moiety might result in rapid clearance and favorable tumor: normal tissue ratios of enzyme activity were pursued in order to optimize and simplify the system [66]. For instance, MFE-CP, a recombinant fusion protein of CPG2 with MFE-23, an anti-CEA single chain Fv antibody variable fragment, was designed for ADEPT and showed effective localization for MFE-CP to CEA-expressing tumors but without clearing rapidly from the normal tissues, however, adding branched mannose to MFE-CP allowed for rapid clearance from the circulation and mediated the uptake of MFE-CP by mannose receptors, and provided MFE-CP in the glycosylated form [66, 67].

Biodistribution studies of radiolabeled MFE-CP using different techniques have shown that MFE-CP is able to penetrate through tumor tissues and showed favored localization in the CEA positive viable regions [67]. Although the glycol-forms have a highly favorable influence on the clearance of the therapeutic from the bloodstream, it should not impair the biological functions of the fusion protein, especially the enzyme localization in the tumor [66].

The second technique used to enhance the clearance of AEC that do not bind to tumor antigen and remained in the blood is anti-PEG IgM antibody, which binds to pegylated antibody-enzyme conjugate and speeds up its clearance causing an increase in the tumor: blood ratio from 3.9 to 29.6 without any reduction of the conjugate at the tumor site [11].

The third reported technique involves two complementary therapies; (1) an antivascular agent, agent such as 5,6-dimethylxanthenone-4-acetic acid (DMXAA) which destroys tumor vasculature that selectively inhibits tumor blood flow causing extensive hemorrhagic necrosis to the central zone, and (2) an antitumor antibody conjugated to therapeutics, which selectively targets tumor cells, able to terminate the surviving outer zone of viable cells as well preserves high levels of conjugate inside the tumor mass but not in normal tissues. This results in retention of high tumor levels of AEC conjugate at the time of prodrug administration, followed by blood vessel destruction by DMXAA which allows for more prodrug to be converted to the active drug leading to enhanced tumor growth inhibition [63].

Another technique described to accelerate the clearance of AEC was based on using anti-idiotypic antibodies. It uses the differences between the prodrug and the active drug in which the active toxic drug might be selectively degraded by an enzyme that does not degrade the prodrug [2].

Supression of Immune Response Against Aec

A number of clinical trials of ADEPT systems on the bacterial enzyme CPG2 has been conducted, and the clinical benefit of the ADEPT method has been proved by these trails [68, 69]. Yet, all patients developed antibodies against the protein components which restricted the rapid repetition. Meanwhile, it is not known if CPG2 contains any T-cell epitopes, still, number of factors could be attributed to the immunogenicity observed in these ADEPT trials [33]. It has been known that chemical conjugates of proteins have high immunogenicity rate and all issued trials used chemical conjugates to connect antibody fragments with carboxypeptidase. In addition, carboxypeptidase is a dimeric enzyme, therefore, any conjugation would have a relative slow plasma clearance, in contrast to β-lactamase which is a monomeric protein and has a fast plasma clearance [33]. Therefore, it is important to find a way to minimize or suppress antibody responses against the enzyme–antibody conjugate and to solve the immunogenicity problem in clinical studies of ADEPT [11, 19, 33].

One approach to reduce the effect of an immune response is to use intracellular enzymes. This approach relies on the limited ability of prodrugs to reach these enzymes in healthy tissues in which a human- derived enzyme is engineered to acquire unique substrate specificity [33]. A mutant human enzyme forms have been used to prevent systemic toxicity raised by the use of a variety of human enzymes. An example is a mutant form of human CPA conjugated to a tumor-associated antibody which was effective in activating different types of prodrugs, such as thymidylate synthase inhibitors, GW 1031 and GW 1843, and the dihydrofolate reductase inhibitor, methotrexate, however, not all of these prodrugs were effective substrates for the endogenous CPA enzyme, but in general, using mutant human enzymes may offer less immunogenicity and systemic toxicity than using endogenous enzymes [1].

Additionally, epitope deletion strategy can be used to generate a deimmunized biotherapy, in which a disruption of the interaction between the immunogenic peptide sequences and MHC II and/or T-cell receptors takes place to prevent any immune response. A new approach for protein deimmunization called Dynamic Programming for Deimmunizing Proteins (DP^2) was constructed to optimize a target protein so as to reduce its immunogenicity as assessed by T-cell epitope prediction while maintaining stability and activity. In this approach, P99βL was chosen as a model system, and the goal was a design and construction of efficient enzyme variants that have good catalytic proficiency, high stability and reduced epitope content [70].

Another method used the immunosuppressive agent cyclosporine A, although not desired in cancer and offers only restricted mitigation of an immune response against the conjugate, but it has shown to delay the host immune response against the murine monoclonal antibodies, however, it did not prevent it [3, 11, 19, 33]. Cyclosporine A was used in a pilot-scale clinical trial of ADEPT and when it was given intravenously, blood levels were controlled permitting three cycles of therapy to be administrated during a 21-day cycle, however, advanced research suggests that immune suppression may not be an advantage in some systems, and that ADEPT and the immune system may work synergistically to give an enhanced therapeutic effect [11, 67].

Another approach to modify the immunogenicity of a foreign protein involves pegylation; attachment of polyethylene glycol chains to the protein. Despite some successful results this approach was not pursued further [11, 19].

Abzymes

Most ADEPT systems incorporate bacterial enzymes which decrease potential associated immunogenicity stemming from the nature of the conjugate components. For eliminating this disadvantage the use of a catalytic antibody which can be humanized by existing technologies to decrease their inherent in vivo mammalian immunogenicity will be recommended [12]. Bagshawe and coworkers have suggested the concept of replacing the enzyme component of ADEPT by humanized catalytic antibodies that can provide targeted therapy enhancement [12]. The mAb–enzyme/prodrug therapy that uses catalytic mAbs (abzymes) is known as antibody-directed abzyme prodrug therapy, ADAPT which has the ability to affect prodrug activation [5, 12].

Normally, creation of abzymes achieved by immunization of mice with the reaction transition state analogue (TSA), followed by mAbs isolation by hybridization techniques [5, 12]. The first reported catalytic mAb was the one that was successful in releasing chloramphenicol from an ester prodrug. Since then, catalytic mAbs have proven their ability to activate prodrugs of 5-fluorodeoxyuridine, a nitrogen mustard, doxorubicin and camptothecin. However, and despite the antibody ability to activate their singular prodrug substrates, the catalytic antibodies transition state analog approach mostly offers catalysts that work only on a precise substrate, and not on structurally related analogs. As a result, such antibodies would be anticipated not to be able to activate drugs for which they were not specifically designed. In addition, each of these acyl transfer activation can theoretically be achieved by endogenous enzymes like esterases or proteases which limit the specificity in the activation step. Moreover, catalytic mAbs efficiencies are orders of magnitude lower than that required to achieve in vitro and in vivo immunological specific prodrug activation [5, 19]. For instance, the catalytic mAb defined for d-valine-5-fluorodeoxyuridine ester activation was shown to activate a prodrug, but with 5% molar equivalents of mAb to the prodrug [5].

Single turnover of the prodrug by each mAb variable region can elucidate the perceived cytotoxic effects of the catalytic mAb/prodrug combination. Therefore, there is no any evidence that mAb acts in a catalytic manner. One of the recent studies revealed that a catalytic mAb activated prodrugs of doxorubicin and camptothecin via a sequential retro-aldol/retro-Michael reaction, however, the needed amount of mAb to reach a substantial drug generation was almost stoichiometric [5].

On the other hand, a new approach to catalytic antibodies that involve a process known as reactive immunization has been recently described. This approach was found to be more efficient when combined with the transition state analog approach [19]. Enhanced catalytic proficiency and expansive substrate scope are the primary advantages of prodrug activation. On the other hand, the study demonstrated that the catalytic antibody efficiency achieved by using reactive immunization for the aldol reaction matches those of the natural aldolase enzymes [19].

First studies involving prodrug activation with aldolase antibodies were conducted and prodrugs of doxorubicin and camptothecin were prepared by a design of drug-masking linker that is activated by antibody 38C2 catalysis of successive retro-aldol retro-Michael reactions. However, and in contrary to natural aldolase enzymes that usually operate on phosphorylated sugar derivatives, antibody aldolase 38C2 was able to catalyze the retro-aldol reactions that involve tertiary aldols where no natural enzyme is known to catalyze such process [19].

In order to extend this approach to other anticancer drugs, a prodrug of etoposide was designed, tested in neuroblastoma mouse model. The masking linker in this study was attached to etoposide at the phenolic oxygen. The results revealed that prodrug **36** has proven to be a substrate for antibody 38C2-catalyzed activation and confirmed superior chemical stability and a profound 100-fold reduced toxicity against the NXS2 neuroblastoma cell line [19].

In order to investigate the concept of localized activation of prodrug **36** in an animal model, the prodrug was systemically delivered by intraperitoneal injection (i.p.), and the study results revealed dramatic tumor growth reduction in animals received both the catalytic antibody and prodrug **36**. However, etoposide administration at the maximal tolerated dose of 40 mg/kg revealed a sign of systemic toxicity. It should be indicated that no systemic toxicity was detected in animals treated with prodrug **36** (1,250 mg/kg) at 30-fold the administered dose of etoposide [19]. The absence of any apparent systemic toxicity of prodrug **36** at high doses is considered as an evidence that the drug masking linker is not readily detached by endogenous enzymes, and the localized activation of the prodrug is superior to systemic application of etoposide, suggesting that the active etoposide concentration at the tumor site produced by antibody-catalyzed activation of prodrug **36** exceeded the concentration of etoposide accessible when it is systemically given at the maximal tolerated dose. However, despite the localized activation of the prodrug after intratumoral injection of the catalyst, it seems that this approach will not be applicable to dispersed metastatic disease that requires a development of targeting devices for catalytic antibody 38C2 [19].

Other murine aldolase catalytic antibodies have recently become available and could be humanized by using this method. These antibodies are 84G3 and 93F3 and they are the most effective catalytic antibodies yet reported, achieving rates up to 2 s^{-1}, and accelerations rate (Kcat/ Kuncat) exceeding 10^8 [19].

This catalytic antibody-based prodrug activation system may offer a new non-immunogenic approach to cancer chemotherapy and HIV-1 disease [19].

Nanobody-Based Conjugates As an Efficient Cancer Therapy

Antibodies have received a significant attention to be used for cancer therapy. Homogeneity, nonexistence of regions inclined to aggregate or vulnerable to proteolysis, affinity and specificity, high solubility, and stability are the most important elements to be taken into consideration during the development of effective conjugates for cancer therapy [22].

Searching for a small fragment of antibody that has the ability to bind to antigens started from full antibody molecules to Fab to recombinant single-chain Fv fragments (scFv) (by cloning the corresponding gene fragments and expression in bacteria) as these small molecules have been shown to change the bio-distribution of these recombinant proteins, often improving their access to places that are difficult to reach by larger entities leading to enhance in tumor penetration. In addition, they accelerate blood clearance, and reduce immunogenicity in contrast to the complete antibody. However, an inadequate yield of functional, monomeric products in heterologous expression systems in scFvs and their conjugates remains an obstacle in the development of scFv derivatives for therapeutic purposes and improvements should be made to enhance their stability, expression yield, protease resistance, and aggregation caused by synthetic linkers [22]. The functional heavy-chain antibodies lacking small chains are naturally occurring in different species like nurse sharks where their antigen-binding site is reduced to a single domain. Their VHH domain creates a new prospect to acquire soluble antigen-binding fragments of minimal size that can be affinity-matured in vivo to yield molecules that interact via one variable domain with an antigen having suitable affinity and specificity. This variable fragment with a molecular mass of 15 kDa and atypical immunoglobulin fold and prolate shape (4.4 nm high; 2.8 nm diameter) is referred to as nanobody [22].

In one study, Virna Cortez-Retamozo and coworkers have isolated a panel of anti-CEA nanobodies from a phage-display library derived from in vivo-matured camel heavy-chain antibodies and they recognize different non-overlapping epitopes on the CEA molecule, allowing for the opportunity of generating biparatopic constructs, and for assessment of potential nanobodies to deliver toxic principles to tumors in a selective manner [22].

β-lactamase from E. cloacae P99 was fused to the high-affinity binder cAb-CEA5, where the former was preferred due to its effectiveness in converting many substrates into potent cytotoxic compounds, whereas llama γ2c hinge was used because the natural flexibility of the immunoglobulin hinge guarantees an independent movement of the connected variable domains in immunoglobulins of the natural antibody [22]. The cAb-CEA5: L βL conjugate was extracted as soluble protein and because the nanobody entity in the conjugate recognizes its antigen with the same affinity as the monomer and because the enzyme reserved full enzymatic activity, the conjugate was functional in all aspects. On the other hand, the biodistribution studies indicated that cAb-CEA5: LβL cleared rapidly from the systemic circulation and localized favorably in tumors without the need for a clearance agent.

It was suggested that the required time between the conjugate and prodrug administrations is quiet short because of the highly specific uptake of the immunoconjugate by the tumor and its rapid clearance from non-target tissue [22].

As a result of these satisfactory biophysical and pharmacological properties of nanobodies and the ease of their construction, nanobodies are considered as a promising new generation of antibody- based therapeutics.

Physiologically Based Pharmacokinetic Model (PBPK) Estimation for Adept

Due to the fact that ADEPT system is a complex system, it would be preferable if ultimate expectations of the therapeutic outcome are undertaken before conducting extended and expensive large-scale preclinical and clinical studies.

Pharmacokinetics (PK) and pharmacodynamics (PD) studies application has been shown to be useful in guiding drug development. Both use mathematical modeling for analyzing a complex system into elementary components which allows for better understanding of ADEPT and optimizing the therapeutic regimen [13]. Limited number of publications has used mathematical modeling methods for ADEPT therapy guidance. Those published studies presumed a simple compartment model for AbE, prodrug, and active drug, and the model used is restricted to pharmacokinetic properties of biological molecules. Therefore, PBPK has been suggested as a good tool to predict pharmacokinetic properties of antibodies [13].

PBPK methodology typically includes physiological parameters, such as blood flow rates, organ volumes, drug-dependent parameters, such drug binding and metabolism rates. Moreover, PBPK modeling is able to integrate ADEPT components, such as FcRn, which has a crucial role in antibody recycling and elimination, and tumor size [13, 71].

AEC, Prodrug and Active Drug Distribution

The distribution of AEC, prodrug, and active drug was analyzed with the baseline physiological, biological, and physical parameters, where the tumor/plasma AbE ratio escalates rapidly before day 4, followed by a slowly rising phase up to day 8 explaining the reason behind choosing 3 days baseline interval between AbE and prodrug injection [13].

The distribution of the prodrug between tumor and normal tissues is relatively nonselective; the concentration of the prodrug is much higher in the plasma than in tumor cells, whereas the distribution of the active drug in tumors is higher than in the plasma, and the active drug's AUC ratio according to the baseline parameters is between 1.5 and 2 [13].

Table 4. Baseline values of the model of AbE, prodrug and active drug

Constant	Baseline value
f up prodrug	1
f up drug	1
Kp- prodrug	1
Kp- drug	1
Mwt prodrug (Dalton)	700
Pprodrug (cm/s)	1.4×10^{-5}
Pdrug (cm/s)	5×10^{-3}
Emax (1/min)	6000
EC50 prodrug (M)	200
Surface area in muscle (cm2)	1.24
PStumor/PSmuscle	10
PSliver/PSmuscle	10
PSorgan/PSmuscle (organs other than liver and tumor)	1
Clint_prodrug (ml/min)	1
Clint_drug (ml/min)	1
Dose_AbE (mol)	10^{-11}
Interval between AbEand prodrug (days)	3

Summary and Conclusion

Antibody directed enzyme prodrug therapy (ADEPT) is a new method for cancer treatment. It is a two-step approach where an antibody-drug activating enzyme conjugate (AEC) is given first to be targeted and localized into the tumor and accumulates predominantly at the tumor cells that have the wanted tumor associated antigen. In the second step a nontoxic prodrug is injected systemically to be converted to its corresponding active form with high tumor concentration by the localized enzyme. This method has advantages over the older cancer therapy and is considered as a promising approach in the area of cancer treatment.

References

[1]   Xu, G. & McLeod HL. (2001) Strategies for enzyme/prodrug cancer therapy. Clinical cancer research : an official journal of the American Association for Cancer Research 7, 3314-24.

[2]   Bagshawe KD. (1995) Antibody-directed enzyme prodrug therapy for cancer: its theoretical basis and application. Molecular medicine today 1, 424-31.

[3]   Bagshawe KD. (1989) The First Bagshawe lecture. Towards generating cytotoxic agents at cancer sites. British journal of cancer 60, 275-81.

[4]   Teicher BA, Chari RV. (2011) Antibody conjugate therapeutics: challenges and potential. Clinical cancer research : an official journal of the American Association for Cancer Research 17, 6389-97.

[5]   Senter PD, Springer CJ. (2001) Selective activation of anticancer prodrugs by monoclonal antibody-enzyme conjugates. Advanced drug delivery reviews 53, 247-64.

[6]   Jain RK. (1989) Delivery of novel therapeutic agents in tumors: physiological barriers and strategies. Journal of the National Cancer Institute 81, 570-6.

[7]   Melton RG, Sherwood RF. (1996) Antibody-enzyme conjugates for cancer therapy. Journal of the National Cancer Institute 88, 153-65.

[8]   Bagshawe KD. (1987) Antibody directed enzymes revive anti-cancer prodrugs concept. British journal of cancer 56, 531-2.

[9]   Bagshawe KD, Sharma SK, Springer CJ, Rogers GT. (1994) Antibody directed enzyme prodrug therapy (ADEPT). A review of some theoretical, experimental and clinical aspects. Annals of oncology : official journal of the European Society for Medical Oncology / ESMO 5, 879-91.

[10] Mayer A, Sharma SK, Tolner B, Minton NP, Purdy D, Amlot P, Tharakan, G. Begent, R. H. Chester, K. A. (2004) Modifying an immunogenic epitope on a therapeutic protein: a step towards an improved system for antibody-directed enzyme prodrug therapy (ADEPT). British journal of cancer 90, 2402-10.

[11] Bagshawe KD, Sharma SK, Begent RH. (2004) Antibody-directed enzyme prodrug therapy (ADEPT) for cancer. Expert opinion on biological therapy 4, 1777-89.

[12] Wentworth P, Datta A, Blakey D, Boyle T, Partridge LJ, Blackburn GM. (1996) Toward antibody-directed "abzyme" prodrug therapy, ADAPT: carbamate prodrug activation by a catalytic antibody and its in vitro application to human tumor cell

killing. *Proceedings of the National Academy of Sciences of the United States of America 93*, 799-803.

[13] Fang L, Sun D. (2008) Predictive physiologically based pharmacokinetic model for antibody-directed enzyme prodrug therapy. *Drug metabolism and disposition: The biological fate of chemicals 36*, 1153-65.

[14] Tietze LF, Feuerstein T. (2003) Highly selective compounds for the antibody directed enzyme prodrug therapy of cancer. *Australian journal of chemistry 56*, 841-54.

[15] Shukla GS, Krag DN. (2006) Selective delivery of therapeutic agents for the diagnosis and treatment of cancer. *Expert opinion on biological therapy 6*, 39-54.

[16] Yuan F, Baxter LT, Jain RK. (1991) Pharmacokinetic analysis of two-step approaches using bifunctional and enzyme-conjugated antibodies. *Cancer research 51*, 3119-30.

[17] de Groot FM, Damen EW, Scheeren HW. (2001) Anticancer Prodrugs for Application in Monotherapy: Targeting Hypoxia,Tumor-Associated Enzymes, and Receptors. *Current Medicinal Chemistry 8*, 1093- 122.

[18] Yoon KJ, Qi J, Remack JS, Virga KG, Hatfield MJ, Potter PM, Lee, R. E.Danks, M. K. (2006) Development of an etoposide prodrug for dual prodrug-enzyme antitumor therapy. *Molecular cancer therapeutics 5,* 1577-84.

[19] Shabat D, Lode HN, Pertl U, Reisfeld RA, Rader C, Lerner RA, Barbas, C. F., 3rd. (2001) In vivo activity in a catalytic antibody-prodrug system: Antibody catalyzed etoposide prodrug activation for selective chemotherapy. *Proceedings of the National Academy of Sciences of the United States of America 98*, 7528-33.

[20] Tietze LF, Krewer B. (2009) Antibody-directed enzyme prodrug therapy: a promising approach for a selective treatment of cancer based on prodrugs and monoclonal antibodies. *Chemical biology & drug design 74*, 205-11.

[21] Zawilska JB, Wojcieszak J, Olejniczak AB. (2013) Prodrugs: A challenge for the drug development. *Pharmacological reports : PR 65*, 1-14.

[22] Cortez-Retamozo V, Backmann N, Senter PD, Wernery U, De Baetselier P, Muyldermans S, Revets, H. (2004) Efficient cancer therapy with a nanobody-based conjugate. *Cancer research 64,* 2853-7.

[23] Springer CJ, Niculescu-Duvaz II. (1997) Antibody-directed enzyme prodrug therapy (ADEPT): a review. *Advanced drug delivery reviews 26*, 151-72.

[24] Chari RV. (2008) Targeted cancer therapy: conferring specificity to cytotoxic drugs. *Accounts of chemical research 41*, 98-107.

[25] Bagshawe KD, Springer CJ, Searle F, Antoniw P, Sharma SK, Melton RG, Sherwood, R. F. (1988) A cytotoxic agent can be generated selectively at cancer sites. *British journal of cancer 58*, 700-3.

[26] Sharma SK, Boden JA, Springer CJ, Burke PJ, Bagshawe KD. (1994) Antibody-directed enzyme prodrug therapy (ADEPT). A three-phase study in ovarian tumor xenografts. *Cell biophysics 24-25*, 219-28.

[27] Senter PD, Saulnier MG, Schreiber GJ, Hirschberg DL, Brown JP, Hellstrom I, Hellstrom, K. E. (1988) Anti-tumor effects of antibody-alkaline phosphatase conjugates in combination with etoposide phosphate. *Proceedings of the National Academy of Sciences of the United States of America 85*, 4842-6.

[28] Senter PD, Schreiber GJ, Hirschberg DL, Ashe SA, Hellstrom KE, Hellstrom I. (1998) Enhancement of the in vitro and in vivo antitumor activities of phosphorylated

mitomycin C and etoposide derivatives by monoclonal antibody-alkaline phosphatase conjugates. *Cancer research 49*, 5789-92.

[29] Kerr DE, Schreiber GJ, Vrudhula VM, Svensson HP, Hellstrom I, Hellstrom KE, Senter, P. D. (1995) Regressions and cures of melanoma xenografts following treatment with monoclonal antibody beta-lactamase conjugates in combination with anticancer prodrugs. *Cancer research 55*, 3558-63.

[30] Eccles SA, Court WJ, Box GA, Dean CJ, Melton RG, Springer CJ. (1994) Regression of established breast carcinoma xenografts with antibody-directed enzyme prodrug therapy against c-erbB2 p185. *Cancer research 54*, 5171-7.

[31] Han HK, Amidon GL. (2000) Targeted prodrug design to optimize drug delivery. *AAPS pharmSci 2*, E6.

[32] Jungheim LN, Shepherd TA. (1994) Design of Antitumor Prodrugs: Substrates for Antibody Targeted Enzymes. *chemistry review 94*, 1553- 66.

[33] Harding FA, Liu AD, Stickler M, Razo OJ, Chin R, Faravashi N, Viola, W.Graycar, T.Yeung, V. P. Aehle, W.Meijer, D.Wong, S.Rashid, M. H.Valdes, A. M.Schellenberger, V. (2005) A beta-lactamase with reduced immunogenicity for the targeted delivery of chemotherapeutics using antibody-directed enzyme prodrug therapy. *Molecular cancer therapeutics 4*, 1791-800.

[34] Rooseboom M, Commandeur JN, Vermeulen NP. (2004) Enzyme-catalyzed activation of anticancer prodrugs. *Pharmacological reviews 56*, 53-102.

[35] Capucha V, Mendes E, Francisco AP, Perry MJ. (2012) Development of triazene prodrugs for ADEPT strategy: new insights into drug delivery system based on carboxypeptidase G2 activation. *Bioorganic & medicinal chemistry letters 22*, 6903-8.

[36] Knox RJ, Friedlos F, Sherwood RF, Melton RG, Anlezark GM. (1992) The bioactivation of 5-(aziridin-1-yl)-2,4-dinitrobenzamide (CB1954)--II. A comparison of an Escherichia coli nitroreductase and Walker DT diaphorase. *Biochemical pharmacology 44*, 2297-301.

[37] Wallace PM, Senter PD. (1991) In vitro and in vivo activities of monoclonal antibody-alkaline phosphatase conjugates in combination with phenol mustard phosphate. *Bioconjugate chemistry 2*, 349-52.

[38] Senter PD. (1990) Activation of prodrugs by antibody-enzyme conjugates: a new approach to cancer therapy. *FASEB journal : official publication of the Federation of American Societies for Experimental Biology 4*, 188-93.

[39] Kerr DE, Senter PD, Burnett WV, Hirschberg DL, Hellstrom I, Hellstrom KE. (1990) Antibody-penicillin-V-amidase conjugates kill antigen-positive tumor cells when combined with doxorubicin phenoxyacetamide. *Cancer immunology, immunotherapy : CII 31*, 202-6.

[40] Satoh T, Hosokawa M, Atsumi R, Suzuki W, Hakusui H, Nagai E. (1994) Metabolic activation of CPT-11, 7-ethyl-10-[4-(1-piperidino)-1- piperidino]carbonyl oxycamptothecin, a novel antitumor agent, by carboxylesterase. *Biological & pharmaceutical bulletin 17*, 662-4.

[41] Smith GK, Banks S, Blumenkopf TA, Cory M, Humphreys J, Laethem RM, Miller, J.Moxham, C. P. Mullin, R. Ray, P. H. Walton, L. M. Wolfe, L. A., 3rd. (1997) Toward antibody-directed enzyme prodrug therapy with the T268G mutant of human carboxypeptidase A1 and novel in vivo stable prodrugs of methotrexate. *The Journal of biological chemistry 272*, 15804-16.

[42]   Azoulay M, Florent JC, Monneret C, Gesson JP, Jacquesy JC, Tillequin F, Koch, M. Bosslet, K. Czech, J. Hoffman, D. (1995) Prodrugs of anthracycline antibiotics suited for tumor-specific activation. *Anti-cancer drug design 10*, 441-50.

[43]   Bakina E, Farquhar D. (1991) Intensely cytotoxic anthracycline prodrugs: galactosides. *Anti-cancer drug design 14*, 507-15.

[44]   Abraham R, Aman N, von Borstel R, Darsley M, Kamireddy B, Kenten J, Morris, G. Titmas, R. (1994) Conjugates of COL-1 monoclonal antibody and beta-D-galactosidase can specifically kill tumor cells by generation of 5-fluorouridine from the prodrug beta-D-galactosyl-5-fluorouridine. *Cell biophysics 24-25*, 127-33.

[45]   Bosslet K, Czech J, Hoffmann D. (1994) Tumor-selective prodrug activation by fusion protein-mediated catalysis. *Cancer research 54*, 2151-9.

[46]   Cheng TL, Wei SL, Chen BM, Chern JW, Wu MF, Liu PW, Roffler, S. R. (1999) Bystander killing of tumour cells by antibody-targeted enzymatic activation of a glucuronide prodrug. *British journal of cancer 79*, 1378-85.

[47]   Vrudhula VM, Svensson HP, Kennedy KA, Senter PD, Wallace PM. (1993) Antitumor activities of a cephalosporin prodrug in combination with monoclonal antibody-beta-lactamase conjugates. *Bioconjugate chemistry 4*, 334-40.

[48]   Rodrigues ML, Presta LG, Kotts CE, Wirth C, Mordenti J, Osaka G, Wong, W. L. Nuijens, A. Blackburn, B. Carter, P. (1995) Development of a humanized disulfide-stabilized anti-p185HER2 Fv-beta-lactamase fusion protein for activation of a cephalosporin doxorubicin prodrug. *Cancer research 55*, 63-70.

[49]   Vrudhula VM, Svensson HP, Senter PD. (1997) Immunologically specific activation of a cephalosporin derivative of mitomycin C by monoclonal antibody beta-lactamase conjugates. *Journal of medicinal chemistry 40*, 2788-92.

[50]   Meyer DL, Jungheim LN, Law KL, Mikolajczyk SD, Shepherd TA, Mackensen DG, Briggs, S. L.Starling, J. J. (1993) Site-specific prodrug activation by antibody-beta-lactamase conjugates: regression and long-term growth inhibition of human colon carcinoma xenograft models. *Cancer research 53*, 3956-63.

[51]   Rodrigues ML, Carter P, Wirth C, Mullins S, Lee A, Blackburn BK. (1995) Synthesis and beta-lactamase-mediated activation of a cephalosporin-taxol prodrug. *Chemistry & biology 2*, 223-7.

[52]   Mauger AB, Burke PJ, Somani HH, Friedlos F, Knox RJ. (1994) Self-immolative prodrugs: candidates for antibody-directed enzyme prodrug therapy in conjunction with a nitroreductase enzyme. *Journal of medicinal chemistry 37*, 3452-8.

[53]   Vrudhula VM, Senter PD, Fischer KJ, Wallace PM. (1993) Prodrugs of doxorubicin and melphalan and their activation by a monoclonal antibody-penicillin-G amidase conjugate. *Journal of medicinal chemistry 36*, 919-23.

[54]   Bignami GS, Senter PD, Grothaus PG, Fischer KJ, Humphreys T, Wallace PM. (1992) N-(4'-hydroxyphenylacetyl)palytoxin: a palytoxin prodrug that can be activated by a monoclonal antibody-penicillin G amidase conjugate. *Cancer research 52*, 5759-64.

[55]   Dahan A, Khamis M, Agbaria R, Karaman R. (2012) Targeted prodrugs in oral drug delivery: the modern molecular biopharmaceutical approach. *Expert opinion on drug delivery 9*, 1001-13.

[56]   Karaman R, Fattash B, Qtait A. (2013) The future of prodrugs – design by quantum mechanics methods. *Expert Opinion on Drug Delivery 10*, 713–729.

[57] Karaman R. (2013) Prodrugs design based on inter- and intramolecular processes. *Chem. Biol. Drug. Des 82*, 643–668.

[58] Webley SD, Francis RJ, Pedley RB, Sharma SK, Begent RH, Hartley JA, Hochhauser, D. (2001) Measurement of the critical DNA lesions produced by antibody-directed enzyme prodrug therapy (ADEPT) in vitro, in vivo and in clinical material. *British journal of cancer 84*, 1671-6.

[59] Francis RJ, Sharma SK, Springer C, Green AJ, Hope-Stone LD, Sena L, Martin, J. Adamson, K. L. Robbins, A. Gumbrell, L. O'Malley, D. Tsiompanou, E. Shahbakhti, H. Webley, S. Hochhauser, D. Hilson, A. J. Blakey, D. Begent, R. H. (2002) A phase I trial of antibody directed enzyme prodrug therapy (ADEPT) in patients with advanced colorectal carcinoma or other CEA producing tumours. *British journal of cancer 87*, 600-7.

[60] Blakey DC, Burke PJ, Davies DH, Dowell RI, East SJ, Eckersley KP, Fitton, J. E. McDaid, J. Melton, R. G. Niculescu-Duvaz, I. A. Pinder, P. E. Sharma, S. K. Wright, A. F. Springer, C. J. (1996) ZD2767, an improved system for antibody-directed enzyme prodrug therapy that results in tumor regressions in colorectal tumor xenografts. *Cancer research 56*, 3287-92.

[61] Tietze LF, Feuerstein T, Fecher A, Haunert F, Panknin O, Borchers U, Schuberth, I. Alves, F. (2002) Proof of principle in the selective treatment of cancer by antibody-directed enzyme prodrug therapy: the development of a highly potent prodrug. *Angew Chem Int Ed Engl 41*, 759-61.

[62] Chen Y, Hu L. (2009) Design of anticancer prodrugs for reductive activation. *Medicinal research reviews 29*, 29-64.

[63] Pedley RB, Sharma SK, Boxer GM, Boden R, Stribbling SM, Davies L, Springer, C. J. Begent, R. H. (1999) Enhancement of antibody-directed enzyme prodrug therapy in colorectal xenografts by an antivascular agent. *Cancer research 59*, 3998-4003.

[64] Kratz F, Muller IA, Ryppa C, Warnecke A. (2008) Prodrug strategies in anticancer chemotherapy. *ChemMedChem 3*, 20-53.

[65] Sharma SK, Bagshawe KD, Burke PJ, Boden JA, Rogers GT, Springer CJ, Melton, R. G. Sherwood, R. F. (1994) Galactosylated antibodies and antibody-enzyme conjugates in antibody-directed enzyme prodrug therapy. *Cancer 73*, 1114-20.

[66] Medzihradszky KF, Spencer DI, Sharma SK, Bhatia J, Pedley RB, Read DA, Begent, R. H. Chester, K. A. (2004) Glycoforms obtained by expression in Pichia pastoris improve cancer targeting potential of a recombinant antibody-enzyme fusion protein. *Glycobiology 14*, 27-37.

[67] Sharma SK, Pedley RB, Bhatia J, Boxer GM, El-Emir E, Qureshi U, Tolner, B. Lowe, H. Michael, N. P. Minton, N. Begent, R. H. Chester, K. A. (2005) Sustained tumor regression of human colorectal cancer xenografts using a multifunctional mannosylated fusion protein in antibody-directed enzyme prodrug therapy. *Clinical cancer research : an official journal of the American Association for Cancer Research 11*, 814-25.

[68] Napier MP, Sharma SK, Springer CJ, Bagshawe KD, Green AJ, Martin J, Stribbling, S. M. Cushen, N. O'Malley, D. Begent, R. H. (2000) Antibody-directed enzyme prodrug therapy: efficacy and mechanism of action in colorectal carcinoma. *Clinical cancer research : an official journal of the American Association for Cancer Research 6*, 765-72.

[69] Martin J, Stribbling SM, Poon GK, Begent RH, Napier M, Sharma SK, Springer, C. J. (1997) Antibody-directed enzyme prodrug therapy: pharmacokinetics and plasma levels of prodrug and drug in a phase I clinical trial. *Cancer chemotherapy and pharmacology 40*, 189-201.

[70] Osipovitch DC, Parker AS, Makokha CD, Desrosiers J, Kett WC, Moise L, Bailey-Kellogg, C.Griswold, K. E. (2012) Design and analysis of immune-evading enzymes for ADEPT therapy. *Protein engineering, design & selection : PEDS 25*, 613-23.

[71] Ferl GZ, Wu AM, DiStefano JJ, 3rd. (2005) A predictive model of therapeutic monoclonal antibody dynamics and regulation by the neonatal Fc receptor (FcRn). *Annals of biomedical engineering 33*, 1640-52.

Index

A

acetaldehyde, 125, 128, 136

acetaminophen, 225

acetic acid, 30, 212, 223, 224, 231, 266

acetone, 124, 125

acetylation, 222, 255

acetylcholine, 7

acid, 2, 4, 13, 15, 18, 20, 22, 23, 25, 27, 28, 29, 30, 37, 38, 41, 42, 45, 46, 47, 48, 52, 54, 55, 56, 57, 58, 59, 60, 61, 67, 68, 69, 70, 71, 72, 74, 75, 78, 80, 81, 83, 99, 104, 106, 110, 111, 115, 116, 119, 122, 123, 124, 126, 128, 129, 130, 136, 140, 141,143, 146, 147, 151, 153, 156, 157, 158, 159, 160, 167, 171, 172, 187, 198, 212, 225, 253, 255, 263

acidic, 4, 10, 42, 46, 52, 58, 59, 67, 81, 120, 122, 135, 146

acidity, 54

acidosis, 106

acne vulgaris, 133

acquired immunodeficiency syndrome (AIDS), 127, 161, 162, 173, 175

activation energy, 28, 30, 42, 44, 45, 47, 48, 49

active centers, 197

active compound, 85, 211, 214

active site, 2, 9, 25, 27, 29, 42, 52, 54, 84, 87, 96, 116, 141, 153

active transport, 108, 163, 188, 215, 256

activity level, 196

acute myelogenous leukemia, 34

acute myeloid leukemia, 72, 91, 143

acute renal failure, 176

acute respiratory distress syndrome, 185

acylation, 42, 117, 122

adenine, 126, 136, 137, 174, 196, 212, 260

adenocarcinoma, 199, 227, 257

adenosine, 195

adenovirus, 178, 185, 187, 189, 193, 194, 200, 201, 202, 203, 205, 208

adenylate kinase, 162

ADP, 196

adrenal gland, 199

adverse effects, 10, 11, 14, 161

aesthetic, 96

aggregation, 175, 270

agonist, 8, 14, 51, 115, 123, 135

alanine, 23, 124, 144, 156, 157, 171, 256

alcohols, 67, 105, 114, 115, 133, 151, 197

aldolase, 268, 269

algorithm, 27

aliphatic amines, 23, 54, 124

alkaloids, 154, 259

alkylation, 86, 248, 261

amine group, 8, 20, 117, 122

amine(s), 4, 8, 10, 12, 18, 20, 21, 23, 27, 35, 44, 46, 54, 58, 61, 67, 68, 70, 82, 103, 117, 118, 119, 120, 121, 122, 123, 124, 125, 133, 134, 135, 222, 223

amino, 5, 6, 11, 12, 13, 18, 21, 51, 54, 55, 57, 64, 66, 67, 70, 75, 79, 89, 91, 99, 111, 119, 120, 130, 134, 135, 143, 145, 157, 164, 167, 172, 173, 198, 200, 212, 225, 246, 248, 252, 253, 255, 263

amino acid(s), 5, 11, 12, 13, 18, 21, 51, 57, 64, 66, 67, 75, 79, 89, 91, 99, 111, 119, 134, 135, 145, 157, 164, 167, 198, 200

amino groups, 6, 51, 111

ammonia, 68, 70, 199, 200

ammonium, 35, 40, 254

anaerobic bacteria, 171

analgesic, 19, 20, 22, 51, 83, 95, 122, 154

androgen, 135, 148, 168

anemia, 184

angiogenesis, 145

angiotensin converting enzyme, 18

280 Index

anhydrase, 116
aniline, 35, 41, 227
annealing, 189
anti-asthma, 10
antibiotic, 86, 94, 96, 143, 260
antibody, viii, 15, 17, 65, 82, 90, 91, 98, 143, 144, 146, 154, 166, 177, 201, 202, 233, 234, 235, 236, 237, 238, 239, 240, 241, 243, 250, 253, 260, 265, 266, 267, 268, 269, 270, 271, 272, 273, 274, 275, 276
anti-cancer, 11, 121, 215, 216, 235, 237, 246, 272
anticancer activity, 265
anticancer drug, 15, 94, 166, 179, 180, 225, 228, 262, 269
anticonvulsant, 23, 114, 123
antigen, 140, 168, 178, 187, 233, 234, 235, 236, 237, 238, 239, 240, 244, 252, 253, 266, 270, 272, 274
antipsychotic, 92, 101, 111
antipsychotic drugs, 101
antipyretic, 18, 28, 61, 80, 95
antisense, 213
antitumor, 135, 151, 167, 181, 194, 195, 196, 197, 198, 208, 213, 217, 230, 245, 248, 253, 258, 266, 273, 274
antitumor agent, 195, 198, 274
antiviral agents, 218
antiviral drugs, 173, 175
apoptosis, 148, 186, 191, 200, 224, 225
aqueous solutions, 59, 136
arabinoside, 147
arginine, 145
aromatic rings, 4
arrest, 224
artery, 187
asbestos, 178
ascorbic acid, 91
aspartic acid, 23, 163
assessment, 64, 175, 213, 270
asthma, 14, 64, 115
atoms, 26, 28
ATP, 89, 140, 145, 196, 206
attachment, 190, 267
avian, 187

B

bacteria, 23, 65, 99, 124, 160, 171, 191, 195, 196, 199, 219, 226, 246, 248, 249, 270
bacterial artificial chromosome, 191
bacterial strains, 243
bacteriophage, 204
barriers, vii, 3, 11, 13, 15, 25, 42, 78, 86, 103, 110, 117, 130, 141, 166, 168, 175, 179, 250, 272

base, 11, 22, 26, 35, 68, 110, 122, 123
base catalysis, 68
basicity, 54, 117
BBB, 104, 117, 118, 123, 140, 153, 154
benefits, 115, 242
benign, 179
benzene, 51, 256
bile, 91, 151, 176, 198
bile acids, 91, 198
binding energy, 25
bioavailability, ix, 12, 16, 20, 22, 28, 35, 37, 38, 40, 41, 45, 46, 47, 57, 59, 61, 62, 73, 75, 77, 84, 86, 87, 89, 91, 92, 94, 95, 97, 100, 107, 108, 112, 118, 125, 126, 128, 129, 130, 132, 139, 141, 145, 154, 155, 159, 160, 161, 162, 164, 197, 198, 214, 250
biochemistry, 62, 64, 67, 73, 75, 131, 134, 168
bioconversion, 17, 24, 99, 100, 133
biological activity, 4, 78, 104, 130
biological behavior, vii, 3
biological systems, 9, 26, 27, 101
biologically active compounds, 12
biosafety, 183, 188
biosynthesis, 145, 196, 198
biotechnology, 166, 170
biotin, 154, 162, 170
bleeding, 15, 19, 51, 57, 61, 66, 71, 75, 99
blindness, 106
blood, 3, 6, 10, 11, 13, 16, 18, 28, 34, 45, 46, 52, 57, 58, 60, 61, 62, 64, 75, 79, 92, 112, 117, 127, 139, 145, 146, 147, 153, 154, 164, 170, 178, 179, 191, 206, 238, 240, 242, 243, 244, 246, 249, 250, 257, 260, 262, 265, 266, 267, 270, 271
blood circulation, 3, 11, 28, 46, 52, 58, 60, 61, 127
blood flow, 147, 250, 262, 266
blood pressure, 45, 164
blood transfusion, 34, 75
blood vessels, 145, 146, 240, 262
blood-brain barrier, 11, 13, 45, 79, 170, 179
bloodstream, 253, 266
body fluid, 162
bonding, 3, 9, 25, 29, 30, 35, 36, 52, 69, 95
bonds, 42, 119, 159
bone, 11, 90, 164, 179, 186, 197, 203
bone marrow, 11, 90, 164, 179
bowel, 141
brain, 13, 45, 50, 79, 117, 134, 139, 140, 153, 154, 155, 170, 175, 187, 190, 191, 195, 199, 201, 202, 230, 248, 264
brain tumor, 230, 264
branching, 18
breakdown, 22, 24, 54, 57, 129
breast cancer, 147, 178

Index

breast carcinoma, 274
bronchodilator, 14
building blocks, 217
by-products, 45, 47
bystander effect, 140, 180, 182, 184, 193, 195, 208, 213, 215, 216, 217, 219, 221, 222, 223, 224, 225, 227, 230, 238

C

Ca^{2+}, 168
caecum, 158
calcium, 38, 73, 140, 148, 168
calcium carbonate, 38
cancer, 11, 21, 63, 64, 65, 72, 90, 101, 121, 122, 130, 133, 135, 140, 142, 143, 145, 147, 148, 150, 151, 165, 166, 167, 168, 177, 178, 179, 180, 181, 182, 184, 185, 186, 191, 192, 193, 199, 200, 202, 203, 205, 206, 207, 208, 209, 211, 213, 214, 215, 216, 217, 218, 220, 223, 225, 228, 229, 231, 233, 234, 236, 237, 238, 239, 242, 250, 260, 262, 264, 267, 269, 272, 273, 274, 275, 276
cancer cells, 11, 121, 122, 130, 142, 143, 145, 147, 151, 165, 168, 178, 179, 180, 181, 184, 199, 200, 206, 213, 216, 217, 235, 236, 238, 239
cancer therapy, 64, 65, 90, 135, 166, 177, 182, 206, 207, 209, 211, 213, 217, 231, 233, 250, 260, 262, 269, 272, 273, 274
cancerous cells, 142, 143, 146, 148, 149, 178
candidates, 12, 66, 208, 250, 261, 275
carbon, 8, 9, 42, 54, 55, 69, 70, 132, 222, 223, 224
carbonyl groups, 18, 103
carboxyl, 4, 6, 18, 30, 41, 45, 54, 55, 103, 120, 148, 151, 256
carboxylic acid(s), 4, 8, 18, 20, 25, 40, 44, 47, 52, 54, 69, 73, 82, 87, 105, 106, 107, 108, 109, 110, 119, 126, 129, 130, 227
carcinogen, 178
carcinogenesis, 178
carcinoma, 178, 186, 200, 207, 219, 227, 244, 245, 248, 249, 253, 254, 258, 275, 276
cardiovascular diseases, 21, 118
catabolism, 198
catalysis, viii, 1, 16, 17, 18, 24, 25, 27, 29, 30, 42, 48, 54, 68, 69, 70, 73, 116, 215, 225, 269, 275
catalyst, 42, 269
catalytic activity, 25, 116, 180, 215
catalytic properties, 73, 169
cation, 222, 223, 224
cDNA, 161, 195
cell culture, 190, 204, 205
cell cycle, 215, 216, 225, 236, 251
cell death, 148, 168, 213, 220

cell division, 142, 179, 218
cell invasion, 175
cell killing, 182, 193, 227, 235, 239, 240, 273
cell line(s), 63, 185, 187, 188, 190, 220, 224, 227, 249, 254, 269
cell membranes, 4, 5, 129, 180, 216, 224, 235
cell surface, 142, 145, 161, 213, 218, 235, 238
central nervous system (CNS), 11, 45, 99, 118, 123, 139, 140, 153, 154, 165, 170, 189, 190, 199, 202
cephalosporin, 8, 67, 243, 259, 275
cervix, 264
cesarean section, 57, 75
challenges, viii, 16, 62, 64, 66, 70, 98, 131, 167, 169, 173, 180, 228, 239, 272
chemical(s), vii, 2, 3, 4, 6, 9, 11, 12, 17, 18, 26, 28, 34, 39, 41, 45, 46, 50, 51, 61, 71, 77, 78, 79, 82, 95, 98, 103, 104, 110, 111, 114, 115, 116, 117, 121, 124, 126, 134, 137, 140, 141, 153, 154, 155, 156, 161, 165, 166, 170, 172, 179, 214, 242, 243, 244, 252, 266, 269, 273
chemical properties, 3, 4, 26
chemical reactions, 77
chemical reactivity, 117, 252
chemical stability, 3, 18, 104, 111, 114, 115, 116, 117, 124, 172, 179, 269
chemical structures, 46, 242, 244
chemotherapeutic agent, 122, 142, 143, 252
chemotherapy, 11, 34, 65, 82, 90, 101, 102, 131, 132, 135, 136, 140, 142, 147, 166, 167, 174, 179, 181, 206, 207, 211, 212, 213, 214, 218, 220, 223, 225, 230, 237, 238, 252, 262, 269, 273, 276, 277
chimera, 135
chiral center, 128
chirality, 128
chlorine, 5
cholesterol, 28, 37, 149
cholinesterase, 24, 116
choriocarcinoma, 246, 252
chorionic gonadotropin, 240
chromatography, 244
chromosome, 189, 193
chronic diseases, 149, 150
chronic lymphocytic leukemia, 264
chymotrypsin, 24, 25, 42, 168
circulation, 14, 17, 23, 46, 82, 83, 114, 157, 159, 162, 180, 201, 215, 216, 266, 270
classes, 17, 82, 142, 202, 216, 222, 262
classification, 74, 82, 83
cleavage, 16, 18, 23, 30, 33, 36, 41, 42, 43, 45, 47, 73, 84, 106, 107, 114, 115, 116, 119, 122, 124, 143, 146, 148, 150, 156, 160, 198, 228, 252
clinical application, 99, 116, 165, 173, 189, 206
clinical oncology, 100, 133, 168

clinical trials, 2, 10, 143, 148, 181, 186, 188, 190, 192, 201, 203, 205, 264, 266

clone, 203

cloning, 195, 221, 270

closure, 70

cobalt, 264

cocaine, 10

coding, 182, 190

coenzyme, 37

colitis, 160, 173

colon, 23, 65, 83, 84, 124, 139, 142, 148, 154, 155, 156, 157, 158, 159, 160, 165, 170, 171, 172, 199, 219, 220, 224, 227, 240, 248, 257, 258, 275

colon cancer, 148, 155, 220, 257

colorectal cancer, 192, 246, 276

combined effect, 25

commercial, vii, 38, 104

complexity, 183, 187, 265

compliance, 23, 50, 51, 77, 89, 92, 95, 98, 111, 114, 161

compounds, 3, 12, 15, 18, 23, 37, 58, 62, 64, 65, 67, 68, 72, 74, 80, 82, 86, 98, 101, 102, 109, 120, 121, 123, 124, 128, 133, 135, 147, 149, 150, 151, 153, 154, 156, 170, 171, 194, 224, 235, 239, 246, 250, 257, 258, 259, 261, 263, 264, 270, 273

condensation, 125

configuration, 51, 105

conjugation, 6, 95, 116, 119, 157, 238, 243, 244, 246, 248, 249, 252, 266

consensus, 25

construction, 187, 267, 270

contaminant, 189

contamination, 191

controversial, 186

conversion rate, 115, 124

COOH, 18, 51, 157

copolymer, 146, 163, 171

correlation(s), 24, 28, 29, 33, 45, 49, 57, 196, 206

correlation function, 28

corticosteroids, 89

cost, 2, 3, 26, 130, 161, 238

cost effectiveness, 3

CPT, 140, 143, 144, 250, 258, 274

cranial nerve, 50

crisis management, 173

crystal structure, 27, 203

cues, 184

culture, 204, 221

culture medium, 221

cure, 2, 34, 142, 161, 221, 228

cures, 274

cyanide, 251

cycles, 161, 267

cycling, 216

cyclodextrins, 159, 172

cyclooxygenase, 134

cyclophosphamide, 86, 224, 225, 226

cyclosporine, 267

cysteine, 146, 147, 162, 167, 244

cystic fibrosis, 186, 190, 208

cytochrome, 6, 16, 18, 22, 24, 63, 66, 121, 147, 149, 150, 169, 200, 224, 226, 248, 262

cytochromes, 4, 169

cytomegalovirus, 127, 132

cytomegalovirus retinitis, 127, 132

cytoplasm, 161, 192

cytosine, 104, 127, 128, 136, 147, 199, 208, 211, 218, 219, 230, 242

cytostatic drugs, 250

cytotoxic agents, 142, 179, 212, 213, 214, 239, 264, 272

cytotoxicity, 63, 65, 135, 142, 144, 172, 180, 194, 200, 215, 216, 218, 223, 228, 235, 244, 248, 249, 250, 254, 257, 259, 260, 261

D

danger, 201

deaths, 57

decomposition, 224

decongestant, 28, 61

deficiencies, 103

deficiency, 139, 187, 201

degradation, 6, 11, 14, 124, 136, 147, 154, 155, 172

degradation process, 147

density functional theory (DFT), ix, 2, 26, 27, 28, 29, 30, 35, 36, 41, 42, 44, 45, 46, 47, 50, 52, 55, 56, 57, 58, 69, 70

dephosphorylation, 115, 130

deposits, 216

deprivation, 148

derivatives, 21, 27, 28, 46, 50, 54, 58, 63, 67, 73, 75, 98, 110, 117, 119, 121, 126, 134, 135, 137, 147, 154, 164, 172, 176, 214, 243, 249, 251, 259, 269, 270, 274

destruction, 121, 187, 266

detectable, 189, 190

developed countries, 57

diabetes, 149, 184

dialysis, 164, 175

diarrhea, 156

dielectric constant, 59

dielectrics, 72

diet, 74

diffusion, 3, 37, 129, 153, 213, 215, 216, 219, 220, 221, 224, 225, 250, 251 digestion, 159

dimerization, 124

dipeptides, 91, 144

disease model, 153

diseases, 45, 77, 101, 133, 153, 154, 155, 186, 187, 190, 191, 197, 205

dispersion, 95

disposition, 30, 36, 67, 99, 100, 101, 132, 134, 136, 137, 171, 273

disseminated intravascular coagulation, 201

distribution, vii, 3, 12, 13, 15, 68, 72, 78, 91, 94, 104, 140, 141, 142, 153, 162, 197, 199, 212, 214, 215, 236, 270, 271

DNA, viii, 17, 72, 91, 121, 122, 135, 142, 161, 162, 167, 174, 178, 179, 181, 185, 186, 187, 191, 192, 193, 199, 203, 204, 205, 209, 212, 218, 220, 221, 222, 224, 225, 246, 248, 250, 255, 256, 260, 261, 263, 276

DNA damage, 167

DNA lesions, 276

DNA polymerase, 91, 218

dogs, 66, 95, 131, 132, 137, 157, 160

DOI, 71

donors, 223

dopamine, 2, 13, 14, 20, 21, 28, 45, 46, 47, 61, 71, 74, 79, 117, 118, 119, 134, 164, 165, 176

dopamine precursor, 176

dopaminergic, 13, 46, 67, 115, 133, 134

dosage, 12, 23, 35, 36, 39, 41, 46, 57, 89, 95, 114, 161

dosing, 34, 57, 58, 92, 116, 206, 213, 216

DPO, 249

drainage, 145, 146

drug action, 14, 237

drug carriers, 153

drug delivery, viii, 1, 12, 13, 15, 20, 37, 63, 64, 65, 67, 68, 73, 79, 86, 87, 98, 99, 100, 101, 102, 125, 126, 127, 130, 131, 135, 149, 150, 166, 169, 170, 171, 172, 173, 272, 273, 274, 275

drug design, viii, 2, 17, 62, 71, 78, 133, 135, 207, 273, 275

drug discovery, 2, 12, 27, 62

drug half-life, 216

drug interaction, 1, 16, 85, 98, 150

drug metabolism, 3, 10, 62, 64

drug reactions, 15

drug release, 23, 124, 159, 251

drug resistance, 166, 179, 235, 237, 239, 258, 262, 264

drug therapy, 244

dystonia, 45

E

ecstasy, 10

edema, 159

elderly population, 153

electrolyte, 164

electron(s), 4, 8, 26, 116, 121, 148, 194, 222, 262, 263

electronic structure, 26, 27

elongation, 218

elucidation, 75

emulsions, 39, 97

encapsulation, 186

encoding, viii, 17, 91, 186, 189, 194, 196, 200, 213, 217, 243, 244, 262

endothelial cells, 145

energy, 25, 26, 28, 30, 42, 44, 47, 48, 49, 50, 53, 55, 56, 72

engineering, 183, 193, 201, 202, 203, 207, 277

entrapment, 126

entropy, 27, 68

environment, 17, 35, 41, 45, 46, 47, 52, 121, 146, 155, 262

environments, 3, 28, 35, 40, 46, 57, 61, 105

enzymatic activity, 155, 238, 244, 270

enzyme inhibitors, 16

epidermis, 89

epinephrine, 110, 132

epithelia, 11, 90, 179

epithelial cells, 91, 111, 175

epithelium, 87, 89, 162, 186

epitopes, 266, 270

EPR, 140, 145, 146, 165

Epstein Barr, 221

equilibrium, 35, 47, 125

erythropoietin, 164, 184

esophageal cancer, 134

ester, 4, 7, 8, 15, 17, 18, 19, 20, 21, 24, 40, 62, 64, 65, 66, 82, 83, 85, 87, 88, 89, 92, 93, 95, 97, 98, 99, 100, 101, 104, 105, 106, 107, 108, 109, 110, 111, 112, 113, 114, 115, 116, 119, 128, 132, 133, 145, 159, 160, 161, 162, 163, 167, 172, 256, 268

estrogen, 95, 102, 116

ethanol, 107, 122

ethers, 69

ethical issues, 185

ethylene glycol, 68, 163, 169

evaporation, 37, 51

exclusion, 226

excretion, 3, 12, 14, 78, 104, 133, 140, 141, 164, 212, 214

experimental condition, 58

exploitation, 118, 189

Index

exposure, 17, 28, 34, 58, 106, 128, 150, 178, 194, 219, 223, 225, 235
extracellular matrix, 147
extraction, 51, 57, 160, 250
extracts, 249
extravasation, 192

F

families, 145, 149, 198
fasting, 58
fat, 4, 198
fatty acids, 198
feces, 157
fertility, 102
fever, 51, 201
fiber, 202
fibrin, 57
fibrosis, 208
first generation, 185, 187, 208, 260
flexibility, 27, 242, 270
fluid, 57, 83, 148, 235
fluorine, 4, 10
folate, 143, 144, 228
folic acid, 143
food, 58, 74, 162, 172
Food and Drug Administration (FDA), 34, 91, 97, 140, 143, 161, 212, 219
force, 25, 27, 28, 29, 47, 49, 54, 72, 213
formaldehyde, 22, 80, 106, 122, 125, 135, 136
formation, 22, 25, 27, 49, 54, 55, 57, 58, 68, 121, 122, 148, 151, 162, 196, 220, 223, 263
fragments, 224, 235, 240, 241, 244, 266, 269
France, 75
free activation energy, 44
free calcium level, 148
free energy, 30, 50, 56
free radicals, 147
freezing, 25
funding, 61
fungal infection, 246
fungi, 199, 219, 246
fusion, 161, 205, 233, 243, 244, 245, 249, 265, 266, 275, 276

G

GABA, 104, 123
gastrointestinal tract, 11, 14, 16, 159, 171, 172
gel, 133
gene combinations, 218

gene expression, 182, 183, 184, 185, 187, 189, 205, 206, 208, 213, 214, 215
gene targeting, viii, 17
gene therapy, 63, 65, 166, 177, 179, 181, 182, 183, 184, 185, 187, 188, 189, 196, 200, 202, 203, 205, 206, 207, 208, 209, 213, 214, 215, 217, 218, 221, 224, 226, 229, 230, 231, 235
gene transfer, 177, 181, 182, 183, 184, 186, 189, 190, 191, 193, 201, 203, 205, 208, 230
genes, viii, 15, 17, 65, 85, 147, 177, 178, 180, 181, 182, 184, 185, 186, 187, 188, 189, 190, 191, 192, 193, 194, 201, 202, 203, 213, 217, 218, 221, 262
genetic disorders, 184, 205
genetic engineering, 183, 193
genetic information, 182, 184, 188, 205
genetics, 193
genome, 182, 183, 185, 186, 187, 188, 189, 190, 191, 192, 193, 201
geometrical parameters, 28, 33
geometry, 28
germ cells, 184
germ line, 185
glial cells, 189
glioblastoma, 220
glioma, 186
glucocorticoid, 172, 173
glucose, 184
glucoside, 158, 171
glutamate, 226, 227, 228, 246, 252
glutamic acid, 158, 171, 212, 218, 225, 246, 247, 252, 253
glutamine, 148, 157, 167
glutathione, 150, 169
glycerol, 176
glycine, 143, 144, 157
glycol, 2, 140, 146, 154, 162, 266, 267
glycoproteins, 147, 188, 190, 203
glycoside, 158, 228, 260
glycosylation, 153, 215, 243, 265
growth, 178, 179, 184, 192, 206, 217, 221, 234, 252, 262, 275
growth factor, 192, 234
guanine, 263

H

hair cells, 179
hair follicle, 11, 90
half-life, 4, 24, 37, 41, 42, 54, 92, 111, 119, 160, 161, 180, 215, 216, 224, 236, 238, 250, 253, 265
Hartree-Fock, 2, 28
H-bonding, 170
HCC, 178

Index

health, 11, 17, 26, 51, 153, 169, 173
health care system, 153
health condition, 17
heart rate, 45
hematocrit, 184
hematopoietic stem cells, 189
heme, 198, 223
hemophilia, 57, 190
hemophilia a, 190
hemorrhage, 57, 75
hepatitis, 63, 150, 169
hepatocellular carcinoma, 196, 207, 221
hepatocytes, 149, 150, 151, 153, 208, 265
hepatoma, 200
hepatotoxicity, 208
heroin, 10
herpes, 61, 91, 101, 177, 190, 193, 196, 203, 211, 213, 217, 218, 230
herpes simplex, 61, 91, 101, 177, 190, 196, 211, 213, 217, 218, 230
herpes simplex virus type 1, 190
herpes virus, 190, 193, 203
heterogeneity, 235, 236
highly active antiretroviral therapy (HAART), 141, 161, 163
histamine, 20, 123, 135
HIV, 67, 100, 114, 132, 133, 140, 160, 161, 162, 163, 164, 165, 173, 174, 178, 187, 189, 269
HIV/AIDS, 173
HIV-1, 173, 269
homeostasis, 129
homocysteine, 200
hormone(s), 142, 168, 179, 198
host, 130, 161, 182, 185, 187, 188, 192, 203, 204, 213, 217, 250, 267
HTLV, 137
human, 2, 3, 11, 51, 63, 64, 65, 66, 74, 100, 112, 116, 132, 139, 142, 148, 152, 157, 159, 168, 169, 171, 172, 174, 180, 181, 184, 185, 186, 188, 189, 190, 191, 192, 194, 195, 196, 198, 199, 200, 201, 204, 205, 208, 213, 217, 218, 220, 221, 223, 224, 225, 227, 228, 230, 236, 238, 239, 240, 241, 242, 243, 244, 245, 246, 248, 249, 252, 253, 254, 257, 258, 260, 265, 266, 272, 274, 275, 276
human body, 112
human genome, 205
human immunodeficiency virus, 66, 174
human kinase, 196
human skin, 100
humoral immunity, 202
hybrid, 28, 189, 193
hybridization, 267
hydrazine, 164

hydrocortisone, 111, 158
hydrogen, 3, 4, 8, 9, 25, 27, 29, 30, 35, 36, 52, 95, 223
hydrogen bonds, 27
hydrogen peroxide, 223
hydrolysis, 6, 7, 8, 16, 17, 18, 20, 21, 25, 27, 42, 44, 53, 54, 55, 56, 58, 59, 60, 67, 68, 69, 70, 73, 75, 85, 92, 110, 112, 115, 116, 118, 119, 120, 122, 135, 137, 147, 151, 158, 159, 171, 172, 197, 198, 199, 246
hydrolysis kinetics, 58
hydrophobicity, 12, 154, 239
hydroquinone, 263
hydroxyl, 6, 8, 9, 18, 23, 27, 28, 37, 40, 51, 52, 61, 89, 95, 103, 105, 110, 111, 112, 113, 114, 115, 116, 125, 130, 160, 172
hydroxyl groups, 114, 172
hypertension, 18, 28, 61, 66
hypothalamus, 45
hypoxia, 121, 142, 165, 167, 214, 262, 263, 264
hypoxic cells, 147, 148, 223, 251, 262

I

ibuprofen, 18, 19, 20, 66
immune reaction, 143
immune response, 184, 185, 187, 201, 202, 204, 205, 213, 217, 218, 221, 266, 267
immune system, 16, 203, 267
immunity, 186, 205, 221
immunization, 217, 267, 268
immunodeficiency, 140, 160, 178, 187
immunogenicity, 143, 183, 185, 201, 235, 238, 239, 241, 242, 266, 267, 270, 274
immunoglobulin, 270
immunoglobulins, 270
immunosuppressive agent, 267
immunotherapy, 192, 274
implants, 153
improvements, 191, 270
impulses, 50
impurities, 183
in vitro, vii, 3, 18, 22, 24, 39, 47, 59, 62, 64, 65, 67, 73, 81, 100, 104, 122, 128, 136, 137, 144, 145, 148, 162, 166, 172, 183, 217, 221, 223, 229, 230, 244, 268, 272, 273, 276
in vivo, vii, viii, 2, 3, 11, 16, 17, 20, 21, 22, 47, 60, 65, 67, 73, 80, 81, 82, 109, 110, 112, 113, 115, 120, 128, 130, 146, 151, 154, 162, 179, 188, 189, 190, 192, 193, 204, 208, 209, 213, 214, 217, 221, 229, 238, 241, 244, 246, 267, 268, 270, 273, 274, 276
India, 75

individuals, 201, 203
induction, 132, 184, 201, 202, 204, 223
industry, 50
ineffectiveness, 252
infection, 67, 92, 100, 133, 163, 174, 182, 185, 186, 187, 189, 190, 193, 195, 202
infectious agents, 208
inflammation, 185
inflammatory bowel disease, 83, 158, 171
inflammatory disease, 156
inflammatory responses, 201
influenza, 92, 107
ingestion, 37, 58
inhibition, 57, 66, 151, 194, 199, 217, 220, 238, 258, 266, 275
inhibitor, 4, 20, 37, 45, 63, 87, 89, 100, 107, 110, 114, 137, 148, 161, 168, 174, 194, 220, 228, 248, 250, 264, 267
injections, 245
injury, 97, 102, 191
innate immunity, 185, 201
insertion, 190, 221
insulin, 184
integrases, 187, 205
integration, 183, 184, 187, 188, 189, 192, 193, 194, 204
interference, 205, 243
internalization, 153, 193, 203, 256
internalizing, 142, 235
intestinal tract, 37, 140, 141, 172
intestine, 3, 6, 28, 35, 40, 41, 46, 59, 61, 129, 158, 199
intracellular calcium, 148
intravenously, 192, 236, 267
ionic solutions, 72
ionizable groups, 98
ionization, 4, 57, 117, 122
ionizing radiation, 148
iron, 223
irradiation, 216
irritable bowel disease (IBD), 141, 155, 158, 160
isolation, 194, 201, 267
isomers, 92
isozymes, 169, 224

J

Japan, 178, 181
Jordan, 66, 132, 166

K

keratinocytes, 65
kidney, 17, 118, 139, 153, 160, 164, 165, 175, 176, 195, 197, 199, 224, 248
kidney failure, 164
kidneys, 6, 164
kill, 179, 180, 182, 193, 213, 215, 216, 253, 274, 275
killer cells, 175
kinase activity, 196
kinetic parameters, 1, 242
kinetic studies, 47, 59
kinetics, 24, 53, 58, 100, 245

L

large intestine, 84, 159
latency, 190, 191
lead, 3, 4, 62, 98, 141, 149, 179, 186, 213, 215, 222, 239, 242, 245
leakage, 202
lecithin, 51
leprosy, 96
lesions, 203
leucine, 141, 163, 170
leukemia, 72, 78, 137, 140, 178, 179, 203, 256
leukocytes, 235
leukopenia, 101
liberation, 112
life cycle, 104, 186
ligand, 11, 142, 202
light, 25, 35, 38, 165
linear polymers, 146
lipids, viii, 17, 51
liposomes, 153, 154, 175, 179, 181, 235
liver, 3, 6, 12, 14, 17, 18, 21, 37, 57, 63, 66, 85, 95, 99, 120, 128, 129, 137, 142, 147, 149, 150, 151, 153, 165, 169, 186, 187, 190, 194, 195, 197, 198, 199, 204, 219, 224, 225, 248, 271
liver cancer, 147, 149, 150, 151, 153, 165, 186
liver enzymes, 224
liver transplant, 57
localization, 153, 217, 236, 238, 240, 243, 265, 266
locus, 191
lumen, 16, 91
lung cancer, 63, 199
Luo, 73
lymph, 178, 186
lymph node, 186
lymphocytes, 162, 188, 195, 248
lymphoid, 100, 155, 235
lymphoid tissue, 155

lymphoma, 166, 249, 264
lysine, 57, 143, 145, 162
lysis, 184, 186
lysozyme, 25, 70

M

mAb, 142, 143, 234, 240, 244, 246, 249, 267, 268
machinery, 183, 188, 192, 193, 204
macrolide antibiotics, 50
macromolecules, 27, 215, 240
macrophages, 163, 165, 175
magnesium, 197
magnitude, 26, 196, 213, 268
malaria, 28, 61
malignancy, 187, 203
malignant cells, 90, 181, 184, 192, 235
malignant mesothelioma, 186
malignant tumors, 179
maltose, 159
mammalian cells, 147, 195, 199, 200, 207, 208, 219, 223, 224, 246
mammalian tissues, 198
mammals, 195, 196, 198, 248
man, 67, 99, 107, 134, 136, 171, 187
management, 12, 67, 75, 100, 133, 174
manipulation, 24
manufacturing, 153, 255
marijuana, 10
marrow, 203
masking, ix, 9, 12, 14, 18, 28, 50, 51, 61, 74, 77, 87, 95, 98, 102, 105, 110, 126, 130, 269
mass, 208, 235, 266
mast cells, 155
matrix, 90, 147
maxillary sinus, 208
measles, 193
media, 35, 41, 46, 53, 58, 159, 162
medical, 167
medication, 39, 45, 58
medicine, 102, 132, 170, 272
melanoma, 21, 146, 186, 229, 244, 246, 248, 274
membrane permeability, 12, 101, 125, 126, 127, 130, 141, 148, 159
membranes, 4, 5, 17, 35, 37, 57, 67, 117, 122, 128, 129, 134, 167, 214, 219
memory, 26
menadione, 194
messenger RNA, 220
metabolic, 8, 9, 83, 174, 274
metabolic disorders, 149
metabolism, vii, 3, 4, 6, 8, 9, 10, 12, 14, 16, 17, 62, 64, 65, 67, 77, 78, 80, 86, 94, 95, 99, 101, 104,
106, 115, 131, 132, 134, 136, 137, 140, 141, 149, 167, 171, 172, 174, 175, 179, 198, 212, 214, 215, 222, 224, 263, 264, 271, 273
metabolites, 3, 6, 10, 11, 18, 37, 64, 82, 99, 106, 154, 159, 162, 213, 216, 218, 220, 225, 228
metabolized, 3, 8, 10, 13, 18, 39, 79, 80, 81, 82, 86, 215, 222
metabolizing, 149, 198
metal complexes, 263, 264
metal ion, 5, 264
metastasis, 179
metastatic disease, 269
methanol, 106, 131
methodology, 139, 271
methyl groups, 7, 8, 9, 12
methylation, 9, 246
methylprednisolone, 160
MHC, 234, 267
mice, 66, 131, 146, 150, 175, 192, 196, 200, 203, 204, 208, 216, 221, 244, 246, 249, 252, 260, 267
microbial cells, 11
microemulsion, 73
microorganisms, 81, 156, 170, 171, 172, 241
microparticles, 175
microsomes, 198
microspheres, 175
migration, 160
mitochondria, 200
mitosis, 142, 143, 179, 188
MNDO, 26, 69
MNDO method, 69
model system, 35, 267
models, 1, 2, 24, 25, 27, 29, 35, 36, 41, 42, 43, 46, 61, 68, 69, 70, 72, 100, 108, 142, 153, 176, 185, 189, 190, 191, 201, 205, 206, 220, 221, 231, 244, 245, 275
modifications, 18, 51, 103, 110, 121, 260
molecular biology, viii, 12, 134
molecular dynamics, ix
molecular mass, 235, 270
molecular oxygen, 147, 198
molecular structure, 141
molecular weight, vii, 3, 104, 157, 160, 163, 194, 215, 234, 249
molecules, 6, 12, 26, 27, 28, 46, 50, 66, 69, 74, 78, 84, 104, 125, 146, 151, 156, 182, 193, 214, 218, 235, 238, 248, 250, 269, 271
monoclonal antibody, 170, 233, 240, 252, 265, 272, 274, 275, 277
Moon, 136
morphine, 11, 154, 159
mortality, 57, 149
mortality rate, 57

mosquito bites, 191
mucosa, 86
multiple sclerosis, 76
mumps, 193
muscular dystrophy, 190
mutagenesis, 184, 185, 249
mutant, 75, 192, 267, 274
mutation, 179, 192
myelodysplastic syndromes, 28, 34, 61, 72
myelosuppression, 253

N

NAD, 135, 195, 255
NADH, 194, 212, 221, 224, 248, 255
nanoparticles, 37, 73, 153, 175
naphthalene, 4
narcotic, 159, 172
National Academy of Sciences, 170, 207, 208, 273
National Institutes of Health, 201, 209
natural compound, 2
natural killer cell, 142, 221
necrosis, 193, 266
nephron, 164
nephrosis, 172
nerve, 50, 191
nervous system, 11, 140, 189
neuroblastoma, 269
neurodegenerative diseases, 153
neurons, 45, 189, 190, 191, 202
neurotransmitter(s), 5, 9, 13, 14, 45, 79
neutral, 12, 41, 42, 45, 68, 73, 128, 222
New England, 132, 173
NH2, 157
nicotinamide, 194
nigrostriatal, 45
nitric oxide, 66
nitrogen, 4, 27, 115, 224, 228, 238, 243, 244, 246,
   251, 252, 253, 254, 255, 263, 268
nitroxide, 121
non-cancerous cells, 179, 213
non-polar, 5
North America, 168
NSAIDs, 2, 20
nuclear membrane, 188
nucleic acid, 11, 182, 213
nucleophilicity, 117, 124
nucleoside analogs, 82
nucleotides, 192
nucleus, 161, 182, 186, 205, 217
nutraceutical, 20
nutrients, 145, 147

O

obstacles, 1, 205, 228, 249
oil, 93, 97, 111
omeprazole, 11
oncogenes, 184, 203
oncogenesis, 203
opioids, 154
opportunities, 15, 262
optimization, 1, 16, 28, 73, 98, 204, 213
organ(s), 11, 13, 15, 16, 79, 90, 139, 142, 149, 153,
   164, 165, 185, 190, 201, 202, 254, 260, 271
organic compounds, 6
organism, 15
ornithine, 201, 208
osteoporosis, 128
ovarian cancer, 179, 186
ovarian tumor, 230, 273
ovaries, 192
overlap, 29, 182
oxidation, 4, 12, 77, 86, 118, 150, 154, 198, 223,
   244, 248, 264
oxidative damage, 150
oxidative reaction, 150
oximes, 6
oxygen, 4, 27, 35, 42, 45, 47, 121, 145, 147, 222,
   269

P

paclitaxel, 242, 244, 250, 264
pain, 15, 28, 51, 61, 93, 95, 97, 98, 179, 191, 214
pancreas, 187
parenchymal cell, 150
participants, 201
partition, 57
pathogenesis, 188
pathology, 172
pathways, 25, 203, 220, 222
PCM, 29, 59, 72
PCT, 74
penicillin, 50, 109, 242, 249, 274, 275
peptidase, 68, 70, 119
peptide(s), viii, 7, 17, 42, 62, 65, 73, 91, 125, 132,
   143, 144, 145, 146, 147, 148, 149, 155, 163, 167,
   168, 175, 181, 202, 203, 228, 256, 267
permeability, 3, 12, 22, 45, 66, 91, 100, 101, 103,
   107, 117, 118, 120, 122, 123, 128, 130, 140, 145,
   154, 159, 179, 213, 222, 234
permeation, vii, 3, 17, 18, 67, 89, 105, 110, 117, 122,
   126, 128, 134
permit, 153, 154

PET, 208
pH, 4, 10, 35, 41, 42, 45, 46, 47, 51, 52, 53, 54, 58, 59, 60, 68, 73, 81, 87, 97, 111, 117, 121, 122, 123, 126, 142, 146, 160, 165, 168, 222, 241, 242, 263
phage, 270
phagocytic cells, 175
phagocytosis, 175
pharmaceutical(s), vii, ix, 3, 13, 26, 50, 51, 74, 77, 86, 98, 103, 104, 110, 131, 132, 133, 135, 136, 171, 172, 179, 237, 239, 261, 274
pharmaceutics, 101, 131, 134, 171, 172
pharmacokinetics, 3, 60, 62, 64, 66, 101, 106, 131, 132, 167, 173, 174, 180, 243, 277
pharmacology, 64, 66, 102, 131, 132, 133, 134, 135, 136, 137, 169, 170, 171, 173, 174, 176, 274, 277
pharmacotherapy, 100
phenol, 24, 27, 248, 253, 274
phenotypes, 51
phenylalanine, 5, 141, 144, 163, 212, 249
phenytoin, 67, 97, 102, 114
Philadelphia, 173
phosphate, 18, 23, 54, 82, 89, 90, 97, 100, 103, 111, 112, 113, 114, 115, 126, 130, 133, 137, 150, 195, 196, 197, 200, 212, 215, 248, 253, 257, 258, 273, 274
phosphates, 12, 91, 126, 150
phospholipids, 153
phosphorus, 195
phosphorylation, 89, 114, 162, 196
physical properties, 4, 26
physicochemical properties, vii, viii, 3, 11, 17, 45, 50, 78, 86, 117, 153, 161, 175, 180, 215
physics, 26
pigs, 171, 172
placebo, 75
plasma levels, 277
plasma membrane, 161, 175
plasmid, 189, 221
plasmid DNA, 221
plasminogen, 57
platelet activating factor, 121
platinum, 151, 169, 251
PM3, 26
polar, 4, 8, 12, 16, 18, 37, 51, 86, 87, 92, 98, 105, 107, 110, 126, 216, 220, 226, 227
polar groups, 5
polarity, 4, 11, 126, 127, 128, 129, 130, 157, 250
polio, 193
polycythemia, 179
polymer(s), 37, 146, 157, 163, 167, 181
polymerization, 125
polymorphisms, 1, 16, 63, 74, 150

polypeptides, 186, 189
polysaccharides, 156, 160
population, 149, 161, 216, 217, 237
potential benefits, 243
precipitation, 97, 114
prevention, 2, 218
primate, 189
principles, 26, 207, 229, 270
probability, 48, 114
progenitor cells, 188
progesterone, 224
prolactin, 45
proliferation, 168, 194, 196, 203, 215
proline, 144
promoter, 179, 184, 186, 191, 229
propagation, 191
prophylactic, 161
propranolol, 111, 132
prostacyclins, 149
prostaglandins, 108
prostate cancer, 21, 135, 147, 148, 149, 165, 168, 186, 219, 230, 248
prostate carcinoma, 168
prostate gland, 21
prostate specific antigen, 90, 148
protection, 115, 221
protein components, 266
protein structure, 145
protein synthesis, 235
proteinase, 168
proteins, viii, 5, 12, 26, 27, 42, 73, 141, 154, 161, 175, 185, 186, 193, 198, 201, 202, 203, 217, 235, 239, 242, 243, 244, 266
proteolysis, 269
protons, 73, 117, 256
proximal tubules, 164
psoriasis, 61, 76
psychiatric patients, 111
psychosis, 132
purification, 146
PVA, 234, 242, 249, 255
pyrimidine, 219

Q

quantum chemistry, 26
quantum dot, 175
quantum mechanics, 26, 27, 62, 98, 131, 166, 207, 230, 275
quaternary ammonium, 120, 121, 148, 167
quinone, 135, 195, 263
quinones, 135, 147, 194, 195, 263

R

radiation, 142, 147, 148, 223, 236
radicals, 121, 256
radio, 246
radiotherapy, 262, 264
reactants, 29, 47, 48, 49, 50, 57
reaction mechanism, 28, 30, 70, 75
reaction medium, 45, 55
reaction rate, 27, 33, 35, 36, 42, 47, 48, 49, 53, 58, 73
reactions, 2, 6, 8, 20, 21, 25, 27, 29, 36, 42, 45, 46, 47, 48, 50, 54, 57, 62, 64, 68, 70, 71, 75, 77, 86, 143, 153, 156, 168, 198, 201, 220, 224, 269
reactive groups, 160
reactivity, 25, 50, 54, 68, 74
receptors, 11, 45, 50, 52, 74, 78, 90, 95, 96, 98, 100, 140, 142, 143, 145, 149, 151, 153, 163, 166, 188, 202, 238, 259, 265
recognition, vii, viii, 149, 185, 187, 242, 244, 254
recombinant proteins, 270
recombinases, 194
recombination, 182, 185, 188
recovery, 116
recreational, 10
recycling, 271
red blood cells, 11, 90, 116, 164
redistribution, 118
regression, 53, 58, 168, 208, 216, 217, 219, 221, 275, 276
regression equation, 53, 58
regulatory changes, 183
relevance, 70
relief, 2, 14, 42, 48
renal cell carcinoma, 221
renin, 164
repair, 179
replication, 161, 179, 181, 182, 184, 185, 186, 187, 189, 190, 191, 192, 193, 207, 208, 218, 219
requirements, 29, 34, 40, 41, 45, 51, 84, 106, 141, 180, 237, 239, 240, 243, 250
residues, 51, 143, 169, 228
resins, 51
resistance, 130, 137, 142, 145, 147, 175, 179, 188, 206, 216, 221, 235, 251, 262, 270
resources, 238
response, 77, 98, 148, 173, 190, 201, 205, 208, 215, 217, 218, 221, 239, 242, 267
restoration, 208
reticulum, 78, 85, 140, 148, 198
retinoblastoma, 186
retrovirus, 160, 174, 195, 202, 203, 204, 205
retroviruses, viii, 17, 177, 187, 188, 203

reverse transcriptase, 161, 162, 174
rewards, 101, 131, 169
RH, 272, 276, 277
ribose, 195, 256
rings, 5, 9, 27
risk(s), 34, 57, 72, 102, 178, 184, 185, 188, 192, 202, 203, 204, 207, 238
risk factors, 102
risk management, 207
rituximab, 143
RNA, 161, 178, 187, 189, 191, 192, 193, 199, 204, 205, 212, 220, 248
RNAi, 205
rodents, 189, 199
rotations, 28
Rouleau, 135
routes, 12, 34, 45, 58
rules, 126

S

safety, 16, 17, 101, 104, 144, 150, 162, 165, 177, 181, 182, 185, 191, 192, 202, 204, 206, 209, 214, 228, 246
saliva, 50
salts, 148
schizophrenia, 92, 101
science, 26, 132, 173
scope, 29, 268
second generation, 185
secretion, 51, 175
segregation, 182
selectivity, vii, 3, 11, 12, 77, 79, 90, 91, 98, 104, 143, 154, 176, 179, 180, 181, 191, 192, 211, 212, 213, 214, 234, 237, 239, 249, 250, 260, 263
sensation, 28, 50, 61, 77, 82, 96, 113, 120
sensitivity, 65, 195, 201, 207, 217, 221, 227
sensitization, 230
sequencing, 205
serine, 42, 116, 151, 168
serum, 148, 149, 168, 170, 188, 196, 254
serum albumin, 170
shape, 170, 179, 270
shock, 178
showing, 33, 43, 148, 181, 237
side effects, 9, 10, 15, 18, 34, 58, 78, 79, 84, 88, 89, 139, 142, 150, 153, 154, 155, 156, 159, 160, 162, 180, 181, 186, 201, 233, 236
signal transduction, 50, 142
signaling pathway, 192
signalling, 168
signals, 191
single chain, 265

skeletal muscle, 187
skeleton, 8, 9
skin, 6, 18, 35, 88, 89, 120, 159, 199
small intestine, 35, 42, 46, 58, 91, 140, 141, 145, 155, 157, 158, 159
smallpox, 192
smooth muscle, 145
sodium, 23, 82, 137, 151
solid tumors, 133, 179, 181, 213, 235, 236, 249, 262
solubility, vii, ix, 3, 4, 12, 17, 21, 22, 23, 24, 35, 37, 38, 40, 41, 45, 46, 51, 62, 64, 66, 67, 82, 86, 89, 95, 97, 98, 103, 108, 111, 112, 113, 114, 115, 117, 119, 121, 122, 128, 130, 141, 159, 160, 161, 162, 179, 214, 260, 264, 269
solution, 3, 26, 42, 54, 68, 73, 114, 136, 160, 223
solvation, 72
species, vii, 3, 99, 132, 182, 186, 188, 189, 197, 204, 214, 216, 220, 224, 226, 227, 263, 270
spleen, 195, 196, 198, 199, 248
SS, 230
stability, 3, 6, 9, 17, 20, 22, 28, 39, 61, 67, 73, 86, 110, 115, 117, 119, 120, 122, 123, 125, 126, 132, 133, 135, 136, 153, 154, 177, 184, 188, 228, 241, 249, 264, 267, 269, 270
stabilization, 8, 69, 70
stasis, 252
state(s), 25, 26, 27, 28, 29, 30, 35, 42, 45, 47, 48, 49, 50, 68, 69, 73, 113, 148, 149, 184, 189, 190, 229, 234, 264, 267, 268
statin, 28, 37, 40, 41, 61
status epilepticus, 97
stem cells, 184
steroids, 158
stimulation, 189, 216
stomach, 3, 22, 28, 46, 52, 58, 61, 122, 155, 158, 199
stomatitis, 188, 208
storage, 111
stromal cells, 186, 193
structural gene, 182
structural protein, 186, 187, 189
structural variation, 25
structure, vii, 2, 3, 4, 5, 8, 15, 19, 20, 23, 25, 26, 30, 41, 50, 51, 63, 64, 67, 69, 75, 81, 82, 89, 92, 93, 94, 95, 106, 111, 117, 121, 122, 123, 124, 125, 126, 127, 128, 129, 135, 141, 145, 146, 151, 158, 195, 196, 198, 202, 250
sub-Saharan Africa, 161
substrate(s), viii, 4, 17, 25, 42, 48, 54, 63, 66, 84, 85, 91, 107, 108, 112, 126, 145, 146, 149, 150, 153, 168, 169, 180, 195, 198, 199, 200, 214, 215, 218, 224, 226, 228, 242, 243, 248, 250, 253, 255, 259, 266, 267, 268, 269, 270

suicide, 63, 65, 181, 185, 207, 211, 213, 215, 217, 229, 230, 231
sulfate, 161
sulfonamides, 11, 81
Sun, 73, 101, 273
suppression, 173, 267
surveillance, 186
survival, 217
susceptibility, 18, 104
suspensions, 37
sweeteners, 50
sympathetic nervous system, 45
symptoms, 92, 161
syndrome, 72, 149, 208, 236
synergistic effect, 20, 110
synthesis, ix, 24, 28, 34, 47, 51, 57, 59, 61, 65, 66, 67, 71, 98, 125, 133, 136, 146, 149, 157, 161, 166, 167, 169, 185, 190, 192, 218, 220, 250
synthetic analogues, 256
systemic immune response, 202, 216

T

target, viii, 3, 5, 11, 12, 13, 14, 15, 17, 58, 79, 90, 91, 126, 127, 129, 135, 139, 141, 144, 145, 151, 153, 154, 163, 164, 165, 166, 170, 181, 182, 183, 184, 185, 186, 187, 188, 193, 203, 204, 205, 213, 214, 218, 223, 225, 233, 235, 236, 238, 243, 250, 260, 262, 264, 267, 270
T-cell receptor, 267
techniques, 51, 206, 262, 266, 267
technology(ies), 2, 51, 74, 95, 102, 154, 170, 173, 182, 205, 213, 244, 267
temperature, 42, 53, 58, 68, 159
testing, 146, 150, 151, 157, 159, 218, 228
testis, 199
textbook, 135, 207
therapeutic agents, 166, 206, 272, 273
therapeutic effects, 245, 249
therapeutic use, 132
therapeutics, vii, 3, 63, 99, 101, 132, 166, 167, 171, 174, 207, 208, 219, 266, 270, 272, 273, 274
therapy, viii, 2, 15, 17, 21, 57, 65, 66, 67, 78, 90, 91, 92, 100, 102, 132, 133, 140, 141, 146, 148, 153, 161, 166, 168, 170, 173, 175, 177, 178, 179, 180, 181, 184, 194, 202, 203, 204, 205, 206, 207, 211, 212, 213, 214, 215, 217, 219, 221, 228, 229, 233, 234, 236, 237, 238, 239, 242, 246, 267, 269, 271, 272, 273, 274, 275, 276, 277
thermodynamic parameters, 29
thermodynamic properties, 30, 35, 56
thoughts, 62, 98, 131
threonine, 244

threshold level, 204
thrombin, 87, 100, 107
thrombosis, 100
thymine, 5
thymus, 196
thyroid, 195, 221, 248
tirapazamine, 63, 121, 167, 264
tissue, vii, 3, 11, 13, 15, 40, 65, 79, 85, 90, 94, 97, 102, 111, 131, 153, 177, 180, 183, 184, 185, 186, 188, 190, 197, 199, 202, 204, 205, 213, 214, 215, 218, 236, 237, 249, 250, 265, 270
tobacco, 178
toluene, 8
tooth, 57
topology, 4
torsion, 27
toxic effect, 11, 90, 145, 148
toxic products, 215
toxic side effect, 10, 142, 201, 202, 203
toxic substances, 10
toxicity, vii, 3, 4, 6, 9, 11, 15, 19, 20, 63, 66, 77, 78, 79, 80, 84, 86, 90, 94, 98, 101, 104, 106, 107, 128, 141, 145, 149, 151, 160, 161, 177, 179, 180, 182, 183, 184, 185, 186, 187, 190, 201, 206, 209, 211, 213, 214, 215, 220, 223, 225, 228, 230, 234, 236, 237, 239, 244, 246, 253, 256, 260, 264, 267, 269
toxicology, 131, 133, 167
toxin, 224, 235, 236
Toyota, 71
trafficking, 135
transcription, 161, 187
transduction, viii, 17, 182, 183, 184, 185, 188, 189, 190, 193, 202, 203, 204, 208, 217
transfection, 175, 208, 217
transferrin, 170
transformation, 34, 109, 120, 128, 203, 220, 257
transfusion, 75
transgene, 177, 185, 187, 189, 190, 191, 193, 200, 201, 204, 205, 207, 208, 209, 213
translation, 179, 183, 213
transmission, 50, 154, 184, 191, 202
transplantation, 34, 164, 203
transport, 5, 11, 12, 65, 86, 89, 91, 98, 107, 108, 112, 151, 153, 154, 155, 170, 176, 205, 219, 220, 240
transportation, 184
trauma, 57, 75, 93
treatment, 2, 5, 18, 21, 23, 28, 34, 45, 47, 57, 61, 63, 64, 66, 67, 71, 72, 75, 76, 77, 80, 83, 91, 92, 96, 97, 100, 101, 110, 118, 124, 127, 128, 130, 134, 136, 142, 143, 147, 148, 153, 159, 161, 162, 166, 167, 171, 173, 174, 179, 181, 186, 190, 191, 192, 193, 196, 206, 207, 211, 213, 214, 217, 219, 220,

221, 223, 225, 229, 230, 233, 234, 235, 238, 244, 246, 248, 249, 252, 262, 265, 272, 273, 274, 276
trial, 2, 72, 75, 132, 157, 174, 185, 201, 207, 246, 253, 263, 265, 267, 276, 277
tropism, 192, 202
trypsin, 24
tryptophan, 51
tuberculosis, 102
tumor cells, viii, 11, 17, 90, 91, 98, 120, 121, 142, 143, 145, 146, 165, 177, 179, 181, 182, 186, 191, 192, 193, 194, 199, 200, 202, 208, 212, 213, 214, 216, 217, 218, 219, 225, 230, 233, 235, 236, 237, 253, 254, 262, 264, 266, 271, 272, 274, 275
tumor growth, 217, 262, 266, 269
tumor resistance, 213, 225
tumor(s), viii, 17, 142, 143, 147, 165, 179, 180, 186, 187, 192, 193, 196, 198, 199, 206, 207, 213, 214, 216, 221, 223, 228, 235, 236, 238, 240, 246, 249, 252, 262, 265, 270, 271, 272
tumours, 230, 276
turnover, 228, 242, 268
tyrosine, 157, 171

U

UK, 10, 69, 100
ulcerative colitis, 23, 67, 83, 124, 136, 155, 159, 171
uniform, 244, 245
United Nations, 173
United States (USA), ix, 68, 70, 71, 131, 169, 170, 208, 230, 273
urea, 66
urethane, 8
urinary bladder, 80
urinary tract infection, 80
urine, 51

V

vaccine, 192
vagus, 50
valence, 8
valine, 91, 92, 111, 268
vapor, 96
variations, 1, 16, 92, 116, 183, 208
vascularization, 193, 250
vasculature, 147, 192, 193, 236, 262, 266
vasodilator, 164, 176
vector, viii, 17, 154, 177, 181, 182, 183, 184, 185, 186, 187, 188, 189, 190, 191, 194, 201, 202, 203, 204, 205, 206, 207, 208, 209, 211, 213, 214, 230
vehicles, 51, 190, 205, 208

versatility, 235
vessels, 145
viral gene, 181, 182, 184, 186, 187, 193, 201
viral infection, 130, 149, 184
viral vectors, viii, 17, 177, 181, 182, 183, 201, 202, 203, 205, 206, 209
virology, 167
virus infection, 101
virus replication, 169, 190
viruses, viii, 17, 175, 177, 178, 181, 183, 184, 185, 187, 188, 189, 190, 191, 192, 193, 196, 202, 203, 204, 205, 206, 207, 208, 209
viscosity, 37
vitamins, 198

W

Washington, 65, 67, 70, 99
waste, 164
water, ix, 6, 22, 23, 27, 28, 30, 40, 42, 44, 50, 55, 57, 62, 65, 67, 73, 82, 89, 97, 98, 102, 110, 111, 114, 117, 121, 122, 128, 130, 133, 148, 151, 160, 161, 174, 198, 214, 260
wettability, 37
wild type, 202, 221
World Health Organization, 173

X

xenografts, 246, 249, 252, 273, 274, 276

Y

yeast, 220, 243, 246
yield, 8, 21, 35, 37, 46, 115, 116, 121, 191, 222, 238, 243, 244, 260, 270

Z

zinc, 130